Fallacies in Medicine and Health

Louise Cummings

Fallacies in Medicine and Health

Critical Thinking, Argumentation and Communication

palgrave
macmillan

Louise Cummings
Department of English
The Hong Kong Polytechnic University
Hung Hom, Kowloon, Hong Kong

ISBN 978-3-030-28512-8 ISBN 978-3-030-28513-5 (eBook)
https://doi.org/10.1007/978-3-030-28513-5

Cover credit: eStudio Calamar/Isaac Ruiz Soler

This Palgrave Macmillan imprint is published by the registered company Springer Nature Switzerland AG
The registered company address is: Gewerbestrasse 11, 6330 Cham, Switzerland

Preface

The decision to write a book that examines arguments and reasoning in medicine and health was motivated by a number of considerations. My academic interests have always straddled philosophy and medical and health disciplines. A book that specifically addresses argumentation in medical and health contexts seemed a natural evolution for someone with interests in public health, logic and reasoning. But equally important was my belief that there have been many significant advances in the treatment of fallacies and argumentation in recent years. However, while these advances have been applied to areas such as politics, law and artificial intelligence, there has been almost total neglect of how new thinking about these aspects of logic might be usefully applied to argumentation in medicine and health. So, logical developments, particularly in fallacy theory, are a major impetus for the current study. But they occur alongside developments in medicine and healthcare that require more than ever that people are able to arrive at informed decisions about medical treatment and make healthy lifestyle choices. The need to equip people with logical skills that will enable them to evaluate the evidential basis of health claims and assess when medical arguments are rationally warranted is a second important impetus for the writing of this book.

As the title indicates, the focus of this book is on the fallacies. A fallacy is a type of weak or invalid reasoning. The fallacies of particular interest to the author are those that go by the name of 'informal fallacies'. They include some familiar names such as slippery slope argument and question-begging argument, as well as some that are less well known like the argument from ignorance and the argument from expertise. Throughout the long history of logic, these arguments have been extensively criticized and even ridiculed by philosophers and logicians. It is a central claim of this book that we must engage with these arguments in a serious way if we want to understand how people reason about the medical problems and health issues that confront them in their daily lives. Specifically, we must move beyond pejorative characterizations of these arguments, and begin to view them as an effective rational resource in our thinking. To this end, the book falls squarely within the approach to the informal fallacies taken by informal logicians and exemplified most clearly by the work of Douglas Walton and John Woods. Woods and Walton have characterized non-fallacious variants of most of the informal fallacies. The positive reorientation of the fallacies that their analyses have made possible is the starting point of the current study.

This book is intended to be used by students of a range of disciplines who want to increase their awareness of how people reason about medical and health issues. To this end, it includes a number of features that will allow readers to develop their practical skills of argument analysis and evaluation.

In dedicated sections, each chapter examines the logical features of a particular argument and the errors that arise when these features are misapplied or deliberately subverted during argumentation. Authentic examples are used to illustrate each feature and logical error or pitfall, with many drawn from actual instances of reasoning in medicine and health. Exercises at the end of sections allow readers to check their understanding of key concepts before proceeding to the next section. Case studies and special topics allow readers to explore certain issues in greater depth. Discussion points create opportunities for student readers to reflect alongside their peers on how they reason about medical and health issues that are often contentious in nature. Annotated suggestions for further reading carefully guide students through a complex literature on the fallacies. A glossary of all the key terms and concepts used in the book allows readers to develop their knowledge without consulting additional sources for clarification of terminology. Questions at the end of each chapter allow readers to consolidate their learning before proceeding to the next chapter. Time-pressed instructors and students who are preparing for exams will benefit from the detailed answers that are provided for all questions. The combination of these features will equip readers to describe and critically evaluate the many different arguments that are used in medical and health contexts.

Finally, a further purpose in writing this book is to convey a sense of the fascination that argumentation in medicine and health has not only for the author but also for a range of other academics in areas such as communication studies, linguistics, psychology and philosophy. Medicine and health are so integral to our daily lives that no-one can afford to relinquish responsibility for judgements and decisions in these areas to others. It is not an exaggeration to say that in examining these deliberations, we are engaging with the very essence of human rationality itself. This examination is a source of immense fascination for any intellectually curious mind. If the book succeeds in conveying to readers the true wonder of this type of inquiry, then it will have achieved another one of its aims.

Louise Cummings
Hung Hom, Hong Kong

Acknowledgements

There are a number of people whose assistance I wish to acknowledge. I particularly want to thank Cathy Scott, Commissioning Editor in Language and Linguistics at Palgrave Macmillan, for responding positively to the proposal for this book. I am grateful to Beth Farrow, Assistant Editor, for her guidance during the preparation of the manuscript. Several other individuals and organizations have given permission for images to be used in this book. I wish to extend my gratitude to them: Amanda Mills; Asian Health Coalition; Australian Associated Press; California Department of Public Health; Centers for Disease Control and Prevention; Debora Cartagena; Department of Health, The Government of the Hong Kong Special Administrative Region; Douglas Walton; Edwin P. Ewing, Jr.; Environmental Protection Agency; Express Newspapers; Health, Safety and Environment Office of The Hong Kong Polytechnic University; HIV Scotland; Informal Logic; James Archer; James Gathany; Jennifer Oosthuizen; Mary Anne Fenley; Massachusetts Department of Public Health; MEN Media; Minister of Health (Canada); Ministry of Health of the New Zealand Government; Moredun Research Institute; National AIDS Trust (UK); National Foundation for Infectious Diseases (USA); New York State Department of Health; PrEPster; Press Association; Private Eye; Road Safety Council of Hong Kong; San Francisco Department of Health; Science Museum; University of Edinburgh; U.S. Department of Agriculture—Animal and Plant Health Inspection Service; U.S. Department of Housing and Urban Development; VisualDx.

Finally, I have been supported by family members and friends who are too numerous to mention individually. I am grateful to them for their kind words of encouragement during my many months of work on this volume.

Contents

Supplementary Information

List of Figures

List of Exercises

Critical Thinking in Medicine and Health

L. Cummings, *Fallacies in Medicine and Health*,
https://doi.org/10.1007/978-3-030-28513-5_1

LEARNING OBJECTIVES: Readers of this chapter will

- appreciate the range of mundane contexts in which we are exposed to medical information and health messages.
- understand the different responses that people have to health messages, ranging from indifference and denial to a high level of critical engagement with the content of messages.
- appreciate the need for robust critical thinking skills in medicine and health in order to expose logical errors and conflicts of interest in the health messages we see and hear, participate in sound decision-making about one's own health, and reduce or eliminate medical errors that put patients at risk of death or serious injury.
- have knowledge of what an informal fallacy is and understand that labels such as 'valid' and 'fallacious' are not inherent properties of arguments but apply only to arguments in certain contexts of use.
- understand the logical tradition that surrounds the fallacies, from Aristotle's challenge to the deceptive or false refutations traded by sophists to present-day pragmatic and cognitive analyses of the fallacies.

1.1 Introduction

Imagine for a moment all the different ways in which you are exposed to medical stories and health messages in a typical day. Over breakfast, you turn on the television and hear that a study has found that coffee consumption reduces the risk of coronary heart disease. As you drive to work, a report about dementia comes over the car radio. You listen closely enough to understand that a lack of exercise significantly increases the risk of developing dementia. You get to your office and learn that one of your colleagues was admitted to hospital overnight with a suspected stroke. You are surprised to hear this news as you know your colleague is only 50 years old and takes good care of his health. So you go online to learn more about stroke and its causes. You have a busy schedule at work and decide to dash out of the office to buy a sandwich. You normally buy a chicken sandwich but you saw a television programme at home the previous evening about salmonella in poultry. So you decide to 'play safe' and opt for a tuna sandwich instead. You finally get out of work at 6 o'clock. As you drive home, you stop at traffic lights and have a couple of minutes to read an advertisement on a billboard at the side of the road. It states the number of units of alcohol that can be safely consumed in a week. You know that you are exceeding these limits, but you quickly put this thought out of your mind as the lights change and you drive off. Your evening at home passes quickly, and it is not long before you are going to bed. You take one of your prescribed sleeping pills and happen to notice a warning on the box that you should not consume alcohol. You know it has been four hours since you had two glasses of wine over dinner and so you do not consider yourself to be at any harm from the drug.

What I have described above is a series of unremarkable events. Most readers will be able to identify with one or more of the circumstances in this scenario. It illustrates the extent to which medical and health messages pervade our daily lives. On some occasions, these messages leave little permanent trace in our minds. We may read the public health advertisement about safe levels of alcohol consumption and then almost instantly forget it. On other occasions, these messages may have increased salience for us. For example, we may listen to a report about dementia with heightened interest if a family member or friend is suffering from the condition, or if we recently participated in a fundraising event in support of a dementia charity. Whatever response we take to these medical stories and health messages, they involve complex cognitive processes such as reasoning, perception, and language decoding. We may reason, for example, that a message has limited relevance to our personal health because we do not engage in a particular behaviour (e.g. alcohol consumption). Alternatively, we may reason that a message is relevant to our health but that we have little or no individual control over a source of risk (e.g. air pollution), and so any modification of behaviour is unlikely to result in health gains. At other times, a health message may encourage us to avoid eating certain foods, or to take more cardiovascular exercise, or to get a flu vaccination or other form of immunisation. The reasoning processes that guide each of these responses are a focus of intellectual curiosity for a wide range of scholars. This book seeks to understand these processes by conducting an in-depth examination of their application to medicine and health.

This book will argue that a special type of reasoning is involved in the mundane scenario outlined above. This reasoning allows us to come to judgement on an issue by means of shortcuts or quick rules of thumb that may be used to bypass knowledge, facts, and evidence about a problem. To this extent, it is a powerful cognitive resource that can serve us well when we are confronted by complex health issues that lie beyond our current state of knowledge. But this resource can also be abused and misused, leading to flawed, defective reasoning. The reasoning in question is best represented by a group of arguments known as the **informal fallacies**. These arguments have occupied a less than auspicious position in the long history of logic. Denigrated for their lack of deductive credentials, these arguments languished in a state of relative neglect until a group of pioneering logicians forced a reconsideration of their logical merits. The work of these so-called informal logicians prompted a sustained effort to characterize non-fallacious variants of most of the informal fallacies. These logicians also pursued a more systematic analysis of the many ways in which these arguments may be used illegitimately during reasoning and **argumentation**. The result of this resurgence of scholarly interest in the fallacies has been new analytical frameworks and theoretical possibilities. The various logical developments that have moved us beyond a wholesale rejection of the fallacies towards a more enlightened approach to the logical merits of these arguments will be examined in ► Sect. 1.4. But first, we must address a more fundamental question. That is the question of why it is important to have a set of rational evaluative skills that can be applied to medicine and health. It is to this question that we now turn.

1.2 Why Think Critically about Medicine and Health?

There are several reasons why it is important to have a set of **critical thinking** skills that can be applied to medicine and health. As the scenario in ▶ Sect. 1.1 illustrates, we cannot evade the relentless exposure to medical and health messages that is part of our daily lives. We would be naïve to think that all, or even most, of these messages are conveying claims that represent some ideal of scientific truth and objectivity. For example, people may not be so ready to accept the claim that coffee consumption reduces the risk of coronary heart disease if they were to discover that a large coffee manufacturer funded the study that produced this finding, or if they were to learn that the study examined a small sample of young, healthy participants over a relatively short period of time. By the same token, a public health advertising campaign about safe levels of alcohol intake loses some of its credibility if a trade association for the alcohol industry has contributed funding to the campaign. It may be legitimately asked if the definition of 'safe' might not have involved a smaller number of weekly units of alcohol if funding for the campaign had not been obtained from the alcohol industry. Each of these conflicts of interest and aberrations of scientific methodology (e.g. the use of a small, unrepresentative sample) passes undetected and unchallenged by people who lack critical thinking skills that can be applied to medicine and health. It is not an exaggeration to claim that medicine and health suffer when citizens, who are deprived of robust critical thinking skills, are unable to hold the individuals, agencies, and organizations responsible for health information and messages to proper rational scrutiny. This point will be emphasized many times in the chapters to follow.

Another reason why it is important to have critical thinking skills about medicine and health is that each of us must make decisions in relation to our personal health. Even negative decisions, for example, the decision *not* to accept an invitation to participate in a cervical screening programme or *not* to take cardiovascular exercise, are still decisions that may be more or less rationally warranted. There can be little doubt that the quality of decision-making in relation to one's personal health deteriorates when critical thinking skills are in short supply. If we use level of formal education as a proxy measure for critical thinking skills,[1] there is clear evidence that individuals with low levels of education experience the poorest health outcomes. Albano et al. (2007) found that black men who completed 12 or fewer years of education had a prostate cancer death rate that was more than double that of black men with more than 12 years of education. The best health outcomes tend to be found in people with college and university education. Loucks et al. (2012) found that individuals with a college degree had substantially lower risk of coronary heart disease after accounting for demographics. These findings hold even when controlling for **confounding variables** such as socio-economic factors. Although we cannot say with certainty that a low level of education (and, by implication, critical thinking skills) *causes* poor health outcomes, we cannot avoid the conclusion that if we want to achieve significant gains in the health of populations, there must be a sustained effort to improve the critical thinking skills that people apply to their own decision-making in matters of health. This would seem to be an inescapable corollary of most studies that have investigated the relationship between education and health.

A further reason why critical thinking skills in relation to medicine and health are essential is related to changes that have occurred in the delivery of medical and health services to patients. In the healthcare systems of mainly developed countries, there has been a move away from a paternalistic approach to medicine, in which doctors make decisions for their patients and patients are expected to defer to those decisions, towards viewing patients as informed decision-makers in their own right. Many patients now expect to make decisions in conjunction with their doctors about the type of treatment that they will receive, and whether or not to pursue treatment in a particular case (e.g. a patient with terminal illness). However, patients cannot participate in this type of decision-making about their medical treatment if they are not equipped with critical thinking skills. These skills will allow them to interrogate doctors about the side effects of pharmacological treatments rather than simply accept the recommendation that a certain prescribed medication represents the best possible medical intervention. Decisions about whether surgery is warranted in the treatment of a patient, or whether some other, less invasive treatment might not also result in an acceptable outcome, can also only be taken by patients who are in possession of critical thinking skills. These skills allow patients to assess the respective merits of different treatment options, based on information from doctors and other sources (e.g. internet), and to arrive at rationally warranted decisions concerning their medical care. Of course, even when involved in decision-making about their health, patients may not select the most effective treatment option. There is certainly scope for improving the quality of patient decision-making (Fowler et al. 2011). The development of robust critical thinking skills is a good place to begin this improvement.

Critical thinking skills are also a vital resource for the medical and health professionals who deliver our healthcare. Notwithstanding significant improvements in the standard of patient care in hospitals, it remains the case that medical errors are alarmingly common, and can result in death and significant patient harm. In the United States each year, medical error results in 44,000 to 98,000 unnecessary deaths and 1 million excess injuries (Weingart et al. 2000). Although there are many different causes of these errors, they most often occur when clinicians are inexperienced and new processes are introduced. Procedures to eliminate and reduce the occurrence of medical errors include improved handovers in patient care between medical staff, avoidance of abbreviations (e.g. QD for 'daily') in written medical communication, and two-person checking of medication infusions for accuracy. These technical procedures and communicative strategies are vitally important in reducing medical errors. However, they must be supplemented by cognitive strategies such as the use of critical thinking skills. These skills can expose the diagnostic errors and defective decision-making of medical professionals. Errors may be related to **cognitive biases** such as **availability**, which is the tendency to attribute a clinical presentation to an obvious, readily available, or recent diagnosis. In their discussion of biases in general medical practice, Coxon and Rees (2015: 14) ask 'Should more time be dedicated to this vital psychology in our training and continual professional development'. The answer to this question must surely be 'yes'. At a minimum, such training must involve exposure of medical and health professionals to the type of critical thinking skills that will be examined in this book (■ Fig. 1.1).

1

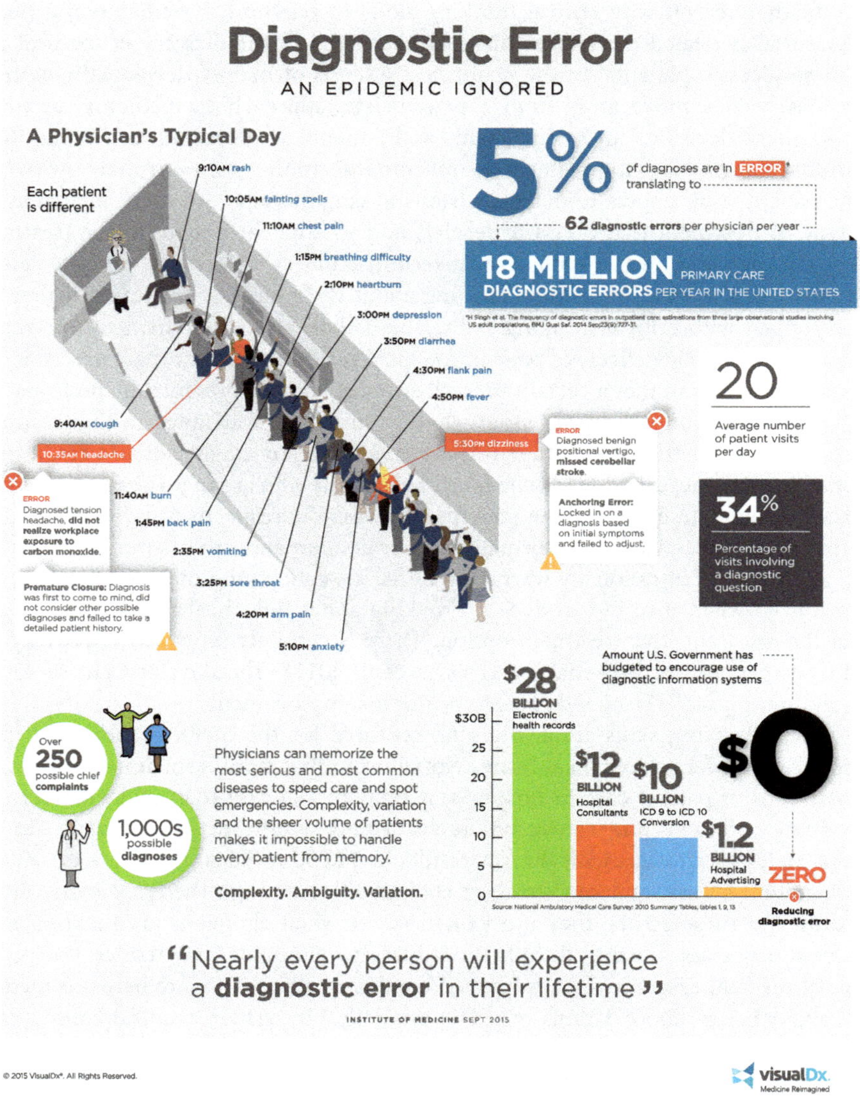

Fig. 1.1 The extent to which diagnostic errors occur in medical practice. Illustration appears with permission from VisualDx (▶ www.visualdx.com)

SPECIAL TOPIC: Errors in medical diagnosis

Much is now known about the frequency and types of errors that occur in medical diagnosis. Many diagnostic errors are related to cognitive biases in the thinking of medical professionals. Improved training in the psychology of these biases in critical thinking courses can help physicians avoid many diagnostic errors. Graber et al. (2005) examined 100 cases of diagnostic error involving internists. Ninety cases involved injury, 33 of which resulted in death. Errors were divided into three categories: no fault errors; system-related errors; and cognitive errors. Only seven cases were judged to be no fault errors. Across the remaining 93 cases there were a total of 548 different system-related or cognitive factors. This equated to 5.9 factors per case. Diagnostic error was related to system-related factors in 65% of the cases. Problems with policies and procedures, inefficient processes, teamwork, and communication were the most common system-related factors.

More significant still were cognitive factors which accounted for 74% of diagnostic errors. The single most common cognitive factor was *premature closure* which is the failure to continue considering reasonable alternatives after an initial diagnosis is reached. For example, a patient was diagnosed with musculoskeletal pain after a car crash, only for a ruptured spleen to be identified. Another common cognitive factor was *faulty context generation* in which there is a lack of awareness or consideration of aspects of a patient's situation that are relevant to diagnosis. For example, a perforated ulcer was missed in a patient who presented with chest pain and laboratory evidence of myocardial infarction (a heart attack). Other common cognitive factors were:

Failed heuristics—failure to apply an appropriate rule of thumb or over-application of such a rule under inappropriate or atypical circumstances. For example, a wrong diagnosis of bronchitis was given to a patient who was later found to have a pulmonary embolism.

Failed perception—a symptom, sign, or finding should be noticeable but is missed by a clinician. For example, a clinician missed a pneumothorax (collapsed lung) on a chest radiograph.

What is interesting is that the factor we commonly attribute errors to—faulty knowledge—was involved in only 11 instances of diagnostic errors related to cognitive factors. For further discussion of cognitive biases and errors in medical diagnosis, the reader is referred to Saposnik et al. (2016) and Croskerry (2003).

1.3 What Is an Informal Fallacy?

Thus far, we have established that there is a need for lay people and experts to have robust critical thinking skills that can be applied to medicine and health. The individual who makes decisions about his or her personal health, and the medical professional who diagnoses and treats patients must both be guided in their deliberations and actions by whatever critical thinking skills are at their disposal. These skills can make the difference between good and poor health outcomes for the person who makes decisions about lifestyle choices such as smoking and exercise. They can also make the difference between safe medical treatment and an error that places a patient at risk of death or serious harm. In short, the importance of the skills that will be explored in this section and in subsequent chapters cannot be overstated. Critical thinking skills can ensure our survival when they work well, and can place us at risk of considerable harm when they are used erroneously. These skills are also the means by which we can undertake a rational evaluation of the informal fallacies. Informal fallacies are arguments that fall short of standards of good or valid reasoning (hence, the term 'fallacies'). Moreover, the manner in which these arguments fall short of these standards cannot be captured by formal (deductive) logic (hence, the term 'informal'). In fact, we will see that we have to look well beyond **formal logic** for an explanation of the fallacious character of these arguments. We will have much to say about the informal fallacies and their role in reasoning in medicine and health in the chapters ahead. But first, we must examine some of the logical flaws that can arise in argument and that may lead to the criticism that a fallacy has been committed.

The date is November 1986. You are listening to a news report on the radio before you set off for work in central London. The report concerns the diagnosis of a new brain disease in British cattle called **bovine spongiform encephalopathy** (BSE). You have been aware for a number of weeks that farmers have been reporting a strange, new illness in some of their herds, but you have been busy at work and have not dwelt on the details of media reports. But there is something about this particular radio report that makes you sit up and take notice of what is said. A government minister is making the following claim with complete confidence: *There is no evidence that BSE transmits to humans*. The certainty with which the minister is expressing this statement leaves you feeling a little disturbed. You know that you and the rest of the listening public are being encouraged to draw the following conclusion: *BSE does not transmit to humans*. The reason you feel disturbed is that you have a friend who is a research scientist at a local university. He has considerable knowledge of **transmissible spongiform encephalopathies** (TSEs) such as **Creutzfeldt-Jakob disease** (CJD) in humans. Your friend told you some time ago that these diseases have a very long incubation period, in some cases of several decades. Based on your recollection of what your friend told you, you wonder how this government minister can possibly be so confident in the reassurances he is offering to the public. You tend to think that his advice to continue eating beef and beef products may not be warranted, particularly at this very early stage in the emergence of a previously unrecognised disease. So you decide that you will exercise caution and avoid eating beef until more is known about this disease in cattle.

Your unease in response to the radio report is fully justified. You and other members of the listening public are being encouraged to accept the logic of the following **argument from ignorance**:

There is *no evidence* that BSE transmits to humans (PREMISE)
Therefore, BSE does *not* transmit to humans (CONCLUSION)

In any argument from ignorance, an arguer reasons from a lack of evidence or knowledge that a proposition P is true to the conclusion that P is false (conversely, from a lack of evidence or knowledge that proposition P is false to the conclusion that P is true). The reason this argument leaves you feeling troubled is that you know that its single premise is a particularly weak basis upon which to draw the conclusion. It may well be the case, as the government minister claims, that there is no evidence to this point in time that BSE transmits to humans. But how can this be a strong basis on which to conclude that BSE does not transmit to humans when so little time has elapsed since the emergence of the disease? Should we not suspend our judgement about the transmissibility of this new disease to humans when the long incubation period of TSEs suggests that it will be some time before transmission can be established? Your questions go straight to the logical flaw in an argument from ignorance—a 'no evidence' statement can only be used to support the truth or falsity of a claim under very specific circumstances. Those circumstances are when a knowledge base in an area is closed (closed world assumption) and has been extensively searched. These circumstances are not satisfied in this particular case. There can be no closed knowledge base when BSE has just emerged in cattle and little is known about this new disease. There is likely to be considerable information about this disease that fell outside of what was known about BSE in November 1986. Your rejection of the logic of the above argument is fully justified as is your decision to avoid any further consumption of beef.

Let us think further about the above scenario. In arriving at your decision that a lack of evidence of the transmissibility of BSE to humans by November 1986 should not be used as grounds that BSE does not transmit to humans, you were influenced by some information about TSEs that was imparted to you by your friend, a research scientist at a local university. You know that your friend has considerable expertise in the area of TSEs. He pursued his PhD in this area and has worked with internationally recognised experts in these diseases. You are inclined to reason as follows:

My friend is an expert in TSEs (PREMISE 1)
My friend asserts that TSEs have long incubation periods (PREMISE 2)
The duration of incubation period falls within my friend's expertise in TSEs (PREMISE 3)
Therefore, what my friend says about the duration of incubation period of this new disease may be taken to be true (CONCLUSION)

You have used what informal logicians call an **argument from authority** or expertise (or *argumentum ad verecundiam*, to give it its Latin name) to arrive at the conclusion that substantial probative weight should be attached to your friend's claim. To the extent that each of the premises in this argument can be supported—for example, that your friend's expertise in premise 1 is real rather than imagined—it is a rationally warranted argument for you to use in your consideration of whether to accept the conclusion of the earlier argument from ignorance.

It emerges that in this single scenario there are two informal fallacies operating alongside each other. But only one of these arguments (the argument from ignorance) is weak or rationally unwarranted (a true fallacy, as it were), while the other argument (the argument from authority) has considerable rational merits. This demonstrates an important feature of the informal fallacies, that they can be more or less rationally warranted in different contexts of use. For that assessment to be made in each individual case, we had to appeal to a wide range of considerations. We had to decide how much evidential weight we could attribute to a friend's expertise in an area and what might constitute an acceptable passage of time for the effects of a new animal disease on human health to become apparent. These are the very judgements that place an evaluation of the informal fallacies well and truly beyond the scope of formal (deductive) logic. They require that we develop new frameworks of analysis that prioritise non-deductive criteria in argument. In the next section, we will consider what some of those criteria look like and the journey that the fallacies have taken en route to them. But before doing so, we return to the issue of when a fallacy is not so fallacious after all.

Let us return to the above scenario. The date is now June 1987. You are listening to the radio again before you leave for work. There is a report on the radio about a recently published epidemiological study that found no evidence of a link between **scrapie** (a TSE in sheep) and CJD in humans. The study involved a 15-year investigation of CJD in France as well as a review of world literature. The reason this report catches your attention is that the number of cases of BSE in cattle is beginning to increase significantly and the disease is now featuring in most major news programmes. Your increased level of attention to the news report on your radio is part of a wider heightened public interest in BSE. The conclusion of the epidemiological study forms the premise of the following argument from ignorance:

There is *no evidence* that scrapie in sheep causes CJD in humans (PREMISE)
Therefore, scrapie in sheep does *not* cause CJD in humans (CONCLUSION)

You feel reasonably confident in accepting the conclusion of this argument. Your confidence stems from the fact that there is extensive knowledge of scrapie and CJD following this long epidemiological study of both diseases. The knowledge base on these diseases may be presumed to be closed (closed world assumption). Also, the investigators who undertook this epidemiological study conducted a review of world literature. This review amounted to an extensive search of the available knowledge of these diseases. With both conditions satisfied, you feel reasonably secure in concluding, like the investigators of the study, that scrapie does not cause CJD in humans.

What this new scenario illustrates is that the rational merits of the argument from ignorance do not inhere in the argument itself. On some occasions of use, the argument is a true fallacy that we are rightly disinclined to accept. On other occasions, the argument has obvious logical strengths and we have little hesitation in accepting its conclusion. The difference lies entirely in the conditions under which the argument is advanced. We will see in the next section that most logicians and philosophers have tended to treat arguments as inherently fallacious or valid. So it is argued that there is something in the very nature of the informal fallacies that distinguishes them as weak or bad forms of reasoning. It is then the task of the logician to identify the logical flaw in question and caution against its use. This view of the fallacies has dominated most of the long history of logic. Against this logical tradition, there is a quite different way of thinking about the fallacies. This involves coming to the task of argument analysis without pre-determined categories of valid and fallacious argument. Rather, the rational merits of arguments emerge from the contexts in which they are advanced. This pragmatic turn in the study of fallacies aims to reconnect arguers to the arguments that they advance. We will see below that this connection had largely been lost in the work of logicians and philosophers who discussed the fallacies. This pragmatic turn has made possible many of the present-day analyses of the fallacies, including an approach to the fallacies that has particular relevance to medicine and health. This is the view that fallacies can serve as facilitative **cognitive heuristics** during medical and health reasoning. It is to an examination of these issues that we now turn.

CASE STUDY: The beef burger incident

The scenarios described above are based on real events, namely, the emergence of BSE or 'mad cow disease' in British cattle in the 1980s. In May 1990, John Gummer, the then UK agriculture minister, attempted to reassure the public about the safety of British beef by feeding a beef burger to his 4-year-old daughter Cordelia in front of the press during a family outing to a boat show. John Gummer was attempting to communicate the following message to the public: *British beef is so safe to eat that I am prepared to feed it to a member of my family. You should follow my lead and do the same.*

Gummer was widely criticised for his actions, and not only because his daughter appeared to be disgusted by the burger and refused to eat it. Many people argued that John Gummer was illegitimately using personal circumstances—the fact that he was prepared to feed beef to one of his own children—to persuade the British public to accept the claim that beef was safe to eat. The use of personal circumstances to support a claim in argument is generally regarded as a weak or flawed form of reasoning. This is particularly true when there is an inconsistency between what an arguer claims and what his personal circumstances suggest he believes. In the latter case, an opponent may rightly charge an arguer with a circumstantial *ad hominem*. But no such inconsistency occurred in the case of John Gummer. He stated that 'beef is safe to eat' and his personal circumstances—encouraging members of his family to eat beef—were entirely consistent with that statement. So was a charge of logical fallacy against him warranted? Or were we simply disturbed by the sight of a young child being coerced into eating a beef burger that she clearly did not want to eat?

Even aside from Gummer's apparent logical consistency between his claim and his personal circumstances, there was still a concern for most people about his choice of argumentative strategy in this case. For some people, the young girl's evident disgust at the beef burger led them to doubt Gummer's claim that his family was eating beef and beef products. In fact, Cordelia looked as if she had never so much as encountered a beef burger. For other people, John Gummer was operating with political motives, and was prepared to defend the interests of the beef industry at all costs, even if this meant putting human health at risk. His sense of political expediency may have trumped all other concerns including any concern for his daughter's well-being. These responses suggested that despite Gummer's evident logical consistency, the public perceived character traits that led them to doubt the veracity of his claim that beef was safe to eat. So while his circumstances withstood logical criticism, his character did less well in this regard. The public had effectively levelled a non-fallacious *ad hominem* argument against John Gummer (◘ Fig. 1.2).

1

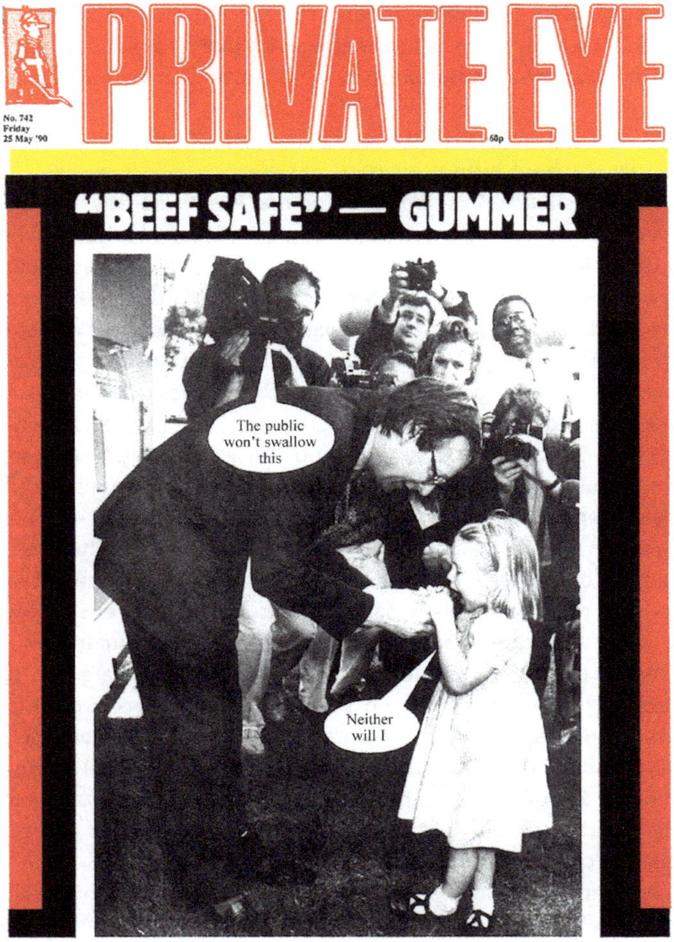
PRIVATE EYE
No. 742
Friday
25 May '90
60p
"BEEF SAFE" — GUMMER
The public won't swallow this
Neither will I

Fig. 1.2 John Gummer and his daughter Cordelia on the front of *Private Eye* in May 1990 (Reproduced by kind permission of PRVATE EYE magazine ▶ www.private-eye.co.uk)

SPECIAL TOPIC: What's in a name?

When it comes to the fallacies, the answer to this question is 'quite a lot, actually'. Many of the terms that you will encounter in this book are found in everyday language where they are used in a way that is not connected to logic and reasoning. An example is the use of the expression 'begging the question'. One begs the question when one assumes the conclusion-to-be-proved in the premise or premises of an argument. An example from recent personal experience illustrates the logical use of this fallacy. In a meeting to discuss student grades, a somewhat frustrated head of department asked those present at the meeting: 'Why did so many of the students get 'A' grades?' To which the reply came: 'Because they did very well'. This logical use of the expression has now been surpassed by a non-logical use in which the term means *raise the question*. In an article in *The Guardian* in May 2010, David Marsh stated that of 32 mentions of 'begging the question' in *The Guardian* and *Observer* over the previous year, all 32 uses had the meaning *raise the question*. This is despite the fact that *The Guardian* style guide advises:

» begs the question is best avoided as it is almost invariably misused: it means assuming a proposition that, in reality, involves the conclusion [...] What it does not mean is 'raises the question', and if you can substitute this phrase, it has been used wrongly. ('Begging the question', *The Guardian*, 24 May 2010)

My point is not one relating to language standards in journalism. It is simply to make readers aware that not every use of words like 'begging the question' relates to logical fallacies. Even the term 'fallacy' is used in ways that are not related to logic and argument. When used in this book, the term means *weak or fallacious argument*. However, in everyday use the term 'fallacy' means a *false belief*, *false claim*, and even a *myth*. These non-logical uses of the term are illustrated below. The underlined word in each example captures the meaning of the word 'fallacy':

» The 10,000 step **fallacy** – and five other health myths to ignore. (*The Telegraph*, 21 February 2017)

There are varying degrees of absurdity in the **fallacies** President Trump peddled during his first week in the Oval Office. Perhaps the most damaging was his insistence that millions of Americans voted illegally in the election he narrowly won. Mr. Trump first made that false claim in late November (*The New York Times*, 27 January 2017).

Just like begging the question, we would do well to recognise these non-logical uses of the term 'fallacy' and be able to set them apart from the logical use of this term that is of interest to us in this book.

1.4 The Logical Journey of the Informal Fallacies

The logical journey of the fallacies begins in Aristotle's *Sophistical Refutations*. For Aristotle (384 BC–322 BC), sophistical refutations had the appearance only of genuine refutations in argument. These illegitimate attempts to appear 'wise' and gain the upper hand in argument became the stock-in-trade of sophists who turned these deceptive techniques into a highly stylized rhetorical practice. Aristotle's disdain for these techniques could not be clearer:

» [I]t is the business of one who knows a thing, himself to avoid fallacies in the subjects which he knows and to be able to show up the man who makes them [...] Those, then, who would be sophists are bound to study the class of arguments aforesaid: for it is worth their while: for a faculty of this kind will make a man seem to be wise, and this is the purpose they happen to have in view. (*Sophistical Refutations*, Section 1, part 1)

Aristotle identified two styles of refutation, one which depends on the language used and the other which is independent of language. In illustration of **amphiboly**, a language-dependent refutation, Aristotle presented this example in which there is play on the 'double meaning' of the expression *sight of*: 'There must be sight of what one sees: one sees the pillar: ergo the pillar has sight'. Aristotle used a refutation that depends upon the consequent to illustrate a refutation that is independent of language: 'since after rain the ground is wet in consequence, we suppose that if the ground is wet, it has been raining; whereas that does not necessarily follow' (Section 1, part 5). For Aristotle, these refutations are simply fallacies employed by sophists whose aim is to achieve 'the semblance of wisdom without the reality'.

Already in Aristotle, we are beginning to see features of the fallacies that would come to define this group of arguments for subsequent generations of logicians and philosophers. For Aristotle, we are under an obligation or duty to avoid fallacies in our own argumentative practice and to expose fallacies wherever they occur. These practices are devoid of any rational merit and should not remain hidden from view. The pejorative character of the fallacies is already firmly established in Aristotle. There is also in Aristotle a feature of the fallacies that was lost to later generations of philosophers but which has more recently been restored. That is the view that these arguments arise in the context of a dialectical exchange between a proponent and an opponent in argument. Against this context, a fallacy is a deceptive dialectical move that is advanced with the aim of prematurely closing down a discussion or confusing an issue to the point where one's opponent in argument accepts a weak or false claim. It is an arguer's failure to advance a claim in argument through legitimate means only that marks out the fallacies as a deviation from rational procedure. This view of the fallacies informs many present-day analyses of these arguments, as we will see in subsequent chapters.

Following Aristotle, a succession of logicians and philosophers expressed their disdain for the fallacies. In the seventeenth century, the Port-Royal logicians Antoine Arnauld (1612–1694) and Pierre Nicole (1625–1695) distinguished between the different ways of reasoning ill (so-called sophisms) and bad reasonings which are common in civil life and ordinary discourse. A fallacy in the former category is **begging the question**. This is 'clearly altogether opposed to true reasoning, since, in all reasoning, that which is employed as proof ought to be clearer and better known than that which we seek to prove' (*Port-Royal Logic*, Third Part, Chap. XIX, Part II, p. 244). Appeals to grounds other than reasons in argument give rise to fallacies in the category of bad reasonings. For the Port-Royal logicians, grounds such as self-love, interest and passion should not convince us in argument: 'what can be more unreasonable than to take our interest as the motive for believing a thing? [...] it is only the truth which must be found in the thing itself, independently of our desires, which ought to convince us' (Third Part, Chap. XX, Part I, p. 263). Clearly, there were no merits in either sophisms or bad reasonings as far as these seventeenth century thinkers were concerned.

This pejorative view of fallacies was continued by John Locke (1632–1704). In Book IV of *An Essay Concerning Human Understanding*, Locke introduced four arguments that will be familiar to present-day readers as the 'ad fallacies'. These arguments were ***argumentum ad verecundiam*** (appeal to modesty), *argumentum ad ignorantiam* (appeal to ignorance), ***argumentum ad hominem*** (appeal to a man's character, principles or practice), and *argumentum ad judicium* (appeal to the foundations of knowledge or probability). It is only the last of these arguments which 'advances us in knowledge and judgment', according to Locke. *Ad verecundiam, ad ignorantiam* and *ad hominem* may dispose us for the reception of truth without helping us to attain it:

> I may be modest, and therefore not oppose another man's persuasion: I may be ignorant, and not be able to produce a better: I may be in error, and another man may show me that I am so. This may dispose me, perhaps, for the reception of truth, but helps me not to it: that must come from proofs and arguments, and light arising from the nature of things themselves, and not from my shamefacedness, ignorance, or error. (Book IV, Chapter XVII: Of Reason)

In his *Logic: or The Right Use of Reason*, Isaac Watts (1674–1748) adds three of his own 'ad fallacies' to Locke's list: *argumentum ad fideum* ('an address to our faith'), *argumentum ad passiones* (an address to the passions), and ***argumentum ad populum*** (an appeal to the people). He also discusses 'several kinds of sophisms and their solution'. These sophisms include Aristotelian sophistical refutations and later additions to the class of fallacies: ***ignoratio elenchi***; ***petitio principii***; *non causa pro causa*; *fallacia accidentis*; ***secundum quid***; **composition** and **division**; ambiguity and imperfect enumeration. Watts continues the pejorative theme about the fallacies which he describes as 'false argumentation'. In his introduction to the sophisms, he states:

> As the rules of right judgment and of good ratiocination often coincide with each other, so the doctrine of prejudice [...] has anticipated a great deal of what might be said on the subject of sophisms: yet I shall mention the most remarkable springs of false argumentation, which are reduced by logicians to some of the following heads. (Part III, Chap. III, Sect. I, p. 266)

In his *Elements of Logic*, Richard Whately (1787–1863) proposes a logical view of the fallacies. The emphasis of this view of the fallacies is 'a scientific analysis of the procedure which takes place in each' (Book III: Introduction, pp. 168–169). Whately divides the fallacies into those 'in the words' (the conclusion does not follow from the premises) and those 'in the matter' (the conclusion does follow from the premises). An argument can be a fallacy even if the conclusion follows from the premises if the premises should not have been assumed (e.g. *petitio principii*) or if the conclusion is not the required conclusion but an irrelevant one (e.g. *ignoratio elenchi*). Whately describes for the first time errors related to the use of analogy. A category of material or non-logical fallacy that deserves special mention is what we have been calling the 'ad fallacies'—the *argumentum ad hominem, argumentum ad verecundiam* and the *argumentum ad populum*, to name just three. In Whately's account, we see the first acknowledgement that certain uses of these arguments are anything but fallacious. He writes:

> There are certain kinds of argument recounted and named by Logical writers, which we should by no means universally call Fallacies; but which *when unfairly* used, and *so far as they are* fallacious, may very well be referred to the present head; such as "*argumentum ad hominem*," [or "personal argument,"] "*argumentum ad verecundiam*," "*argumentum ad populum*," &c. (Book III, Sect. 15, pp. 236–237; italics in original)

Whately makes the point in relation to the *argumentum ad hominem* but he intends it to apply to the other arguments in this category. Essentially, he argues that there are occasions in which a man should be prepared to admit a conclusion which is 'in conformity to his principles of Reasoning, or in consistency with his own conduct, situation, &c.' (pp. 237–238). A conclusion so admitted is not fallacious but is 'allowable and necessary':

> Such a conclusion is often both allowable and necessary to establish, in order to silence those who will not yield to fair general argument; or to convince those whose weakness and prejudices would not allow them to assign to it its due weight. (Book III, Sect. 15, p. 238)

The point about the non-fallaciousness of these arguments remains somewhat undeveloped in Whately's account. However, his discussion nevertheless marks an important break with the hitherto dominant view of these arguments as invariably weak or fallacious forms of argument or reasoning.

John Stuart Mill (1806–1873) devotes the whole of Book V of *A System of Logic* to a discussion of the fallacies. Mill believes that no philosophy of reasoning can be complete without a theory of bad as well as good reasoning. Bad reasoning involves our being seduced into not observing the 'true principles of induction':

> It is, however, not unimportant to consider what are the most common modes of bad reasoning; by what appearances the mind is most likely to be seduced from the observance of true principles of induction. (Book V, Chapter I, Sect. 1)

Given this emphasis on induction, it is unsurprising that inductive fallacies are the focus of Mill's classification system. As Mill expands his system, we see the names of a number of familiar fallacies beginning to appear. For example, under Fallacies of Generalization Mill includes ***post hoc, ergo propter hoc***. This arises 'when the investigation takes its proper direction, that of causes, and the result erroneously obtained purports to be a really causal law' (Book V, Chapter V, Sect. 5). Under Fallacies of Confusion, Mill discusses the fallacy of ambiguity, *petitio principii* and *ignoratio elenchi*. The 'confusion' in these fallacies consists in misconceiving the import of the premises, in forgetting what the premises are, and in mistaking the conclusion which is to be proved, respectively. It is in Mill that we find the most explicit description yet of **false analogy**. For Mill, false analogy does 'not even simulate' an induction:

> This Fallacy stands distinguished from those already treated of by the peculiarity that it does not even simulate a complete and conclusive induction, but consists in the misapplication of an argument which is at best only admissible as an inconclusive presumption, where real proof is unattainable. (Book V, Chapter V, Sect. 6)

Mill also discusses deductive fallacies under Fallacies of Ratiocination. These cases are 'provided against by the rules of the syllogism'. Under Fallacies of Ratiocination, Mill addresses *à dicto secundum quid ad dictum simpliciter*. This fallacy is committed 'when, in the premises, a proposition is asserted with a qualification, and the qualification lost sight of in the conclusion' (Book V, Chapter VI, Sect. 4). In general, although Mill achieves an expansion of the class of fallacies, his account does little to challenge the logically dominant view that these arguments are flawed forms of reasoning.

And so this view of the fallacies as aberrations of logic and reasoning persisted unchanged until the latter half of the twentieth century. In 1970, Charles Hamblin published his groundbreaking text *Fallacies*. Hamblin's frustration with the weaknesses of what he called the 'standard treatment' of the fallacies in introductory logic textbooks is evident in some early remarks in this book:

> And what we find in most cases, I think it should be admitted, is as debased, worn-out and dogmatic a treatment as could be imagined – incredibly tradition-bound, yet lacking in logic and historical sense alike, and almost without connection to anything else in modern logic at all. This is the part of his book in which a writer throws away logic and keeps his reader's attention, if at all, only by retailing traditional puns, anecdotes, and witless examples of his forbears. (Hamblin 1970: 12)

By way of illustration, Hamblin considers the treatment of amphiboly in the textbooks. He argues that many of the examples of this fallacy offered by textbook authors are not arguments at all. Moreover, even if these examples of the use of ambiguous verbal constructions could be made into arguments, they would have little prospect of persuading anyone that they are valid. Hamblin believed that the way to address the weaknesses in the standard treatment was to institute a more systematic approach to the study of fallacies. He aimed to achieve this through the development of a formal dialectic, a formal analysis of rules of dialogue that may be used to capture the dialectical flaws of different fallacies. In illustration of this approach, let us consider how Hamblin analyses the fallacy of *petitio principii* or begging the question within formal dialectic. Hamblin begins with a brief description of the structure of two dialectical forms of this fallacy:

> The simplest possible such argument is 'Why A? *Statements* A, A⊃A'; and, if S and T are statements equivalent by definition, another is 'Why S? *Statement* T. Why T? Statement S'. (1970: 271; italics in original)

Hamblin aims to prohibit these argument sequences by means of the following rules:

> 'Why S?' may not be used unless S is a commitment of the hearer and not of the speaker. The answer to 'Why S?', if it is not 'Statement – S' or 'No commitment S', must be in terms of statements that are already commitments of both speaker and hearer. (1970: 271)

In relation to the argument sequence 'Why S? Statement T. Why T? Statement S', the second of these rules guarantees that where statement T is offered as a justification of S, both T and T⊃S must already be among the commitments of the speaker and the hearer of the dialogue. In such a case, however, the further question Why T? is prohibited by the first of these rules—the questioner is prohibited from asking a question about a statement to which he is already committed.

The details of Hamblin's formal dialectic are less important than what it reveals about his view of the fallacies. It is clear that for Hamblin the type of **circular reasoning** that occurs in *petitio principii* is to be prohibited in formal dialectic. So, even as Hamblin seeks a more systematic approach to the analysis of the fallacies, he remains committed to the largely pejorative characterization of these arguments that dominated historical accounts. It would take later logicians to lay siege to the **deductivism** that is implicit in Hamblin's analysis, and that leads Hamblin to develop increasingly sophisticated formal dialectical rules with which to prohibit the fallacies.

Deductivism is the widely held, though often implicit, view that the only way to conduct logical analysis is to resort to deductive techniques and norms. The norms implicit in the deductivist attitude to the study of logic are captured by the soundness doctrine, the idea that a good argument is one that is deductively valid and has true premises. Johnson (2011: 30) observes that deductivism is deeply entrenched in the history of philosophy. From this position, its effect on the analysis of the fallacies has been particularly profound. For if the soundness doctrine is the standard of a good argument, then most of the arguments that people use in their daily affairs (indeed, in philosophy itself) are fallacies. As soon as we commit to deductivism, we are prejudiced from the outset to find these arguments weak when, in fact, all we have done is apply an incorrect (that is, deductive) standard to their evaluation. Historically, this has been the fate of the arguments we are calling informal fallacies. But while most logicians and philosophers were blind to, or unwilling to challenge, their own deductivism, a new generation of philosophers was not prepared to uphold the deductive ideals of their predecessors. A significant catalyst for this change was developments in the teaching of logic. In the 1970s, undergraduate students in North American universities began to question the relevance of formal deductive logic to the evaluation of the social, moral, and political arguments that they were confronting in their lives. Logic instructors too were finding it increasingly difficult to defend the prominence given to **deductive logic** in the curriculum. Howard Kahane (1971: v) recalls the moment when it became clear to him that instructors could no longer continue to teach deductive logic as the only, or even the most important, form of logic:

> » In class a few years back, while I was going over the (to me) fascinating intricacies of the predicate logic quantifier rules, a student asked in disgust how anything he'd learned all semester long had any bearing whatever on President Johnson's decision to escalate again in Vietnam. I mumbled something about bad logic on Johnson's part, and then stated that Introduction to Logic was not that kind of course. His reply was to ask what courses did take up such matters, and I had to admit that so far as I knew none did. He wanted what most students today want, a course relevant to everyday reasoning, a course relevant to the arguments they hear and read about race, pollution, poverty, sex, atomic warfare, the population explosion, and all the other problems faced by the human race in the second half of the twentieth century.

A new approach to logic that could respond to the concerns of these students was beginning to take shape. This approach examined the use of arguments in context over formal relations between propositions in deductive logic. So-called **informal logic**, as the 'new' logic became known, had significant implications for the study of fallacies. When assessed in the contexts in which they were advanced, many previously weak or fallacious arguments appeared not so fallacious after all. Logicians began in earnest to characterize non-fallacious variants of most of the informal fallacies. Two logicians in particular, John Woods and Douglas Walton, were particularly prolific in this regard, publishing many papers on non-fallacious variants of the fallacies that has continued to the present day (Walton 1985a, b, 1987, 1991, 1992; Woods 1995, 2004, 2007, 2008).

As the following remarks of Walton (1996: 153) demonstrate, models of reasoning that are based on presumption lay at the heart of these new analyses of the fallacies. **Presumptive reasoning** provides a reasonable, but tentative basis for decision-making in those circumstances where knowledge is incomplete, and deductive validity and soundness are not in contention:

> Presumptive reasoning [...] is closely related to a type of argument called the *argumentum ad ignorantiam* (argument from ignorance), traditionally held to be a fallacy. However, arguments from ignorance are not always fallacious. In many cases, absence of knowledge to prove a proposition constitutes good presumptive grounds for tentatively accepting that proposition as a commitment [...] Presumptive reasoning enables practical reasoning to go ahead in variable circumstances where knowledge is incomplete.

Non-fallacious variants of several informal fallacies, including the argument from ignorance, have been analysed in the context of public health reasoning (Cummings 2002, 2004, 2009, 2010, 2011, 2012a). Their use in this context is warranted by the fact that we often need to take urgent health measures in a context where evidence and knowledge are lacking. But as we might suspect with the informal fallacies, their remarkable journey does not end with the characterization of non-fallacious variants of these arguments. For when analysts began to uncover the epistemic virtues of the fallacies, it was not long before they started to conceive of these arguments in terms of facilitative cognitive heuristics during reasoning (Walton 2010). Four of these fallacies-as-heuristics were recently experimentally tested in a large-scale study of public health reasoning (Cummings 2012b, 2013a, b, 2014a, b, c, d, e). Findings from this study have been discussed at length elsewhere (Cummings 2015). On the model of fallacies-as-heuristics that was central to this work, the informal fallacies are mental shortcuts that can bypass expert knowledge that lies beyond the cognitive grasp of the lay person. They are an adaptation of our cognitive resources to a lack of knowledge in domains such as public health. A quite different conception of fallacies-as-heuristics is to be found in Walton (2010). For Walton, the informal fallacies represent shortened or abridged versions of the extended critical questions that can be posed of arguments. We will have more to say about both these conceptions in subsequent chapters. Suffice it to say, the view of fallacies that they represent is a far cry from the pejorative characterizations of these arguments that have dominated most of the history of logic.

CASE STUDY: Health experts warn...

In most health messages we are exposed to, argumentation is usually interspersed among other types of discourse (e.g. explanatory discourse). To the extent that a health argument is present, it can be difficult to identify it and reconstruct it in terms of its component premises and conclusion. Some premises may be missing altogether and have to be supplied by the argument analyst. Those premises that are present can have a number of different functions. Some may report claims made by health experts who are often affiliated with universities or research institutes. Other premises may describe facts and research findings about the health issue that is the focus of the message. The conclusion usually takes the form of a recommendation, either to avoid or modify a risky behaviour (e.g. smoking) or to adopt protective health measures (e.g. immunization). To illustrate these components of a health message, consider the following story about coconut oil that appeared in various media outlets in 2017:

> **Health experts warn against coconut oil**
>
> *Coconut oil raises cholesterol just like other saturated fats do, warns the American Heart Association.*
>
> The health benefits of coconut oil have been questioned, with US authorities warning it raises cholesterol in the same way as other saturated fats.
>
> A new paper released by the American Heart Association urges consumers to ditch coconut oil and instead opt for polyunsaturated fats.
>
> "Because coconut oil increases LDL cholesterol, and has no known offsetting favourable effects, we advise against the use of coconut oil", the association advised.
>
> The advice is in line with the 2013 Australian Dietary Guidelines that says foods predominantly containing saturated fat such as butter, cream and coconut oil must be limited.
>
> Kellie Bilinski, an accredited practising dietitian and spokesperson for the Dietitians Association of Australia says the bottom line is that coconut oil is a saturated fat and there is not enough evidence to suggest using it.
>
> "We know saturated fats are linked with cardiovascular disease", she said.
>
> There is also a large body of evidence showing that polyunsaturated fatty acids (PUFAs), found in foods like salmon and walnuts, reduce cholesterol and can even raise 'good' cholesterol, she said.
>
> A recent study by researchers at the University of Georgia even suggested a PUFA-rich diet may help to control a person's appetite by influencing hormones associated with hunger.
>
> Participants who regularly consumed foods high in PUFAs had a significant decrease in the hormone ghrelin, responsible for increasing hunger.
>
> They also had a significant increase in peptide YY (PYY)—a hormone that increases fullness or satiety. Participants saw increases in PYY while fasting and after consuming a meal.
>
> Ms Bilinski recommends cooking with either olive oil or vegetable oil.
>
>

AAP's prior written permission. AAP and its licensors are not liable for any loss, through negligence or otherwise, resulting from errors or omissions in or reliance on AAP content. The globe symbol and "AAP" are registered trademarks)

SBS News is reporting recent research findings about coconut oil that suggest this oil may not have the beneficial health effects that many people believe it does. It is the way in which these findings are reported that suggests they carry probative weight as premises in an argument. Each statement or claim is associated with a source of expertise and authority. We are not just told, for example, that coconut oil raises cholesterol, but that a reputable body, the *American Heart Association*, is warning the public that this is the case based on findings from one of its research studies. American expertise assumes an international dimension when the advice on coconut oil is said to conform to Australian Dietary Guidelines. A spokesperson for the Dietitians Association of Australia, Kellie Bilinski, who is also an accredited practising dietician, adds yet further authority to the claims that coconut oil is a saturated fat and should not be consumed for this reason. These claims from different expert sources form premises in the following argument from authority:

The *American Heart Association* and the *Dietitians Association of Australia* are expert organizations (PREMISE 1)
These organizations assert that coconut oil is a saturated fat that should not be consumed (PREMISE 2)
If the *American Heart Association* and the *Dietitians Association of Australia* are expert organizations, and these organizations assert that coconut oil is a saturated fat that should not be consumed, then it is true that coconut oil is a saturated fat that should not be consumed (PREMISE 3)
Coconut oil is a saturated fat that should not be consumed (CONCLUSION)

To this point, we have reconstructed only half of the argumentation used in this health story. The focus of argument then shifts from the negative health effects of coconut oil to the beneficial health effects of polyunsaturated fatty acids in foods like salmon and walnuts. These beneficial effects include a reduction of cholesterol and appetite. Once again, these claims are developed as premises in an argument from authority:

The *University of Georgia* and the *Dietitians Association of Australia* are expert institutions (PREMISE 1)
Individuals affiliated with these institutions assert that polyunsaturated fatty acids reduce cholesterol and appetite (PREMISE 2)
If the *University of Georgia* and the *Dietitians Association of Australia* are expert institutions, and individuals affiliated with these institutions assert that polyunsaturated fatty acids reduce cholesterol and appetite, then it is true that polyunsaturated fatty acids reduce cholesterol and appetite (PREMISE 3)
Polyunsaturated fatty acids reduce cholesterol and appetite (CONCLUSION)

Argumentation in this health story unfolds in two stages, with each stage supporting its respective conclusions about coconut oil and polyunsaturated fatty acids by means of an argument from authority. We will have occasion to examine this particular informal fallacy many times in the chapters that lie ahead. Its dominance in medical and health stories reflects the extent to which we defer to expertise in our reasoning about health.

Note

1. The use of formal education as a proxy measure for critical thinking skills is problematic in a number of respects. It assumes, for example, that formal education aims to develop critical thinking skills and that these skills are directly taught in schools when in fact neither may be the case.

Chapter Summary

Key points

- Medicine and health have tended to be overlooked in the critical thinking literature. And yet robust critical thinking skills are needed to evaluate the large number and range of health messages that we are exposed to on a daily basis.
- An ability to think critically helps us to make better personal health choices and to uncover biases and errors in health messages and other information. An ability to think critically allows us to make informed decisions about medical treatments and is vital to efforts to reduce medical diagnostic errors.
- A key element in critical thinking is the ability to distinguish strong or valid reasoning from weak or invalid reasoning. When an argument is weak or invalid, it is called a 'fallacy' or a 'fallacious argument'.
- The informal fallacies are so-called on account of the presence of epistemic and dialectical flaws that cannot be captured by formal logic. They have been discussed by many generations of philosophers and logicians, beginning with Aristotle.
- Historically, philosophers and logicians have taken a pejorative view of the informal fallacies. Much of the criticism of these arguments is related to a latent deductivism in logic, the notion that arguments should be evaluated according to deductive standards of validity and soundness. Against deductive standards and norms, many reasonable arguments are judged to be fallacies.
- Developments in logic, particularly the teaching of logic, forced a reconsideration of the prominence afforded to deductive logic in the evaluation of arguments. New criteria based on presumptive reasoning and plausible argument started to emerge. Against this backdrop, non-fallacious variants of most of the informal fallacies began to be described for the first time.
- Today, some argument analysts characterize non-fallacious variants of the informal fallacies in terms of cognitive heuristics. During reasoning, these heuristics function as mental shortcuts, allowing us to bypass knowledge and come to judgement about complex health problems.

Suggestions for Further Reading

(1) Sharples, J. M., Oxman, A. D., Mahtani, K. R., Chalmers, I., Oliver, S., Collins, K., Austvoll-Dahlgren, A., & Hoffmann, T. (2017). Critical thinking in healthcare and education. *British Medical Journal, 357*: j2234. ► https://doi.org/10.1136/bmj.j2234.

The authors examine the role of critical thinking in medicine and healthcare, arguing that critical thinking skills are essential for doctors and patients. They describe an international project that involves collaboration between education and health. Its aim is to develop a curriculum and learning resources for critical thinking about any action that is claimed to improve health.

(2) Hitchcock, D. (2017). *On reasoning and argument: Essays in informal logic and on critical thinking*. Cham: Switzerland: Springer.

This collection of essays provides more advanced reading on several of the topics addressed in this chapter, including the fallacies, informal logic, and the teaching of critical thinking. Chapter 25 considers if fallacies have a place in the teaching of critical thinking and reasoning skills.

(3) Hansen, H. V., & Pinto, R. C. (Eds.). (1995). *Fallacies: Classical and contemporary readings*. University Park: The Pennsylvania State University Press.

This edited collection of 24 chapters contains historical selections on the fallacies, contemporary theory and criticism, and analyses of specific fallacies. It also examines fallacies and teaching. There are chapters on four of the fallacies that will be examined in this book: appeal to force; appeal to ignorance; appeal to authority; and *post hoc ergo propter hoc*.

Questions

(1) Diagnostic errors are a significant cause of death and serious injury in patients. Many of these errors are related to cognitive factors. Trowbridge (2008) has devised twelve tips to familiarize medical students and physician trainees with the cognitive underpinnings of diagnostic errors. One of these tips is to explicitly describe heuristics and how they affect clinical reasoning. These heuristics include the following:

Representativeness—a patient's presentation is compared to a 'typical' case of specific diagnoses.

Availability—physicians arrive at a diagnosis based on what is easily accessible in their minds, rather than what is actually most probable.

Anchoring—physicians may settle on a diagnosis early in the diagnostic process and subsequently become 'anchored' in that diagnosis.

Confirmation bias—as a result of anchoring, physicians may discount information discordant with the original diagnosis and accept only that which supports the diagnosis.

Using the above information, identify any heuristics and biases that occur in the following scenarios:

Scenario 1: A 60-year-old man has epigastric pain and nausea. He is sitting forward clutching his abdomen. He has a history of several bouts of alcoholic pancreatitis. He states that he felt similar during these bouts to what he is currently feeling. The patient states that he has had no alcohol in many years. He has normal blood levels of pancreatic enzymes. He is given a diagnosis of acute pancreatitis. It is eventually discovered that he has had acute myocardial infarction.

Scenario 2: A 20-year-old, healthy man presents with sudden onset of severe, sharp chest pain and back pain. Based on these symptoms, he is suspected of having a dissecting thoracic aortic aneurysm. (In an aortic dissection, there is a separation of the layers within the wall of the aorta, the large blood vessel branching off the heart.) He is eventually diagnosed with pleuritis (inflammation of the pleura, the thin, transparent, two-layered membrane that covers the lungs).

(2) Many of the logical terms that were introduced in this chapter also have non-logical uses in everyday language. Below are several examples of the use of these terms. For each example, indicate if the word in italics has a *logical* or a *non-logical* meaning or use:
(a) University 'safe spaces' are a dangerous *fallacy*—they do not exist in the real world (*The Telegraph*, 13 February 2017).
(b) The MRI findings *beg the question* as to whether a careful ultrasound examination might have yielded some of the same information on haemorrhages (*British Medical Journal: Fetal & Neonatal*, 2011).
(c) The youth justice system is a *slippery slope* of failure (*The Sydney Morning Herald*, 26 July 2016).
(d) The EU countered with its own gastronomic *analogy*, saying that "cherry picking" the best bits of the EU would not be tolerated (*BBC News*, 28 July 2017).
(e) As Ebola spreads, so have several *fallacies* (*The New York Times*, 23 October 2014).
(f) Removing the statue of Confederacy Army General Robert E. Lee no more puts us on a *slippery slope* towards ousting far more nuanced figures from the public square than building the statue in the first place put us on a *slippery slope* toward, say, putting up statues of Hitler outside of Holocaust museums or of Ho Chi Minh at Vietnam War memorials (*Chicago Tribune*, 16 August 2017).
(g) We can expand the *analogy* a bit and think of a culture as something akin to a society's immune system—it works best when it is exposed to as many foreign bodies as possible (*New Zealand Herald*, 4 May 2010).
(h) The Josh Norman Bowl *begs the question*: What's an elite cornerback worth? (*The Washington Post*, 17 December 2016).
(i) The intuition behind these *analogies* is simple: As a homeowner, I generally have the right to exclude whoever I want from my property. I don't even have to have a good justification for the exclusion. I can choose to bar you from my home for virtually any reason I want, or even just no reason at all. Similarly, a nation has the right to bar foreigners from its land for almost any reason it wants, or perhaps even no reason at all (*The Washington Post*, 6 August 2017).

(j) Legalising assisted suicide is a *slippery slope* toward widespread killing of the sick, Members of Parliament and peers were told yesterday (*Mail Online*, 9 July 2014).

(3) In the Special Topic 'What's in a name?', an example of a question-begging argument from the author's recent personal experience was used. How would you reconstruct the argument in this case to illustrate the presence of a fallacy?

(4) On 9 July 2017, the effect of coconut oil on health was also discussed in an article in *The Guardian* entitled 'Coconut oil: Are the health benefits a big fat lie?' The following extract is taken from that article. (a) What type of reasoning is the author using in this extract? In your response, you should reconstruct the argument by presenting its premises and conclusion. Also, is this argument valid or fallacious in this particular context?

» When it comes to superfoods, coconut oil presses all the buttons: it's natural, it's enticingly exotic, it's surrounded by health claims and at up to £8 for a 500 ml pot at Tesco, it's suitably pricey. But where this latest superfood differs from benign rivals such as blueberries, goji berries, kale and avocado is that a diet rich in coconut oil may actually be bad for us.

The article in *The Guardian* also makes extensive use of expert opinion. Two such opinions are shown below. (b) What *three* linguistic devices does the author use to confer expertise or authority on the individuals who advance these opinions?

Christine Williams, professor of human nutrition at the University of Reading, states: "There is very limited evidence of beneficial health effects of this oil".

Tom Sanders, emeritus professor of nutrition and dietetics at King's College London, says: "It is a poor source of vitamin E compared with other vegetable oils".

The author of the article in *The Guardian* went on to summarize the findings of a study by two researchers that was published in the British Nutrition Foundation's Nutrition Bulletin. The author's summary included the following statement: *There is no good evidence that coconut oil helps boost mental performance or prevent Alzheimer's disease.* (c) In what type of informal fallacy might this statement be a premise?

Answers

(1)

Scenario 1: An anchoring error has occurred in which the patient is given a diagnosis of acute pancreatitis early in the diagnostic process. The clinician becomes anchored in this diagnosis, with the result that he overlooks two pieces of information that would have allowed this diagnosis to be disconfirmed—the fact that the patient has reported no alcohol use in many years and the presence of normal blood levels of pancreatic enzymes. By dismissing this information, the clinician is also showing a confirmation bias—he attends only to information that confirms his original diagnosis.

Scenario 2: A representativeness error has occurred. The patient's presentation is typical of aortic dissection. However, this condition can be dismissed in favour of conditions like pleuritis or pneumothorax on account of the fact that aortic dissection is exceptionally rare in 20-year-olds.

(2) (a) non-logical; (b) non-logical; (c) non-logical; (d) non-logical; (e) non-logical; (f) logical; (g) logical; (h) non-logical; (i) logical; (j) logical

(3) The fallacy can be illustrated as follows. The head of department asks the question 'Why did so many of these students get 'A' grades'? He receives the reply 'Because they did very well'. But someone might reasonably ask 'How do we know that they did very well?' To which the reply is 'Because so many students got 'A' grades'. The reasoning can be reconstructed in diagram form as follows:

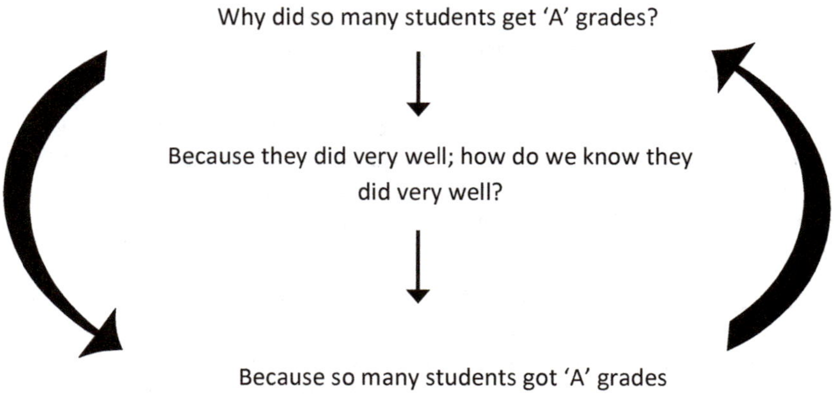

(4)

(a) The author is using an analogical argument, which has the following form:

P1: Blueberries, goji berries, kale, avocado and coconut oil are natural, exotic, pricey and surrounded by health claims.
P2: Blueberries, goji berries, kale and avocado have health benefits.
C: Coconut oil has health benefits.

This is a false analogy, or a fallacious analogical argument, because coconut oil does not share with these other superfoods the property or attribute <*has health benefits*>.

(b) The author uses academic rank, field of specialization, and university affiliation to confer authority or expertise on individuals who advance expert opinions.
(c) This statement could be a premise in an argument from ignorance.

References

Albano, J. D., Ward, E., Jemal, A., Anderson, R., Cokkinides, V. E., Murray, T., et al. (2007). Cancer mortality in the United States by education level and race. *Journal of the National Cancer Institute, 99*(18), 1384–1394.

Coxon, J., & Rees, J. (2015). Avoiding medical errors in general practice. *Trends in Urology & Men's Health, 6*(4), 13–17.

Croskerry, P. (2003). The importance of cognitive errors in diagnosis and strategies to minimize them. *Academic Medicine, 78*(8), 775–780.

Cummings, L. (2002). Reasoning under uncertainty: The role of two informal fallacies in an emerging scientific inquiry. *Informal Logic, 22*(2), 113–136.
Cummings, L. (2004). Analogical reasoning as a tool of epidemiological investigation. *Argumentation, 18*(4), 427–444.
Cummings, L. (2009). Emerging infectious diseases: Coping with uncertainty. *Argumentation, 23*(2), 171–188.
Cummings, L. (2010). *Rethinking the BSE crisis: A study of scientific reasoning under uncertainty*. Dordrecht: Springer.
Cummings, L. (2011). Considering risk assessment up close: The case of bovine spongiform encephalopathy. *Health, Risk & Society, 13*(3), 255–275.
Cummings, L. (2012a). Scaring the public: Fear appeal arguments in public health reasoning. *Informal Logic, 32*(1), 25–50.
Cummings, L. (2012b). The public health scientist as informal logician. *International Journal of Public Health, 57*(3), 649–650.
Cummings, L. (2013a). Public health reasoning: Much more than deduction. *Archives of Public Health, 71*(1), 25.
Cummings, L. (2013b). Circular reasoning in public health. *Cogency, 5*(2), 35–76.
Cummings, L. (2014a). Informal fallacies as cognitive heuristics in public health reasoning. *Informal Logic, 34*(1), 1–37.
Cummings, L. (2014b). The 'trust' heuristic: Arguments from authority in public health. *Health Communication, 29*(10), 1043–1056.
Cummings, L. (2014c). Coping with uncertainty in public health: The use of heuristics. *Public Health, 128*(4), 391–394.
Cummings, L. (2014d). Circles and analogies in public health reasoning. *Inquiry, 29*(2), 35–59.
Cummings, L. (2014e). Analogical reasoning in public health. *Journal of Argumentation in Context, 3*(2), 169–197.
Cummings, L. (2015). *Reasoning and public health: New ways of coping with uncertainty*. Cham, Switzerland: Springer.
Fowler, F. J., Jr., Levin, C. A., & Sepucha, K. R. (2011). Informing and involving patients to improve the quality of medical decisions. *Health Affairs, 30*(4), 699–706.
Graber, M. L., Franklin, N., & Gordon, R. (2005). Diagnostic error in internal medicine. *Archives of Internal Medicine, 165*(13), 1493–1499.
Hamblin, C. L. (1970). *Fallacies*. London: Methuen.
Johnson, R. H. (2011). Informal logic and deductivism. *Studies in Logic, 4*(1), 17–37.
Kahane, H. (1971). *Logic and contemporary rhetoric: The use of reason in everyday life*. Belmont, CA: Wadsworth Publishing Company.
Loucks, E. B., Buka, S. L., Rogers, M. L., Liu, T., Kawachi, I., Kubzansky, L. D., et al. (2012). Education and coronary heart disease risk associations may be affected by early life common prior causes: A propensity matching analysis. *Annals of Epidemiology, 22*(4), 221–232.
Saposnik, G., Redelmeier, D., Ruff, C. C., & Tobler, P. N. (2016). Cognitive biases associated with medical decisions: A systematic review. *BMC Medical Informatics and Decision Making, 16,* 138. ▶ https://doi.org/10.1186/s12911-016-0377-1.
Trowbridge, R. L. (2008). Twelve tips for teaching avoidance of diagnostic errors. *Medical Teacher, 30,* 496–500.
Walton, D. N. (1985a). Are circular arguments necessarily vicious? *American Philosophical Quarterly, 22*(4), 263–274.
Walton, D. N. (1985b). *Arguer's Position*. Westport, CT: Greenwood Press.
Walton, D. N. (1987). The ad hominem argument as an informal fallacy. *Argumentation, 1*(3), 317–331.
Walton, D. N. (1991). *Begging the question: Circular reasoning as a tactic of argumentation*. New York: Greenwood Press.
Walton, D. N. (1992). *Plausible argument in everyday conversation*. Albany: SUNY Press.
Walton, D. N. (1996). *Argumentation schemes for presumptive reasoning*. Mahwah, NJ: Erlbaum.
Walton, D. N. (2010). Why fallacies appear to be better arguments than they are. *Informal Logic, 30*(2), 159–184.

1

Weingart, S. N., Wilson, R. M., Gibberd, R. W., & Harrison, B. (2000). Epidemiology of medical error. *Western Journal of Medicine, 172*(6), 390–393.

Woods, J. (1995). Appeal to force. In H. V. Hansen & R. C. Pinto (Eds.), *Fallacies: Classical and contemporary readings* (pp. 240–250). University Park: The Pennsylvania State University Press.

Woods, J. (2004). *The death of argument: Fallacies in agent-based reasoning*. Dordrecht: Kluwer Academic.

Woods, J. (2007). Lightening up on the ad hominem. *Informal Logic, 27*(1), 109–134.

Woods, J. (2008). Begging the question is not a fallacy. In C. Dégremont, L. Keiff, & H. Rükert (Eds.), *Dialogues, logics and other strange things: Essays in honour of Shahid Rahman* (pp. 523–544). London: College Publications.

Arguing from Ignorance

L. Cummings, *Fallacies in Medicine and Health*,
https://doi.org/10.1007/978-3-030-28513-5_2

LEARNING OBJECTIVES: Readers of this chapter will

- be able to discern when ignorance is an undesirable state or disposition that should be avoided, and when ignorance can be gainfully employed in our various deliberations.
- be able to recognize the conditions under which a knowledge base may be said to be closed, and the linguistic markers of this closure.
- be able to recognize the conditions under which a knowledge base may be said to be extensively searched, and the linguistic markers of this search.
- be able to identify when a knowledge base has been closed prematurely, for example, in advance of an investigation, often with a view to forcing the hearer's acceptance of the conclusion of an argument from ignorance.
- be able to identify when a knowledge base has been only partially searched, and understand the implications of an inadequate search for the rational warrant of the resulting argument from ignorance.
- be able to understand the epistemic gains that derive from the use of the argument from ignorance as a cognitive heuristic in our thinking and reasoning.

2.1 Introduction

The word 'ignorance' has some rather negative connotations. In general, ignorance is a mental state or condition of existence that most people want to avoid. We undertake study at school, college, and university with a view to acquiring knowledge and ridding ourselves of ignorance. We watch television programmes about astronomy, politics, and history because we want to be well informed and knowledgeable about the world around us. We experience affirmation when we are told that we have extensive knowledge of a topic or discipline, and embarrassment or even shame when our lack of knowledge or ignorance in an area is exposed. Ignorance can cause us to fail an examination, prevent us from obtaining an academic or professional qualification, and lead to negative appraisal from an employer. With such negative consequences related to a lack of knowledge, it seems strange for anyone to claim that ignorance can be a valuable resource, particularly when we are engaged in **reasoning** and decision-making in medicine and health. Yet, that is exactly what I will claim in this chapter. It will be argued that ignorance is too often disparaged when it is, in fact, central to many of the deliberations that we engage in on a daily basis. By way of illustration, consider the following scenario. I want to attend a cousin's wedding in Dublin and decide that I should make the trip by train. I walk into the train station on my way home from work and pick up a timetable. It shows that there are two stops on the journey from Belfast to Dublin. These stops are at Dundalk and Drogheda. A friend later enquires if she can travel with me on the train as she wants to attend a music festival in Newry. She asks me if the Dublin train stops at Newry. I reply that it does not.

This scenario will not strike the reader as remarkable in any way. In fact, it is typical of the many everyday interactions that each of us undertakes with little effort or reflection. But there is a real sense in which my response does reveal something significant. What it reveals is the ease with which I am able to employ ignorance to answer my friend's question. The reasoning that resulted in my response can be reconstructed as follows:

> I have *no evidence or knowledge* that the train stops in Newry.
> Therefore, the train does *not* stop in Newry.

I have used an argument from ignorance to answer my friend's question. The **premise** of this argument lays bare my lack of knowledge or ignorance. I use this lack of knowledge to conclude that the train does not stop in Newry. Moreover, I draw this **conclusion** quite legitimately. After all, if the train did stop in Newry, this should be shown in the timetable. The fact that Newry does not appear in the timetable is all the grounds I need to conclude that the train does not stop at Newry. In the next section, it will be shown that this argument satisfies two conditions on the use of the argument from ignorance, or at least the non-fallacious use of this argument. We will see in this chapter that there are many other circumstances where an argument from ignorance is not rationally warranted. But first, let us consider another scenario where this argument is employed, this time in an issue related to medicine and health. A new cholesterol-lowering drug is undergoing clinical trials before it is launched onto the market. The pharmaceutical company that is developing the drug has tested it on 10,000 human subjects with elevated blood cholesterol in centres in the USA, UK, France, Australia, and China. The purpose of the trials is to establish that the drug is effective in lowering blood cholesterol, and that it can do so without causing harm in the form of adverse reactions or side-effects. A panel of independent experts in pharmacology is brought together to examine the results of these trials. After a wide-ranging review of the evidence, the panel concludes as follows:

> There is *no evidence* that drug *X* causes harm.
> Therefore, drug *X* does *not* cause harm.

This argument has the same form as the 'train' argument above. The panel has argued from a lack of evidence (or knowledge) that the drug causes harm to the conclusion that it does not cause harm. Like the 'train' argument, this use of the argument from ignorance is also warranted. After all, a large multi-site trial involving 10,000 participants has been conducted. Also, the results of the trial have been reviewed by a panel of experts in the area. If the drug did cause harm, the trial and subsequent review would reveal that to be the case. Because there is no evidence of harm, the panel can safely conclude that the drug does not cause harm. This argument illustrates yet again that there are certain contexts in which arguing from a state of ignorance or lack of knowledge (or evidence) is warranted. Moreover, these contexts are as likely to involve expert scientific issues such as drug safety as they are more mundane issues like planning a train journey. The logical merits of the argument remain the same regardless of whether the argument is advanced by scientific experts or lay people. This fundamental observation will resonate throughout the chapters in this book.

The sections in this chapter will unfold as follows. In ▶ Sect. 2.2, we consider some of the reasons logicians, philosophers, and others have given for rejecting the use of the argument from ignorance. It will be argued that the characterization of this argument as a weak, fallacious, or invalid form of reasoning usually betrays certain assumptions about what it means to *know* something. These assumptions contain hyperbolical standards for knowledge which, it is claimed, no practically-situated rational agent can attain. In ▶ Sect. 2.3, we examine the logical and epistemic conditions under which use of the argument from ignorance is rationally warranted. These conditions—a *closed world assumption* and an *extensive search criterion*—were fulfilled in the arguments from ignorance examined above. There are many situations, however, where these conditions are not fulfilled and the argument is unwarranted in consequence. In ▶ Sect. 2.4, we examine some of those situations within a wider assessment of the use of the argument from ignorance in medical and health contexts. Finally, in ▶ Sect. 2.5, we consider some of the ways in which reasoning in medicine and health can be facilitated by use of the argument from ignorance. On these occasions, it is useful to conceive of the argument as a cognitive heuristic or a mental shortcut that bridges gaps in our knowledge. An examination of the features of this heuristic—we will call it an *ignorance heuristic*—will conclude the discussion of this chapter.

2.2 Attitudes to Ignorance

We do not need to search far to find negative attitudes towards ignorance. Comments about a person's state of ignorance are one of the most common forms of personal insult or abuse. Expressions such as "You are an *ignorant* idiot!" and "What *ignorant* twit forgot to lock the door?" are part of everyday language use. Politicians attack the ignorance of their opponents with predictable regularity. During a parliamentary debate on energy price in the House of Commons in the UK, Conservative Member of Parliament, Sir Alan Duncan, addressed his Labour opponent in the following terms:

> The idea that a regulator can suddenly say, "Oh, there's the wholesale price, therefore there is the retail price", is total lunacy and *ignorance*, of which the right honourable Lady should be ashamed. (House of Commons, 14 January 2015)

Sometimes, the target of a political attack on ignorance is implied rather than explicitly stated. During his commencement address at Rutgers University in May 2016, Barack Obama made the following pointed remarks. They were clearly aimed at presidential challenger Donald J. Trump:

> Class of 2016, let me be as clear as I can be. In politics and in life, *ignorance* is not a virtue. It's not cool to not know what you're talking about. That's not keeping it real or telling it like it is. That's not challenging political correctness. That's just not knowing what you're talking about. And yet we've become confused about this.

Ignorance is also widely credited as the cause of discrimination and prejudice in society. Intolerance towards other people on grounds of race, gender, sexuality, and religion, it is argued, results from a lack of knowledge or ignorance about cultures, identities, and ways of life that differ from our own. Conflict between peoples and nations is also attributed to ignorance. The role of ignorance in these seemingly intractable human problems is clearly identified in the Constitution of the United Nations Educational, Scientific and Cultural Organization (UNESCO). The opening paragraphs to the Constitution, which was signed on 16 November 1945 and ratified by 20 countries on 4 November 1946, read as follows:

> The Governments of the States Parties to this Constitution on behalf of their peoples declare:
> That since wars begin in the minds of men, it is in the minds of men that the defences of peace must be constructed;
> That *ignorance* of each other's ways and lives has been a common cause, throughout the history of mankind, of that suspicion and mistrust between the peoples of the world through which their differences have all too often broken into war;
> That the great and terrible war which has now ended was a war made possible by the denial of the democratic principles of the dignity, equality and mutual respect of men, and by the propagation, in their place, through *ignorance* and prejudice, of the doctrine of the inequality of men and races.

Beyond politics, social equality, and international relations, ignorance is at the heart of many of the most pressing challenges in public health. The emergence of the AIDS epidemic in the 1980s prompted governments around the world to launch public health campaigns. In the UK, the Conservative government led by Margaret Thatcher responded to the growing threat of this new infectious disease by launching the 'AIDS Don't Die of Ignorance' campaign. A leaflet bearing these words was sent to every household in the UK (see Fig. 2.1). It was accompanied by an extensive television campaign that also warned of the risks posed by this new disease. Worldwide, ignorance of AIDS was costing many thousands of people their lives. The only public health tool available to stem the rapidly growing number of new cases was to increase people's knowledge of how the disease was transmitted and of the preventative measures that could be taken. Consequently, the battle against ignorance was to become the central theme of HIV/AIDS public health campaigns around the world, and is still the case today (see Fig. 2.2).

In short, ignorance has little to commend it. It contributes to human conflict, discrimination and prejudice, and is a significant factor in the spread of infectious disease. With ignorance as the source of so much human suffering, it will seem strange to the reader that I should now propose that ignorance be positively embraced under certain circumstances. Those circumstances are represented by the 'train' argument in ▸ Sect. 2.1. There is a general expectation that a train timetable will be complete, that is, that it will show all the stops that the train makes in a particular journey. It is accordingly reasonable to conclude that if stop *X* is not indicated on the timetable, then the train does not take in stop *X* on its route. The reasoning in this case is a deductively valid **modus tollens inference**:

If *P*, then *Q*	If the train stops at *X*, then *X* would appear in the timetable.
Not-*Q*	But *X* does not appear in the timetable.
Therefore, not-*P*	Therefore, the train does not stop at *X*.

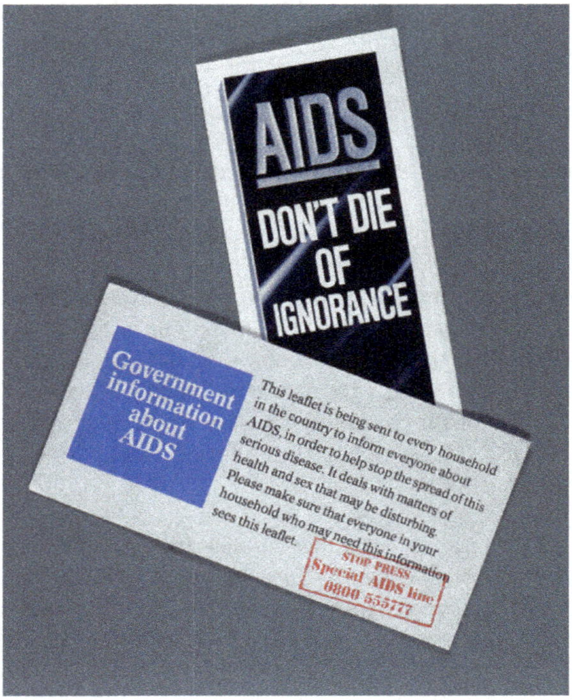

Fig. 2.1 UK Government AIDS awareness leaflets, 1987 (Science Museum, 1986–1987. Object No. 1994-75.

But neither of the premises from which this **inference** is drawn mentions ignorance or a lack of knowledge. So where does ignorance enter into this two-premise argument? Ignorance is the source of the rational warrant for the two premises in this argument. In ▶ Sect. 2.1, we said that two conditions needed to be fulfilled for use of an argument from ignorance to be rationally warranted. Those conditions are a closed world assumption and an extensive search criterion. The closed world assumption is an assumption to the effect that a knowledge base is complete in the sense of containing all relevant information in a particular domain. This assumption provides rational warrant for the first premise above—the train timetable is a complete knowledge base of all train journeys and the stops within those journeys. The extensive search criterion requires that the knowledge base in a particular domain is extensively searched. That criterion is satisfied when I open the timetable, locate the particular journey I want to undertake, and search all the stops that will be made as part of that journey. This criterion provides rational warrant for the second premise above. It is because the closed world assumption and the extensive search criterion are so robust in the case of the 'train' argument that they can provide the strongest possible rational warrant for the premises in this **deductively valid argument**. But let us be under no illusion about either of these conditions. The only reason they have any leverage at all in the above argument is because there is a complete, extensively searched knowledge base

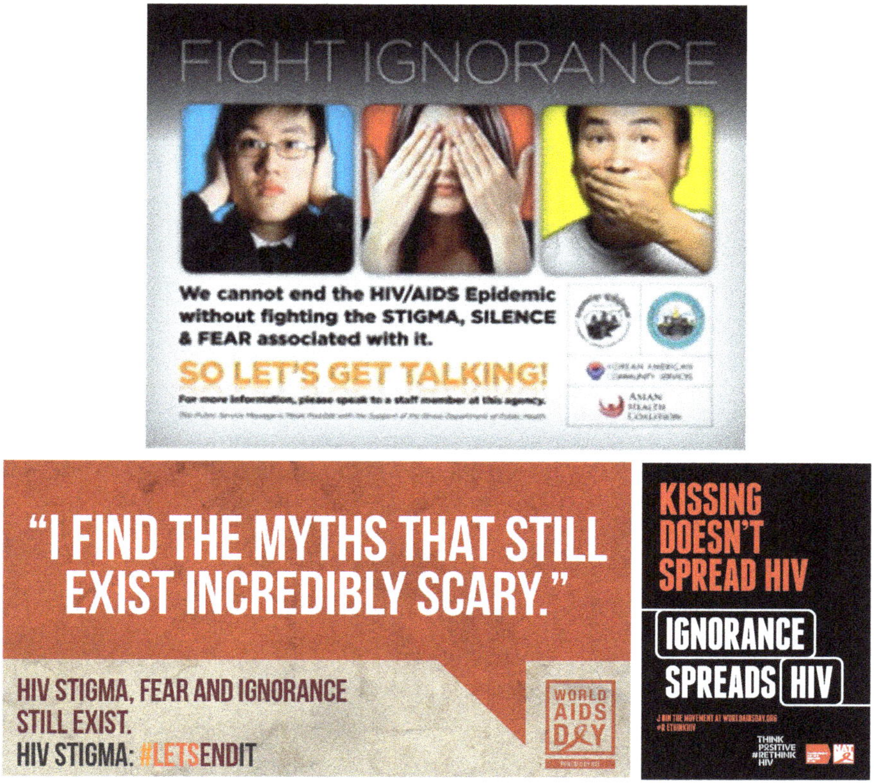
FIGHT IGNORANCE
We cannot end the HIV/AIDS Epidemic without fighting the STIGMA, SILENCE & FEAR associated with it.
SO LET'S GET TALKING!
For more information, please speak to a staff member at this agency.
"I FIND THE MYTHS THAT STILL EXIST INCREDIBLY SCARY."
HIV STIGMA, FEAR AND IGNORANCE STILL EXIST.
HIV STIGMA: #LETSENDIT
WORLD AIDS DAY
KISSING DOESN'T SPREAD HIV
IGNORANCE SPREADS HIV
THINK POSITIVE #RETHINK HIV

Fig. 2.2 The emphasis on fighting ignorance is evident in these campaign posters. The Asian Health Coalition launched the 'Fight Ignorance' campaign in 2011–2012 with the aims of reducing misinformation and stigma surrounding HIV/AIDS in Asian American communities (reproduced with the permission of the Asian Health Coalition). Ignorance is also the target of the 'Think Positive: Rethink HIV campaign' (2015) and the 'Let's End It' campaign (2017) of the National AIDS Trust in the UK (Copyright NAT [National AIDS Trust])

that does not contain knowledge of *X* or *Y* (where *X* and *Y* could be **propositions** in a knowledge base). The ignorance at the centre of an argument from ignorance is exactly this 'missing' or 'absent' knowledge.

The idea that the absence of knowledge (i.e. ignorance) can be grounds on which to draw a conclusion in argument strikes many observers as a decidedly weak form of reasoning. This was clearly demonstrated in an experimental investigation of reasoning that was conducted in 879 members of the general public in the UK (Cummings 2015). The argument from ignorance was one of four types of reasoning investigated in this study (Cummings 2014). Among some of the responses made by participants was the following remark about a food additive that had been used for 40 years without consequences for human health. The absence of ill health effects during this time, it was commented, did not constitute *proof* that the additive was safe:

> The additive has been widely used for 40 years and during that time numerous tests have been undertaken. That suggests safety, but doesn't constitute proof of it (62-year-old, university educated, white British man)

Statements based on a lack of evidence were judged by some participants to be an inadequate basis for *knowledge*. In such cases, it was considered that *doubt* still remained:

> The text states "there is no evidence that scrapie was transmissible to humans". This statement leaves me with doubt, therefore, I don't know (50-year-old, university educated, white British woman)

> The statement "there is no evidence that the asthma drug is unsafe" leaves some doubt that it is generally safe to all groups (59-year-old, university educated, white British woman)

The absence of evidence left some participants with a sense of *uncertainty* that something was or was not the case. This was variously expressed, with some participants reporting a lack of *confidence*, while others said they were not *sure* about what to conclude:

> 'No evidence that the vaccine was unsafe' doesn't instil me with confidence that it is safe (30-year-old, university educated, white British woman)

> I personally am not 100% sure it was safe (45-year-old, secondary school educated, white British man)

For these participants, notions such as proof, knowledge, doubt, and certainty are bound up with epistemic standards that are not satisfied by an absence or lack of evidence. For this reason, any claim based on such evidence should be rejected or at least treated with great caution and even suspicion. The opinions of these lay participants are not dissimilar from those expressed by professional philosophers and logicians, many of whom reject an absence of knowledge or evidence as anything but the weakest possible grounds upon which to accept a claim in argument. Robinson (1971) is unambiguous about the lack of merit in an argument based on ignorance. He states:

> The argument from ignorance is bad. Ignorance is not one of the sources of knowledge; and premises about our ignorance do not reasonably give conclusions about our knowledge. Ignorance is a good ground for suspending judgement, but not for taking a side. (102)

Toulmin et al. (1984) are no less negative in their rejection of the argument from ignorance. This argument, they claim, leaves us that "we cannot certainly infer anything at all" (145). In fact, they go even further in their dismissal of this argument when they claim that it 'trivializes' the notion of evidence itself:

> To provide backing for such a warrant, we should have to argue that *lack of proof* is itself a kind of evidence, and this would trivialize the concept of *evidence* beyond recognition. (1984: 146, italics in original)

LeBlanc (1998) also sees little merit in the argument from ignorance, which she describes as "not very informative". She goes further when she states:

> From a premise of ignorance, we cannot conclude anything but mere possibility, and many things are possible. (191)

Most recently, Kelley (2014) queries whether any judgement can be reasonably based on a lack of knowledge or evidence. He argues that:

> The absence of evidence usually means that we simply don't know enough to make a judgement. Such ignorance cannot be transmuted into knowledge, any more than brass can be transmuted into gold. (130)

These views of lay people and professional philosophers have something important in common. It is a belief that concepts such as knowledge, proof, and evidence should be held to exacting epistemic standards. Moreover, it is against these standards that the argument from ignorance is judged to be inherently weak as a form of reasoning. But where exacting epistemic standards can become problematic is when they lead us to reject all sorts of rational inquiries according to which we can claim to know that something is true. In other words, exacting epistemic standards can sometimes be allowed to run amok and become standards that are so hyperbolical in nature that no practically-situated rational agent could possibly attain them. I contend that this has been the fate of the concept of knowledge. Knowledge has become so imbued with inflated epistemic standards that it seems that there are no circumstances in which we can rightfully say that *X* knows that *p*. So construed, knowledge is not an exacting epistemic concept but an unattainable concept. Nicholas Rescher (1980) captures this same inflation in the concept of certainty that leaves us with a pervasive scepticism in which we can never truly be said to know anything at all:

> One must distinguish between *mundane* or *practical* (or "effective") certainty on the one hand and *transcendental* or *categorical* (or "rigid") certainty on the other. The former is certainty "beyond any *reasonable* doubt", the latter certainty "beyond any *possible* doubt at all – be it reasonable or otherwise". And the certainty we claim for our knowledge is of the former, and not necessarily of the latter kind. (1980: 37, italics in original)

Hyperbolical epistemic standards such as transcendental certainty serve only to distort the concept of knowledge. If we can reclaim knowledge from these standards, as I believe we can, then we have a reasonable prospect of acknowledging all the different ways in which we can claim to know that something is true. One of those ways is to use the absence of knowledge or evidence of a proposition within an appropriately circumscribed domain as a basis of a claim to knowledge. This is, in effect, the type of reasoning that occurs in an argument from ignorance. When evaluated against appropriate epistemic standards, as I am proposing should be the case, an argument from ignorance is a productive source of claims that can be used in decision-making and other types of judgement. In some cases, these claims have the rational warrant of knowledge itself. But even when the conclusion of an argument from ignorance is not a *known* thesis, but a *presumed* thesis, it is not because the conclusion falls short of some hyperbolical standard of what it means to know that something is true. Rather, it is simply that on a particular occasion of use, the argument lacks some of the rational warrant that is present on other occasions of use. This is the position that has been taken by Douglas Walton, one of many informal logicians who have adopted a more benign view of the rational merits of the argument from ignorance. Walton (1996) has been explicit about the need to develop frameworks of **argument evaluation** that fall within the rational resources of practically-situated arguers. Within these frameworks, many so-called fallacies appear not so fallacious after all. This is also the case for the argument from ignorance:

> Presumptive reasoning […] is closely related to a type of argument called the *argumentum ad ignorantiam* (argument from ignorance), traditionally held to be a fallacy. However, arguments from ignorance are not always fallacious. In many cases, absence of knowledge to prove a proposition constitutes good presumptive grounds for tentatively accepting that proposition as a commitment […] Presumptive reasoning enables practical reasoning to go ahead in variable circumstances where knowledge is incomplete. (1996: 153)

This is the view of the argument from ignorance that will inform the rest of this chapter. There is nothing inherently fallacious about this argument. Rather, it is more or less rationally warranted in certain contexts of use. Many of those contexts relate to medicine and health. The task of each of us as we attempt to evaluate an argument from ignorance is to establish the features of the context in which it is used that make it more or less rationally warranted. We will see in ▶ Sect. 2.3 that this task is not as easy as it sounds. It can involve background knowledge of a topic or discipline and some quite sophisticated logical and epistemic judgements.

SPECIAL TOPIC: Ignorance and health

It is worth adding a cautionary note at this stage. In advocating the use of ignorance in argument, I am not suggesting that people should actively avoid acquiring knowledge about the many different things they experience in their lives. My stance is not a call to reject education and learning, and to live in a state of self-imposed ignorance. It is quite the opposite, in fact. The use of ignorance in argument is proposed as a means of *increasing* our knowledge. There is no contradiction between advocating that we use ignorance during reasoning and recommending that we undertake efforts to eradicate ignorance through education and learning. Accepting one of these positions does not require that we reject the other position.

If we think for a moment about health, the serious consequences of ignorance can be very clearly demonstrated. We saw earlier that ignorance can expose us to risk from infectious diseases like HIV and hepatitis. It can also lead us to adopt lifestyles that damage our health, and prevent us from engaging with health checks and screening programs (e.g. bowel cancer screening). Indicators of ignorance about health are easy to find. Jalloh et al. (2017) interviewed 1413 randomly selected respondents from 9 out of 14 districts in Sierra Leone about their knowledge of Ebola three months into the 2014 outbreak. Only 42% of respondents linked Ebola to a virus. A further 41% falsely believed that they could protect themselves from Ebola by washing with salt and hot water, while 30% expressed the mistaken view that Ebola is transmitted by air (■ Fig. 2.3).

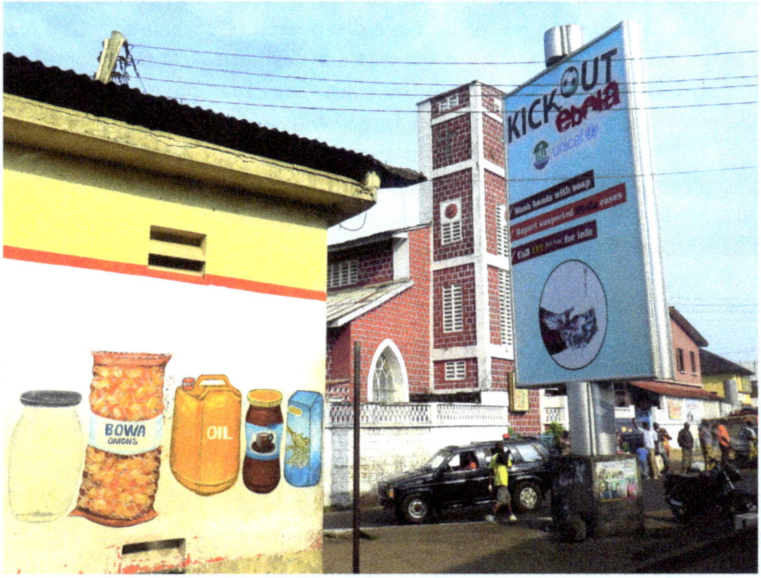

■ **Fig. 2.3** A street scene in the capital city of Freetown, Sierra Leone, during the 2014 West African Ebola virus outbreak. The 'Kick Out Ebola' message was used to raise awareness of the disease (Photo by Angela J. Sanchez, M.S., M.T. is reproduced courtesy of CDC)

Some 26% of Jalloh et al.'s respondents had no formal education. However, even in better educated subjects, there are still high levels of ignorance about matters related to health. Between February and April 2008, Inungu et al. (2009) examined knowledge of HIV/AIDS in 650 students enrolled at a Midwestern University in the United States. Although 98.2% of respondents knew that the chances of contracting HIV/AIDS were reduced by having only one partner who was not infected, and by using condoms consistently during sex, 19.9% did not know if mosquitoes transmitted HIV/AIDS. A further 14.4% thought that mosquitoes did represent a route of transmission. Even in individuals who were receiving tertiary-level education, gaps in knowledge about this prominent infectious disease were still very much in evidence.

2.3 Logic and Ignorance

We have already seen that not every appeal to ignorance in argument is rationally warranted. If I tell you that the Dublin train does not stop in Newry because I found *no evidence* when I examined the timetable that Newry is one of the stops, then you may be reasonably confident in concluding that the train does not stop in Newry. However, imagine for one moment that you discover I was consulting an old timetable or a timetable that had a few pages missing. Would you be so inclined under these conditions to accept my claim that the Dublin train does not stop in Newry? Of course you would not. That is because you would have discovered circumstances that lead you to doubt that the knowledge base upon which I am basing my claim is complete. If I am consulting an old timetable, the route the train takes may have been altered so as to include Newry as one of the stops on the journey. If one of the missing pages lists some of the stops that the Dublin train makes, then Newry could conceivably be one of the stops on a missing page. In both scenarios, you have discovered something that leads you to query if the *closed world assumption* holds in this particular case. This assumption can be stated as follows:

> ***Closed world assumption:***
>
> An assumption to the effect that all information that is relevant to a particular domain *D* is contained in a knowledge base *K*.

In our example above, we tend to doubt that all information that relates to the train journey between Belfast and Dublin (domain *D*) can be contained in knowledge base *K*, represented here by the timetable, when we discover that the timetable is old or that the copy I am consulting has missing pages. This simple example of how the closed world assumption can fail to hold in a particular case powerfully illustrates that there are certain conditions on the use of ignorance in argument. Not just *any* absence of knowledge or evidence can provide logical grounds for a conclusion. Moreover, the conditions under which the closed world assumption may not be presumed to hold are as numerous as the different types of knowledge bases at the centre of this assumption. On some occasions, there may be information that is relevant to a particular domain *D* but that cannot be contained in our knowledge base *K* because inadequate time has elapsed for this to occur. Just such a scenario arose in the 1980s during the BSE epidemic in the UK, when the public was encouraged to continue eating beef and beef products because there was *no evidence* that BSE transmitted to humans. It was known at the time that BSE was a spongiform encephalopathy and, as such, would have a lengthy incubation period. It would take many years before scientists would know if BSE could transmit to humans. Certainly, the absence of evidence of BSE transmission to humans in the early months of the epidemic could not be used as grounds on which to conclude that BSE does not transmit to humans. The closed world assumption did not hold in this case because information about the transmission properties of BSE was not present in our knowledge base about this new disease, and could not possibly be present in the early months following the emergence of BSE.

So the closed world assumption does not hold in the case where there has been inadequate time for investigators to establish if a proposition *P* is the case. This raises the question of what constitutes adequate time. For a disease like BSE with a lengthy incubation period, the passage of just a few months was certainly inadequate. But this judgement becomes more difficult to make as we encounter longer periods of time. Would we also be inclined to describe 10 years or 20 years as inadequate? Would the failure of BSE to transmit to humans after 30 years be sufficient grounds on which to conclude that BSE does not transmit to humans? We are beginning to see some of the complex judgements that arguers must make as they attempt to evaluate the rational merits of different arguments. Moreover, time is not the only condition that may affect whether the closed world assumption holds in a particular case. If investigators have not had at their disposal the resources that are required to establish if a certain proposition *P* is true, then we can conclude nothing at all from the fact that there is no evidence that *P*. Imagine the proposition that we are interested in is the claim that restaurant workers in a certain large city are carriers of **hepatitis A**. However, due to budget cuts, there is a lack of trained staff to take blood samples from restaurant workers and to test these samples for the presence of hepatitis A in the laboratory. We certainly could not say under such circumstances that the lack of evidence that there are restaurant workers who are carriers of hepatitis A leads us to conclude that such workers do not exist. The closed world assumption does not hold in this case because investigators have been constrained by budget cuts from adding any information about the hepatitis A status of restaurant workers to the knowledge base *K*.

When trying to establish if the closed world assumption holds in a particular case, there are linguistic markers that arguers can use to assist them. For example, if we are told that a particular pesticide has been in extensive use for the last 50 years and there is no evidence that it has caused ill health in humans, then we can be reasonably certain that it does not cause ill health in humans. The two markers that lead us to believe that the closed world assumption obtains in this case are the fact that the pesticide has been in *extensive use* and that it has been in use for *50 years*. The former marker—we will call it the *dose marker*—lets an arguer see that there has been widespread exposure of humans to the pesticide in question. The latter marker—we will call it the *temporal marker*—lets an arguer see that a sufficient period of time has elapsed in which adverse health effects, if they were to occur, would have become evident. Other linguistic markers capture the size of an investigation and the expertise of investigators. Imagine for a moment that you are told that 10,000 restaurant workers in New York are tested for hepatitis A in an epidemiological investigation that is conducted by public health experts in the city's health department, and there was no evidence that restaurant workers are carriers of hepatitis A. Then you would feel reasonably certain in concluding that restaurant workers are not carriers of hepatitis A. In this case, the two markers that are the basis of your certainty are the fact that there has been a large investigation—10,000 restaurant workers were tested—and that the investigators had the requisite expertise to conduct the investigation. We will call the former marker the *scope marker*, and the latter marker the *expertise marker*. These markers may occur singly or in combination. They can each influence positively and negatively the extent to which the closed world assumption may be presumed to hold in a particular case.

EXERCISE 2.1: Closed world assumption

We have seen that a number of linguistic markers may be used by arguers to determine if the closed world assumption holds in a particular case. We called these markers *dose, temporal, scope* and *expertise markers*. The following statements are taken from the press releases of a number of public health agencies. Imagine that each of these statements exists in the background of an argument from ignorance. For each statement, indicate the type of markers that may be used by arguers to decide if the closed world assumption is warranted in a particular case.

(A) *The Department of Health, Australia, 3 April 2017*

» Perfluoroalkyated substances have been used since the 1950s in industrial processes, in a range of common household products, and some types of firefighting foams. (Press release: Australian guidance values for assessing exposure to perfluorooctane sulfonate (PFOS) and perfluorooctanoic acid (PFOA))

(B) *Centers for Disease Control and Prevention (CDC), USA, 25 January 2018*

» CDC looked at nearly 1 million births in 2016 in 15 U.S. states and territories [...] About three out of every 1000 babies born in 15 states and territories in 2016 had a birth defect possibly associated with Zika virus infections in the mother. (Press release: More birth defects seen in parts of U.S. with local Zika spread)

(C) *Public Health England, UK, 3 August 2017*

» Public Health England (PHE) has run a surveillance system with partners since 2010. This now includes surveillance at more than 30 UK sea and airports and at the largest used tyre importers. Since invasive mosquitoes have become more widespread in France, surveillance has been conducted by PHE at motorway service stations in the south east of England on the main routes from the south coast ferry ports and Eurotunnel (since 2014). The surveillance system combines a number of traps that detect mosquito eggs, host-seeking and blood-fed mosquitoes and larval sampling. (Press release: Mosquito treatment in Ashford, Kent)

Where the closed world assumption holds in a particular case, it can increase the rational warrant of the conclusion of an argument that is based on ignorance. But another condition must also be fulfilled for ignorance to have proper logical standing in an argument. We have been calling that condition the *extensive search criterion*. This criterion can be stated as follows:

Extensive search criterion:

The search of a knowledge base *K* is conducted to the fullest extent possible, using every reasonable means available.

A knowledge base *K* can be complete in the sense of containing all relevant information in a particular domain *D*. However, if the base is not extensively examined, then little logical weight can be attached to any ignorance claim that is based upon it. Imagine that a knowledge base contains the blood test results of the 10,000 restaurant workers in New York who were tested for hepatitis A in the above scenario. However, the scientists who are reviewing the results from the epidemiological study decide to examine only 2500 blood test results from restaurant workers who are employed at establishments in the north of the city. We would be very much disinclined to accept any claim based on what was not found during such a limited search of the knowledge base. By the same token, we would also be unlikely to accept a claim based on a search of the knowledge base, even a very extensive search of the knowledge base, if that search were conducted by non-expert reviewers. Even medically qualified or scientifically trained individuals may not have the requisite expertise to assess the epidemiological implications of a large number of blood test results for hepatitis A. So while we are prepared to accept the verdict of a panel of infectious disease epidemiologists who have conducted an extensive review of the knowledge base, we are much less likely to do so if we are told that gastroenterologists or astrophysicists undertook the review. The judgements that are required to decide if the extensive search criterion is satisfied in a particular case are no less complex than those needed to determine if the closed world assumption holds in a certain context. But as with the closed world assumption, there are linguistic markers that can guide us in making these judgements.

To get a sense of what these markers look like, we return to the BSE epidemic that occurred in the UK. Shortly after the first cases of BSE emerged in British cattle, a group of investigators published a significant article in the journal *Neurology*. The article concerned a spongiform encephalopathy in sheep called scrapie. The question of interest to the investigators, Brown et al. (1987), was whether there was any epidemiological evidence to suggest that scrapie had transmitted to humans. Brown et al. concluded that there was no evidence that scrapie in sheep had transmitted to humans. The basis of their ignorance claim was a review of the world literature on CJD as well as an examination of the results of a 15-year epidemiological study of CJD and scrapie in France. In other words, the available evidence was very extensively examined by Brown and his colleagues. Moreover, these investigators were expertly qualified to make an assessment of the evidence. The lead author, Paul Brown, and two of his co-authors were based at the Laboratory of Central Nervous System Studies at the U.S. National Institutes of Health in Bethesda, Maryland. A further co-author, Richard Raubertas, was affiliated with the Division of Biostatistics at the University of Rochester Medical Centre in New York. We will call these features the *comprehensiveness marker* and the *expertise marker*, respectively. A search of a mundane knowledge base, such as the journeys in a train timetable, does not need to be undertaken by experts. In this case, an expertise marker may be superseded by a *competence marker*—the individual who is examining the timetable is presumed to have a certain minimum level of competence. Alone or in combination, these markers can influence our assessment of whether the extensive search criterion is satisfied in a particular case.

EXERCISE 2.2: Extensive search criterion

To give you practice at identifying linguistic markers related to the extensive search criterion, you should examine the following statements. They are taken from press releases from a number of public health agencies around the world. Each statement describes an investigation. You should identify key features of the investigation using terms such as *expertise marker* and *comprehensiveness marker*:

(A) *The Department of Health, Australia, 26 February 2015*

» As each case was notified they were investigated by state health authorities in Victoria like all cases of Hepatitis A [...] after investigation of cases and detailed analyses of food consumption histories, the Victorian authorities confirmed a possible association with frozen berries on Thursday 12 February 2015. (Media statement: Hepatitis A linked to frozen berries)

(B) *Department of Health, Hong Kong, 2 April 2010*

» The Centre for Health Protection (CHP) of the Department of Health today received notification from the Queen Elizabeth Hospital about a 70-year-old man presenting with neurological symptoms and history of human swine influenza (HSI) vaccination. A CHP spokesman said "CHP will closely monitor the clinical progress and further laboratory results of the patient. Information about the case will be reviewed by the Expert Group in due course for determination of diagnosis and etiology". The Expert Group has earlier reviewed Guillain-Barré syndrome (GBS) cases with HSI vaccination history and concluded that no causal relationship could be established on the basis of the observed GBS incidence. (Press release: Centre for Health Protection investigates a patient with lower limb symptoms and history of human swine influenza vaccination)

(C) *Department of Health, South Africa, 5 December 2017*

» In July 2017 doctors from neonatal units in Chris Hani Baragwanath and Steve Biko Academic hospitals alerted the National Institute for Communicable Diseases (NICD) about an unusually high number of babies with listeriosis. This triggered a review by NICD of all cases diagnosed in both public and private hospitals. (Media statement: Minister of Health, Dr Aaron Motsoaledi, on the outbreak of listeriosis in South Africa)

This section has demonstrated that when employed under certain conditions, ignorance can have logical standing in an argument. Those conditions are represented by the closed world assumption and the extensive search criterion. Of course, whether or not an argument fulfils these conditions in a particular case is a task for the argument analyst. In the context of medicine and health, the argument analyst could be each one of us—the parent who is deciding whether or not to vaccinate a child, the doctor who wants to recommend a course of treatment to a patient, or the public health official who is issuing advice on how to limit the transmission of an infectious disease. For each of us must evaluate the logical role of ignorance in argument in deliberations about our own health and the health of others. In the next section, we examine a number of ignorance arguments used in medical and health contexts. We will see that conditions such as the closed world assumption and extensive search criterion are not always fulfilled in these contexts.

SPECIAL TOPIC: 'No evidence' statements in systematic reviews

One context in which 'no evidence' statements are used extensively in medicine and health is in the conclusions of systematic reviews. When we consider what these reviews involve, it is not difficult to see why this is the case. A systematic review is a review of all research studies and their findings relating to a particular question. In undertaking such a review, investigators aim to identify all studies in an area, select those studies that satisfy certain criteria for inclusion in the review, assess the quality of the studies and the evidence that they produce, synthesise their findings, and arrive at a balanced interpretation of their significance. Upon completion of a systematic review, a knowledge base may be said to be closed (at least at a particular point in time) and extensively searched. A 'no evidence' statement is then used to characterise any proposition that is not contained in the knowledge base.

The issue that concerns us is whether a systematic review can be used to transform a 'no evidence' statement into the premise in a strongly warranted argument from ignorance. On some occasions, a systematic review appears to do just that. Where a review has included only the most rigorously conducted studies that produce high-quality evidence, then there are very strong grounds for drawing a conclusion based on an absence of evidence. Such studies are typically randomized controlled trials (RCTs) like those referred to by Pennington et al. (2016) in the conclusion of a systematic review of the use of speech and language therapy (SLT) to treat children with dysarthria (a motor speech disorder) that is acquired before three years of age:

> This review found no evidence from randomised trials of the effectiveness of speech and language therapy interventions to improve the speech of children with early acquired dysarthria.

The 'no evidence' statement in the conclusion to this review can be used as a premise in a strongly warranted argument from ignorance:

Strongly warranted argument from ignorance:
There is *no evidence* that SLT is effective in the treatment of children with early acquired dysarthria.
Therefore, SLT is *not* effective in the treatment of children with early acquired dysarthria.

A RCT produces high-quality evidence. A systematic review of other types of studies can also give rise to 'no evidence' statements. However, to the extent that these statements are based on reviews of studies other than RCTs, they may provide weaker warrant in an argument from ignorance. Tsoumanis et al. (2018) conducted a systematic review of uncontrolled observational studies of the prevalence of chlamydia and gonorrhoea in men who have sex with men (MSM). This systematic review concluded that there was an absence of evidence that screening of MSM for chlamydia and gonorrhoea achieved a lowering of the prevalence of these infections:

> Our study was not able to provide evidence that screening for chlamydia and gonorrhoea lowers the prevalence of these infections in men who have sex with men.

This conclusion can certainly provide *some* rational warrant for the claim that screening does *not* achieve a lowering of prevalence of chlamydia and gonorrhoea in MSM. But this rational warrant is altogether weaker than the rational warrant in our first example, on account of the fact that it is based on a systematic review of observational studies and not RCTs:

Weakly warranted argument from ignorance:
There is an *absence of evidence* that screening for chlamydia and gonorrhoea lowers the prevalence of these infections in MSM.
Screening for chlamydia and gonorrhoea does *not* lower the prevalence of these infections in MSM.

Variants of these 'no evidence' statements are also commonly used in the conclusions of systematic reviews. Sometimes, the evidence that is lacking from the knowledge base is described as 'strong' or 'significant'. This implies that there is evidence available but that it is weak or insignificant. It would be an interesting empirical question to consider if the addition of these adjectives to the noun 'evidence' has the effect of deterring an arguer from drawing an inference based on ignorance. In this way, an arguer may reason that there is *some* (weak) evidence that *p* and that it cannot therefore be concluded that *not-p*. These variants are illustrated by the following examples. In the first example, the 'no evidence' claim relates to the effectiveness of non-speech oral motor treatments in the management of children with developmental speech sound disorders:

> Currently **no strong evidence** suggests that non-speech oral motor treatments are an effective treatment or an effective adjunctive treatment for children with developmental speech sound disorders. (Lee and Gibbon 2015)

In the second example, the absence of evidence relates to the effectiveness of dysphagia interventions (swallowing treatments) in the management of clients with hereditary ataxia:

> There is an **absence of any significant evidence** supporting the use of dysphagia intervention in hereditary ataxia. (Vogel et al. 2015)

These 'no evidence' and 'absence of evidence' statements appear to provide the weakest basis of all the statements that we have examined for a conclusion based on ignorance. For while there is *some* evidence that *p*, even some weak evidence that *p*, there appears to be little rational warrant for drawing the conclusion that *not-p*.

DISCUSSION POINT: Systematic reviews in academic journals

In an article in the *British Medical Journal*, Alderson and Roberts (2000) pose the question: 'Should journals publish systematic reviews that find no evidence to guide practice?' The authors argue that journals should make a point of publishing such reviews rather than waiting for reviews that show marked benefit or harm. However, some experts disagree, arguing that inconclusive systematic reviews simply reinforce the message that there is clinical uncertainty. What do you think journals should do with systematic reviews that report no evidence?

2.4 Arguing from Ignorance in Medicine and Health

We have already seen some of the ways in which ignorance can be used to positive and negative effect in argument. If I argue that proposition *p* is *not* the case because there is no evidence that *p* is the case, and I have based my 'no evidence' claim on a closed knowledge base that has been extensively searched, then I have very strong grounds indeed for claiming that not-*p* is true. This was effectively the position of Brown and his colleagues in 1987 when they argued that scrapie does not transmit to humans because there was no evidence based on a review of the world literature and a 15-year epidemiological study that scrapie transmits to humans. But very often in medicine and health, arguments from ignorance can go badly awry. In these cases, we do not have a rationally warranted claim that we can use in reasoning and decision-making, but an unwarranted, possibly false claim that gets us nowhere at all. When a knowledge base is closed prematurely, as it was in the case of the BSE epidemic in the UK, we can base almost nothing at all on ignorance. The claim that BSE does not transmit to humans because there was no evidence that it had transmitted to humans was not only rationally unwarranted when it was advanced, but has since also been tragically shown to be false. Also, when a knowledge base, even a complete knowledge base, is only partially examined, we can base nothing at all on a claim that a particular proposition is not in the base. Ignorance achieves nothing for us if a search of a base has been incomplete, or has not been competently or expertly conducted. In this section, we will see how arguers in medical and health contexts navigate these conditions on the logical use of ignorance in argument.

Consider the following extract from a press release on 25 March 2014 from Public Health England (PHE). The extract describes the findings of a report by PHE into the health effects of water fluoridation schemes:

> Children in local authorities with water fluoridation schemes have less tooth decay than those in local authorities without such schemes, says a new report by Public Health England (PHE). The report says there is no evidence of harm to health in fluoridated areas. PHE has found no differences between fluoridated and non-fluoridated areas in their rates of hip fracture, osteosarcoma (a form of bone cancer), cancers overall, Down's syndrome births or all-cause mortality (all recorded causes of death). (Press release: Fluoride monitoring report finds lower levels of tooth decay in fluoridated areas and no evidence of harm to health)

Imagine that you are the parent of a young child and that you live in a water fluoridation area. You have had concerns for some time about the potential health effects of fluoridation. You have read stories online and in the local newspaper about this issue, and have also discussed it with some of your friends. You hear on the television that Public Health England has published a significant report on the issue. You head to the PHE website where you read the above press release. You have no scientific or technical expertise to draw on, and you certainly do not believe you have the knowledge to read and understand the full report. So you try to make the best assessment possible of the findings of the report based on the press release from PHE. You feel reasonably convinced on the basis of the press statement that water fluoridation does not cause ill health effects in humans. Three factors lead you to this conclusion. The first factor is the finding of lower levels of tooth decay in children who live in local authorities that have water fluoridation schemes. This positive finding suggests that there are health benefits to be derived from fluoridation. The second factor is the finding that a number of cancers, congenital disorders, and other conditions do not have an elevated prevalence in fluoridated areas. The logical pull of these factors is clearly in the direction of the conclusion that fluoridation does not cause ill health effects. The third factor is the use of a 'no evidence' statement. When interpreted against the backdrop of the rest of the PHE press release, and particularly the logical pull of the first two factors, this statement leads you to reason along the following lines:

> There is *no evidence* that water fluoridation causes harm to humans.
> Therefore, water fluoridation does *not* cause harm to humans.

You believe the conclusion of this argument from ignorance is rationally warranted given some additional information that PHE has included in its press release. This information conveys two key facts about fluoridation that were not previously part of your knowledge:

» Currently, around 6 million people live in areas with fluoridation schemes. Many schemes have been in operation for over 40 years.

These facts provide the rational warrant you need to support the closed world assumption at the heart of your argument from ignorance. The fact that around 6 million people have been exposed to fluoridation is an important *dose marker* that gives you confidence that the knowledge base on the health effects of fluoridation may be assumed to be closed. Also, the fact that many fluoridation schemes have been in operation for over 40 years is an important *temporal marker* that the knowledge base may be treated as closed. The closed world assumption appears strongly warranted to you in this particular case on the basis of these two markers. Your attention then turns to the extensive search criterion. You want to determine if this is as strongly warranted as the closed world assumption. Additional information in the press release once again helps you make a decision. The press release from PHE states that this is the first report on the health of people living in fluoridated areas since PHE came into existence in April 2013. However, you have sufficient trust in the expertise of this body to conclude that the authors of the report will have conducted the fullest review possible of all the available evidence on the health effects of fluoridation. So you use an *expertise marker* as rational warrant for the extensive search criterion. With both the closed world assumption and the extensive search criterion strongly warranted in this case, you feel there is sufficient rational justification to draw the conclusion of the above argument from ignorance. You come away from reading the PHE press release with the firm belief that water fluoridation does *not* cause harm to humans.

This scenario has all the hallmarks of a rationally warranted use of the argument from ignorance. First, the argument does not stand alone as the sole means of rational persuasion of readers. Rather, the conclusion of the argument from ignorance—fluoridation does *not* cause harm to humans—is also supported by two other findings that are independent of the argument from ignorance. These are the findings of reduced levels of tooth decay in children who live in fluoridated areas, and similar prevalence of cancers and congenital disorders in fluoridated and non-fluoridated areas. Second, PHE provides sufficient background information for readers to determine if the two conditions on the rationally warranted use of the argument from ignorance—the closed world assumption and the extensive search criterion—hold in this particular case. The press release clearly indicates for readers that a large number of people have been exposed to fluoridation over a period of at least 40 years. Readers can readily identify a dose marker and a temporal marker in this information, which may be used to support the closed world assumption. That PHE is a reputable body of public health experts provides readers with an expertise marker that they can use to support the extensive search criterion. Third, although this is the first water fluoridation report that PHE has produced since it came into existence in April 2013, the Chief Knowledge Officer at PHE, Professor John Newton, is reported in the press release to have said that PHE is required by legislation to produce a similar report every four years. This information recognizes the possibility that new evidence may be forthcoming in the future. This evidence may substantially change the knowledge base that is the basis of our current conclusion that fluoridation does not cause harm to humans. The PHE press release acknowledges that this conclusion, like the conclusion of any ignorance argument, is defeasible in the presence of contrary evidence. A less responsible form of public health communication may not have countenanced the possibility of such revision.

This last point is sufficiently important to warrant further discussion. Any claim based on an argument from ignorance is defeasible in the sense that it can be overturned if contrary evidence emerges at some later point in time. In the above scenario, that possibility is explicitly signalled by Professor John Newton when he states that there will be continuous monitoring of the human health effects of fluoridation in subsequent reports by PHE. But very often, the defeasible nature of a claim that is based on ignorance can be indicated through the use of language rather than by the provision of additional information as in this particular case. There are linguistic markers of **defeasibility** in the same way that there are linguistic markers of a closed knowledge base and an extensively searched knowledge base. To illustrate some of these markers, consider the following 'no evidence' statements in press releases from the Department of Health in Hong Kong:

- *No scientific evidence* to date has confirmed a link between Zika virus and microcephaly or Guillain-Barré syndrome. (Press release on 15 February 2016: Centre for Health Protection closely monitors latest WHO Zika epidemiological updates)
- 'It is also safe to eat pork, provided it is well-cooked. At present, there is *no evidence* that Hong Kong is at high risk of an outbreak. However, we will continue to monitor closely the situation as well as the latest developments in Sichuan', said Dr York Chow, the Secretary for Health, Welfare and Food. (Press release on 1 August 2005: Streptococcus suis to become notifiable disease)

The underlined temporal markers in these statements indicate that the emergence of new evidence may necessitate a revision of the knowledge base upon which these 'no evidence' claims are based. In some cases, these markers may have the effect of dissuading a reader from drawing an inference based on ignorance altogether. But in those cases where an inference is drawn based on the absence of evidence, these markers provide a note of caution to the effect 'Reader beware, what holds now may be overturned at a later point in time'. In drawing the reader's attention to the defeasibility of a claim that is based on the absence of evidence, these temporal markers are doing important logical work. Like the other markers we have examined, they are highlighting the epistemic conditions that are integral to the rationality of the argument from ignorance.

EXERCISE 2.3: Defeasibility of the argument from ignorance

We have seen that there are linguistic markers of defeasibility in the same way that there are linguistic markers of other logical features of the argument from ignorance. The following 'no evidence' statements are taken from press releases of three public health agencies, Public Health England and the Department of Health and Social Care in the UK, and the Department of Health in Hong Kong. For each statement, identify a temporal marker that suggests the defeasibility of claims that are based on an absence of evidence:

(a) *Department of Health, Hong Kong, 10 June 2016*

- 'We have no evidence at this stage that patients of the five recent cases so far had received injections in the same premises. Epidemiological investigations are ongoing', a spokesman for the Department of Health said. (Press release: Centre for Health Protection investigates additional case of suspected botulism following botulinum toxin injections)

(b) *Department of Health and Social Care, UK, 23 December 2011*

- Chief Medical Officer Dame Sally Davies said: 'While we respect the French Government's decision, no other country is taking similar steps because we currently have no evidence to support it. Because of this, and because removing these implants carries risk in itself, we are not advising routine removal of these implants.' (Press release: Chief Medical Officer statement on breast implants)

(c) *Public Health England, UK, 26 November 2015*

» A range of surveillance indicators are used to measure flu activity in the UK. At the moment these remain low across the UK, suggesting there is presently no evidence of community transmission of influenza. (Press release: Improved vaccine uptake for children, pregnant women and older people)

(d) *Department of Health, Hong Kong, 18 January 2010*

» In response to media enquiries concerning a 66-year-old woman with a history of human swine influenza (HSI) vaccination who passed away yesterday, a spokesman for the Centre for Health Protection of the Department of Health said that as clarified with the hospital, 'So far, no evidence shows that the death was related to HSI vaccination'. (Press release: No evidence suggests linkage of fatal case with human swine influenza vaccination)

(e) *Public Health England, UK, 11 February 2015*

» Dr Dipiti Patel, joint director at the National Travel Health Network and Centre, said: 'Birds can carry a wide variety of avian flu viruses and most of these do not cause human illness. The two types of avian flu viruses currently causing the greatest concern for human health are H5N1 and H7N9. These infections are typically seen in people who have had close contact with birds. To date there has been no evidence of sustained human-to-human spread of avian flu viruses.' (Press release: Travel safely this Chinese New Year)

The 'fluoridation' argument is an example of the rationally warranted use of ignorance in extended argumentation. Moreover, Public Health England directly engaged the rational resources of readers by providing the type of information that could achieve closure of the knowledge base at the heart of the argument. This is an example of public health communication that was responsibly conducted *and* rationally warranted. Instances of the sound or rationally warranted use of the argument from ignorance are, however, quite rare in medical and health contexts. Fallacious arguments from ignorance are relatively common in these contexts. In the remainder of this section, an equally detailed analysis will be conducted of the fallacious use of the argument from ignorance in public health. The issue on this occasion concerns the safety of Poly Implant Prothèse (PIP) breast implants following an announcement on 23 December 2011 that the French Government was recommending women to have these implants removed as a precautionary, but non-urgent measure. Recognizing that this announcement would cause widespread concern among the thousands of British women who had also received PIP implants, the Chief Medical Officer, Professor Dame Sally Davies, released a press statement to the public and wrote a letter to general practitioners, Medical Directors in the National Health Service (NHS), and cancer and plastic surgeons. The press release and letter, which were issued by the Department of Health in the UK on the same day as the French Government's announcement, made extensive use of 'no evidence' statements. Two examples of these statements are shown below:

» Chief Medical Officer Dame Sally Davies said: 'Women with PIP implants should not be unduly worried. We have no evidence of a link to cancer or an increased risk of rupture. If women are concerned they should speak to their surgeon.' (Press statement: Chief Medical Officer statement on breast implants)

» In the UK, the Medicines and Healthcare products Regulatory Agency (MHRA) is not [...] recommending routine removal because they have no evidence of any disproportionate rate of implant rupture. Moreover, there is no evidence of any increase in incidence of cancer associated with these implants. (Letter to NHS staff: PIP silicone gel breast implants)

The Chief Medical Officer used 'no evidence' statements on six occasions in these communications to the public and to staff in the NHS. The thrust of these statements was clear. The public and medical professionals alike were being strongly encouraged to draw the conclusions that PIP implants are *not* associated with a disproportionate rate of implant rupture, and are *not* associated with an increase in incidence of cancer. These were undoubtedly reassuring messages for women with these implants to be given. The question that concerns us is whether the claims at the centre of these messages are rationally warranted. These claims are derived by means of the following arguments from ignorance:

There is *no evidence* that PIP implants have a disproportionate rate of implant rupture.
PIP implants do *not* have a disproportionate rate of implant rupture.

There is *no evidence* that PIP implants are linked with an increase in incidence of cancer.
PIP implants are *not* linked with an increase in incidence of cancer.

As with the 'fluoridation' argument, we need to establish if there are grounds for presuming that the closed world assumption and the extensive search criterion hold in this case. The closed world assumption looks decidedly weak on this occasion. The Chief Medical Officer made her remarks on 23 December 2011. This was some six months before the expert group that was tasked with examining the safety of PIP implants produced its final report on 18 June 2012. This group was chaired by Sir Bruce Keogh, NHS Medical Director. An interim report was produced by Sir Bruce and his colleagues on 6 January 2012. However, even the findings of the interim report were not available to the Chief Medical Officer when she embarked on providing reassurance to the public about the safety of PIP implants on 23 December 2011. The haste with which reassurance was offered about the safety of PIP implants was later found to be misguided. In its final report, the expert group chaired by Sir Bruce concluded:

» PIP implants are significantly more likely to rupture or leak silicone than other implants, by a factor of around 2-6. (Keogh 2012: 1)

The Chief Medical Officer did not have access to the interim or final reports of the expert group at the point when she was using 'no evidence' statements to provide reassurances about the safety of PIP implants to the public. These reports, particularly the final report, would have been strong grounds to suppose that the closed world assumption was warranted in this case. But in the absence of these reports, the Chief Medical Officer was basing her 'no evidence' statements on a very limited knowledge base indeed. Clearly, there would be no evidence of any rupture risk or cancer risk associated with these implants *in advance of* the inquiry that was supposed to establish if these risks existed. Of course, the Chief Medical Officer was basing her 'no evidence' statements on some grounds. She set out what these grounds were, both in her press statement and in her letter to key NHS staff on 23 December 2011:

> The Medicines and Healthcare products Regulatory Agency (MHRA) has previously commissioned toxicity testing on the filler, including genotoxicity and chemical toxicity, discussed this with their experts and concluded that there is no associated safety issue. The MHRA have also reviewed available evidence for association of cancers of women with breast implants in consultation with the relevant UK professional bodies for breast surgery and surgical oncology and with the Cancer Registry, and have concluded there is no evidence to indicate any association. (Letter to NHS staff: PIP silicone gel breast implants)

The MHRA regulates medicines, medical devices and blood components for transfusion in the UK. On 29 March 2010, the French medical device regulatory authority—Agence Française de Sécurité Sanitaire des Produits de Santé (AFSSAPS)—informed MHRA that it had suspended the marketing, distribution, export, and use of PIP implants following an inspection of the PIP manufacturing plant. AFSSAPS had established that breast implants manufactured since 2001 had been filled with a silicone gel with a composition different from that which had been approved. In April 2010, AFSSAPS initiated testing of affected implants to look at genotoxicity (potential for cancer), cellular toxicity and irritation to biological tissues. At the end of June 2010, AFSSAPS told the MHRA of delays to their product testing. At that point, the MHRA decided to commission a specific series of tests (the Ames tests) to measure the genotoxic activity of chemicals in PIP silicone. These are the tests that the Chief Medical Officer describes in her letter to NHS staff. The results of these tests were uniformly negative. However, these tests and their results really tell us nothing at all about the claims that are central to the Chief Medical Officer's 'no evidence' statements. It will be recalled that one of those claims concerns the rate of rupture of PIP implants relative to other types of implants. No amount of genotoxicity and chemical toxicity testing could address this concern. This issue could only be addressed by the investigation led by Sir Bruce Keogh as part of the work of his expert group.

As a result of the urgency to provide public reassurance about the safety of PIP implants, the Chief Medical Officer made fallacious use of the argument from ignorance. Her repeated use of 'no evidence' statements suggested that a closed knowledge base was already available to investigators when this was in fact not the case. Toxicity tests of PIP silicone certainly contributed important information to the knowledge base. But these tests could not address questions about the rupture rates of PIP implants that were at the heart of the messages of reassurance offered by the Chief Medical Officer. Answers to these questions awaited the final report of the expert group led by Sir Bruce Keogh. However, this group did not publish its report until 18 June 2012, some six months after the advice given to the public and medical professionals by Professor Dame Sally Davies. This advice was misleading and, on the question of PIP implant rupture rates, was shown ultimately to be inaccurate. The argument from ignorance was 'overplayed' by the Chief Medical Officer in an effort to reassure PIP implant recipients in the UK that there was no need to adopt the precautionary approach taken by French authorities. There was no closed knowledge base or extensively searched knowledge base, as the Chief Medical Officer's statements appeared to suggest. Both awaited the findings of the investigation conducted by Sir Bruce Keogh's expert group. The knowledge base on PIP implant safety did contain information about the toxicity of chemicals in PIP silicone. But this information was erroneously used by the Chief Medical Officer to force the closure of the knowledge base, and draw a reassuring conclusion about PIP implant safety based on the absence of any evidence relating to the rupture of implants (◘ Fig. 2.4).

It has taken considerable work to expose the fallacious argument from ignorance at the centre of the Chief Medical Officer's claims. The knowledge base on PIP implant safety has been subjected to extensive scrutiny. This has necessitated an examination of the type of information that was contributed to the base, as well as an assessment of how and when this information was obtained, and whether it relates to the claims advanced by the Chief Medical Officer. Needless to say, this level of scrutiny exceeds the interest and intellectual curiosity of most members of the public, perhaps even most PIP implant recipients. This is exactly why fallacious uses of the argument from ignorance are so dangerous. They can easily strike us as a persuasive form of argument when further analysis reveals that they are anything but rationally warranted. Some logical protection is afforded if we keep the closed world assumption and extensive

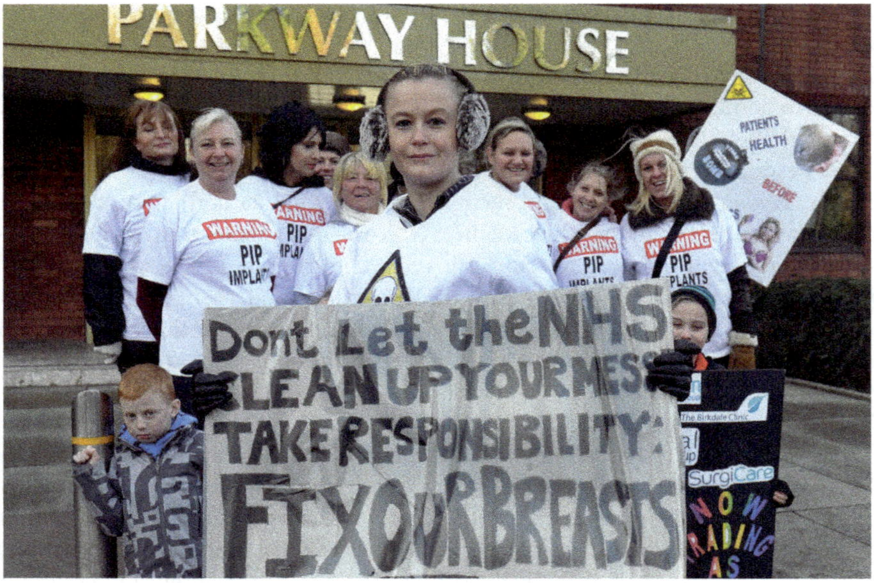

◘ **Fig. 2.4** Protest at Surgicare Medical Group clinic in Northenden, south Manchester, by women with faulty PIP breast implants including Laura Costello (centre, front), January 22, 2012 (Reproduced with kind permission of MEN Media)

search criterion at the centre of our attention. In this case, it became apparent quite quickly that the Chief Medical Officer was overstating the closure of the knowledge base on PIP implant safety. Repeated use of 'no evidence' statements did little to disguise the fact that the knowledge base lacked information relating to the rupture rates of PIP implants. And the results of toxicity tests, which did form part of the knowledge base, were unable to address this critical aspect of PIP implant safety. Alongside the overuse of 'no evidence' statements, another feature of this scenario that should have alerted us to a potentially fallacious use of the argument from ignorance was the timing of the Chief Medical Officer's statements. These statements were a hasty reaction to the precautionary measures taken by the French Government. They were not arrived at in a reflective way and in full consideration of the conclusions of the expert group led by Sir Bruce Keogh. Only the latter could truly be said to close the knowledge base on PIP implant safety.

CHECKLIST: How to use the argument from ignorance

Features to observe…

- There must be good reasons to suppose that the closed world assumption holds in a particular case. Information that can help an arguer close a knowledge base should be provided. Dose markers and temporal markers are effective proxies for a closed knowledge base.
- There must be good reasons to suppose that the extensive search criterion holds in a particular case. Information that can help an arguer establish the extent of the search of a knowledge base should be provided. The expertise of a scientific review panel is one marker of a rigorous, comprehensive search process.
- An argument from ignorance can provide strong rational warrant for a conclusion or a claim. But it should not be made to carry an excessive evidential burden. This can be avoided by bringing forward other evidence that is independent of the argument from ignorance in support of a claim.
- An argument from ignorance is a defeasible form of argumentation that can be overturned as new evidence emerges. To this end, information should be conveyed and language should be adopted that conveys openness to the possibility of revision.

Features to avoid…

- Forced closure of the knowledge base is a common reason why the argument from ignorance fails. Quite often, closure can occur before an investigation or inquiry has even taken place, in which case it will be inevitable that there will be no evidence relating to a claim.
- Even when there is evidence in the knowledge base, this evidence may not relate to a proposition or a claim that is central to a 'no evidence' statement. However, the presence of this unrelated evidence may be used to force the closure of the knowledge base and present the base as complete.
- Fallacious arguments from ignorance are most often used to provide reassurances about the safety of food or a medical product when there is a

breaking medical or health story that is likely to cause widespread public alarm. The overuse of 'no evidence' statements to frame reassurances about safety is often an indication that the argument is being used fallaciously.

- The absence of linguistic markers that suggest defeasibility is often a sign that the argument from ignorance is being used fallaciously. Markers such as *at the present time* and *from the available evidence* suggest that any claim based on a 'no evidence' statement is subject to revision should new evidence emerge. When these markers are noticeably absent, it should raise suspicion of a fallacious argument from ignorance.

2.5 Ignorance as a Cognitive Heuristic

It has been argued throughout the chapter that there is nothing inherently fallacious about the argument from ignorance. Rather, the argument is more or less rationally warranted under certain conditions. When there is a closed knowledge base and an extensively searched knowledge base, the absence of evidence that *p* is true is reasonable grounds for concluding that *p* is false. In this final section, we examine non-fallacious uses of the argument from ignorance in more detail. A proposition that cannot be located in a knowledge base following investigation of a question or issue and an extensive search of the base can quite legitimately be claimed to be false. But what makes us want to terminate an investigation and draw a conclusion based on ignorance rather than leave an inquiry open on an indefinite basis? After all, some evidence may be forthcoming that might definitively address an issue one way or another and avoid the need to draw an inference based on an absence of knowledge or evidence. The reason we do not allow investigations and other forms of inquiry to be continued on an indefinite basis is that reasoning is not a purely theoretical exercise. Rather, it is conducted within the practical sphere of action. In this sphere, we are all practically-situated cognitive agents who must make decisions and take courses of action in order to thrive and survive. None of us can afford the luxury of interminable cognitive deliberation, especially not if we want to find food and shelter and protect ourselves from various threats in our environment. Each of these goals requires actions to be performed within certain time constraints. And for this to occur, deliberation must come to an end.

Nowhere is the demand for action more keenly felt than in medicine and health. An infectious disease outbreak will not await the conclusion of exhaustive investigations by scientists and public health officials before it takes its grim toll on the lives of human beings. Preventative measures must often be taken in advance of the completion of an investigation and on the basis of scarce evidence. Decision-making in the absence of complete evidence is not an unusual state of affairs in medicine and health. Just such a scenario characterized the early public health response to HIV/AIDS before scientists had even succeeded in identifying a blood-borne virus as the causal agent of this novel disease. It was also the basis of the human Specified Bovine Offal (SBO) ban that was instituted in November 1989 and that was to prove a decisive measure in protecting human health from BSE. But even decision-making in the absence of evidence must be guided by some type of rational procedure. The argument from ignorance, I contend, is just such a procedure. Its function is that of a mental shortcut or cognitive heuristic that allows us to bridge gaps in our knowledge and arrive at a warranted claim that can become a basis for action. As events unfold and new evidence emerges, the claim in question may need to be rejected. The inherent defeasibility of the argument from ignorance means that its conclusion may be subject to revision. But until this is necessary, its conclusion can provide a tentative basis for action in a context where inaction could have serious consequences for human health. Inaction in the presence of extended deliberation can certainly avert an erroneous decision and course of action. But it is a poor pro-survival cognitive policy by any reasonable standard.

So the use of ignorance as a heuristic is motivated by the action orientation of the practical sphere, and particularly the need to terminate deliberation and pursue a course of action. Inquiry and other forms of deliberation place considerable demands on the resources, including attention and memory, of cognitive agents. These resources are finite in nature and must be sparingly deployed. Deliberation is also a time-intensive process as agents interrogate all aspects of a problem or issue. Through its termination of deliberation, the ignorance heuristic is achieving important economies in terms of time and resources for cognitive agents. This is the hallmark of all heuristics. They are 'fast and frugal' procedures that do not expend the resources of their more systematic counterparts in reasoning (Gigerenzer and Goldstein 1996). The scientist or health worker who must respond to an emerging infectious disease or other health problem can employ heuristics as a rational strategy for managing decision-making under the pressure of the practical sphere. The termination of deliberation and subsequent acceptance of a claim that the ignorance heuristic makes possible gives investigators some epistemic foothold in an incomplete evidential base. That foothold permits decisions and actions to be taken in the absence of evidence, such as when the human SBO ban was instituted in advance of any knowledge of the transmissibility of BSE to humans. The epistemic and practical gains that accrue from action in the absence of evidence outweigh the costs associated with error, and the costs associated with total inaction until such times as evidence becomes available. Against these alternatives, the ignorance heuristic is an effective use of our rational resources, and is not the 'fallacy' that many commentators have argued is the case.

Chapter Summary

Key points

- An argument from ignorance contains a premise that expresses a lack of knowledge or evidence that *p* is true (alternatively, *not-p* is true). From this premise, it is concluded that *p* is false (alternatively, *not-p* is false).
- The standard view of the argument from ignorance is that it is a fallacy, a type of weak, invalid, or bad reasoning. This has been its characterization by most philosophers throughout the long history of logic.

2

- Informal logicians take a different view of the argument from ignorance. They claim that the argument is more or less rationally warranted in certain contexts of use or under certain conditions.
- Two conditions on the use of a rationally warranted argument from ignorance are the *closed world assumption* and the *extensive search criterion*. The closed world assumption requires that all information relevant to domain *D* is contained in a knowledge base *K*. The extensive search criterion requires investigators to have conducted an exhaustive search of *K*.
- During argument evaluation, a number of linguistic markers can serve as proxies for the closed world assumption and extensive search criterion. They can help an arguer decide if the closed world assumption and extensive search criterion are fulfilled in a particular case.
- Other linguistic markers include expressions like *currently*, *at this stage* and *to date*. These temporal markers remind us that the argument from ignorance is a form of defeasible reasoning. We may need to reject the conclusion of an argument from ignorance as new evidence emerges.
- The argument from ignorance can function as a cognitive heuristic. It allows investigators to gain an epistemic foothold in an incomplete evidential base and accept a claim (albeit tentatively) that may be used as a basis for action. This is especially important in medicine and health where preventative measures to protect human health may need to be taken in the absence of evidence, or before the conclusion of an investigation or inquiry.

Suggestions for Further Reading

(1) Walton, D. (1995). *Arguments from ignorance*. University Park: Pennsylvania State University Press.

This is the only book-length treatment of the argument from ignorance. Walton examines everyday conversations in which the argument is used as a respectable form of reasoning and also situations in which it is fallacious. There is discussion of prominent cases such as the Salem witchcraft trials and McCarthy hearings. One of Walton's case studies examines the issue of the safety of silicone breast implants.

(2) Krabbe, E. C. W. (1995). Appeal to ignorance. In H. V. Hansen & R. C. Pinto (Eds.), *Fallacies: Classical and contemporary readings* (pp. 251–264). University Park: Pennsylvania State University Press.

Krabbe examines two variants of the argument from ignorance. The first is a dialectical move that amounts to an unacceptable attempt to shift the burden of proof. The second is a principle for evaluating the outcome of a dialogue—forcing the proponent who fails to prove *p* to accept *not-p*. Krabbe finds both these variants problematic. But he does not thereby conclude that all appeals to ignorance in dialogue are inherently fallacious. The chapter examines reasonable appeals to ignorance in the context of persuasion dialogue.

(3) Cummings, L. (2015). *Reasoning and public health: New ways of coping with uncertainty*. Cham, Switzerland: Springer.

▶ Chapter 3 in this volume examines the argument from ignorance. The results of an experimental study involving 879 members of the public in the UK are reported. These subjects were asked to assess arguments from ignorance in which the closure of the knowledge base and the search of the knowledge base were varied. The argument is characterized as a cognitive heuristic that facilitates reasoning in contexts of uncertainty.

Questions

(1) An argument from ignorance contains a distinctive premise that uses a particular form of words. It states that there is *no knowledge or evidence* that *X* is the case (alternatively, there is *no knowledge or evidence* that not-*X* is the case). The following passages are taken from a number of different health sources. Identify the ignorance statement in each passage. Attempt to reconstruct this statement as the premise in an argument from ignorance:

(A)

Title Continuation of whooping cough vaccination programme in pregnancy advised

Source Press release, Department of Health and Social Care, United Kingdom, 16 July 2014

These findings are supplemented by the first large study of the whooping cough vaccine safety in pregnancy, published by the Medicines and Healthcare Products Regulatory Agency in the British Medical Journal. Reviewing data from around 18,000 vaccinated women from the Clinical Practice Research Datalink, the research found no evidence of risk from the vaccine to pregnancy or the developing baby, and rates of normal, healthy births were similar to those seen in unvaccinated women.

(B)

Title Response level for Middle East Respiratory Syndrome (MERS) lowered to "Alert"

Source Press release, Department of Health, Hong Kong, 1 August 2015

"According to the World Health Organization, the epidemiological pattern of the outbreak in Korea was similar to hospital-associated outbreaks that have occurred in the Middle East and there is no evidence of sustained community transmission of MERS-Coronavirus (MERS-CoV) in Korea", a spokesman for the Department of Health said.

(C)

Title No evidence of Gouléako and Herbert virus infections in pigs, Côte d'Ivoire & Ghana

Source Academic article, Emerging Infectious Diseases, volume 21, issue 12, 2190–2193

A recent report suggested that two novel bunyaviruses discovered in insects in Côte d'Ivoire caused lethal disease in swine in South Korea. We conducted cell culture studies and tested serum from pigs exposed to mosquitoes in Côte d'Ivoire and Ghana and found no evidence for infection in pigs.

2

(2) Temporal markers such as *so far, currently* and *at the present stage* can be used to indicate that a closed knowledge base may have to be revised if contrary evidence emerges at a later date. They are accordingly important markers of the defeasibility of claims that are based on an absence of evidence or knowledge. However, not all uses of these expressions suggest the defeasibility of claims that are based on an absence of evidence. The following statements are taken from the press releases of public health agencies in the UK and Hong Kong. They each contain the expression *so far*. For each instance of this expression, state if it is used to indicate the defeasibility of a claim that is based on an absence of evidence:

(A)

Title	E-cigarettes around 95% less harmful than tobacco estimates landmark review
Source	Press release, Public Health England, UK, 19 August 2015

An expert independent evidence review published today by Public Health England concludes that e-cigarettes are significantly less harmful to health than tobacco and have the potential to help smokers quit smoking. Key findings of the review include: There is no evidence so far that e-cigarettes are acting as a route into smoking for children or non-smokers.

(B)

Title	Hong Kong's readiness to fight avian influenza under review
Source	Press release, Department of Health, Hong Kong, 26 October 2005

The Permanent Secretary for Health, Welfare and Food, Mrs Carrie Yau, convened an interdepartmental meeting this afternoon to review Hong Kong's readiness to fight avian influenza amid fears that migratory birds might spread the virus with the approach of winter.
"The recent avian flu outbreak among birds and poultry is a cause for concern. However, there is no evidence to date confirming that the H5N1 virus is capable of efficient human-to-human transmission. So far, the series of preventive measures we adopted on local poultry farms, wholesale and retail markets are largely effective in countering the threat of avian flu", she said.

(C)

Title	Mosquito treatment in Ashford, Kent
Source	Press release, Public Health England, UK, 3 August 2017

Enhanced surveillance is being conducted at the site and in the vicinity, including the deployment of additional traps and larval sampling. So far, no further evidence of A. albopictus has been found, and there is no evidence so far that it has become established.

(3) The reconstruction and evaluation of any argument from ignorance requires knowledge of the conditions under which such an argument is more or less rationally warranted. Use your knowledge of these conditions to answer questions about the following extract from the Public Health Agency of Canada:

Title Outbreak of E. coli infections linked to romaine lettuce

Source Press health notice, Public Health Agency of Canada, 9 February 2018

The Public Health Agency of Canada collaborated with provincial public health partners, the Canadian Food Inspection Agency and Health Canada to investigate an outbreak of Escherichia coli 0157, commonly called E. coli. The outbreak involved five eastern provinces. Based on the investigation findings during the outbreak, exposure to romaine lettuce was identified as the source of the outbreak, but the cause of contamination was not identified. No individuals have had illness onset dates beyond December 12, 2017. As a result, the outbreak appears to be over, and the investigation has been closed [...] In total, there were 42 cases of E. coli 0157 illness reported in five eastern provinces: Ontario (8), Quebec (15), New Brunswick (5), Nova Scotia (1), and Newfoundland and Labrador (13). Individuals became sick in November and early December 2017. Seventeen individuals were hospitalized. One individual died. Individuals who became ill were between the ages of 3 and 85 years of age. The majority of cases (74%) were female. There was no evidence to suggest that provinces in western Canada were affected by this outbreak.

(a) This extract contains a claim that is a potential premise in an argument from ignorance. What is that claim?
(b) Use the claim that you identified in response to (a) to construct an argument from ignorance.
(c) Does the argument from ignorance that you constructed in response to (b) have strong rational warrant? Provide a justification of your response.
(d) Can you identify any other claim apart from that in your response to (a) that expresses a lack of knowledge or ignorance?
(e) What information in the passage suggests that the knowledge base about the E. coli outbreak is unlikely to undergo revision at a later point in time?

Answers

Exercise 2.1

(A)
Temporal marker: Perfluoroalkyated substances have been used *since the 1950s*.
Dose marker: People have had considerable exposure to these substances *in a range of common household products* as well as *industrial processes* and *firefighting foams*.

(B)
Expertise marker: The epidemiological investigation was conducted by the Centers for Disease Control and Prevention in the United States, a body of experts in infectious disease control.
Scope marker: The study took in a large geographical region (15 states and territories) as well as a large number of births (nearly 1 million).

(C)
Temporal markers: Mosquito surveillance has been conducted *since 2010* at UK sea and airports and at motorway service stations *since 2014.*
Expertise marker: Surveillance has been conducted by an expert body, namely, Public Health England.
Scope marker: Surveillance has been conducted at more than 30 UK sea and airports and at motorway service stations in south east England.

Exercise 2.2

(A)
Expertise marker: The investigation was conducted by state health authorities in Victoria, Australia.
Comprehensiveness marker: The investigation involved a detailed analysis of all food consumption histories.

(B)
Expertise marker: Two expert bodies were involved in an assessment of a potential relationship between human swine influenza vaccination and Guillain-Barré syndrome. They are the Centre for Health Protection and the Expert Group.
Comprehensiveness marker: The Expert Group reviewed all earlier cases of Guillain-Barré syndrome with a history of human swine influenza vaccination.

(C)
Expertise marker: Review of cases of listeriosis was conducted by an expert body, the National Institute for Communicable Diseases.
Comprehensiveness marker: All cases of listerioris in both private and public hospitals were examined as part of the review.

Exercise 2.3

(a) at this stage; so far; (b) currently; (c) at the moment; presently; (d) so far; (e) to date

End-of-chapter questions

(1)
Part (A):
There is *no evidence* that the whooping cough vaccine poses a risk to a developing baby.
Therefore, the whooping cough vaccine does *not* pose a risk to a developing baby.

Part (B):
There is *no evidence* of sustained community transmission of MERS-Coronavirus in Korea.
Therefore, sustained community transmission of MERS-Coronavirus in Korea does *not* occur.

Part (C):
There is *no evidence* that pigs exposed to mosquitoes are infected with bunyaviruses. Therefore, mosquitoes do *not* transmit bunyaviruses to pigs.

(2)
Part (A): In this extract, *so far* is used to indicate the defeasibility of the following claim based on an absence of evidence: E-cigarettes do not act as a route into smoking for children and non-smokers.

Part (B): In this extract, *so far* is not used to indicate the defeasibility of a claim based on an absence of evidence. That role is performed by the expression *to date*, which indicates that the following claim may have to be revised at a later point in time: The H5N1 virus is not capable of efficient human-to-human transmission.

Part (C): In this extract, there are two instances of the expression *so far*. The first instance is used to indicate the defeasibility of the following claim: A. Albopictus does not exist. The second instance is used to indicate the defeasibility of the following claim: A. albopictus has not become established.

(3)
(a) There is no evidence that provinces in western Canada were affected by the outbreak.
(b) There is *no evidence* that provinces in western Canada were affected by the outbreak. Therefore, provinces in western Canada were *not* affected by the outbreak.
(c) The argument from ignorance does have strong rational warrant. This is because it is based on a closed knowledge base (the investigation into the outbreak is closed) that has been extensively searched (presumably) by the investigators of the outbreak.
(d) At the conclusion of the investigation, the cause of the contamination is not known.
(e) The extract says that no individuals experienced illness onset after 12 December 2017. This suggests that the outbreak is over and there is unlikely to be any need to revise the knowledge base at a later point in time.

References

Alderson, P., & Roberts, I. (2000). Should journals publish systematic reviews that find no evidence to guide practice? Examples from injury research. *British Medical Journal, 320,* 376.

Brown, P., Cathala, F., Raubertas, R. F., Gajdusek, D. C., & Castaigne, P. (1987). The epidemiology of Creutzfeldt-Jakob disease: Conclusion of a 15-year investigation in France and review of the world literature. *Neurology, 37*(6), 895–904.

Cummings, L. (2014). Informal fallacies as cognitive heuristics in public health reasoning. *Informal Logic, 34*(1), 1–37.

Cummings, L. (2015). *Reasoning and public health: New ways of coping with uncertainty*. Cham, Switzerland: Springer.

Gigerenzer, G., & Goldstein, D. G. (1996). Reasoning the fast and frugal way: Models of bounded rationality. *Psychological Review, 103*(4), 650–669.

Inungu, J., Mumford, V., Younis, M., & Langford, S. (2009). HIV knowledge, attitudes and practices among college students in the United States. *Journal of Health and Human Services Administration, 32*(3), 259–277.

Jalloh, M. F., Sengeh, P., Monasch, R., Jalloh, M. B., DeLuca, N., Dyson, M., et al. (2017). National survey of Ebola-related knowledge, attitudes and practices before the outbreak peak in Sierra Leone: August 2014. *BMJ Global Health, 2,* e000285. ▶ https://doi.org/10.1136/bmjgh-2017-000285.

Kelley, D. (2014). *The art of reasoning: An introduction to logic and critical thinking* (4th ed.). New York: W. W. Norton.

Keogh, B. (2012). *Poly Implant Prothèse (PIP) breast implants: Final report of the expert group*. London: Department of Health.

LeBlanc, J. (1998). *Thinking clearly: A guide to critical reasoning*. New York: W. W. Norton.

Lee, A. S.-Y., & Gibbon, F. E. (2015). Non-speech oral motor treatment for children with developmental speech sound disorders. *Cochrane Database of Systematic Reviews*, Issue 3, Art. No.: CD009383.

Pennington, L., Parker, N. K., Kelly, H., & Miller, N. (2016). Speech therapy for children with dysarthria acquired before three years of age. *Cochrane Database of Systematic Reviews*, Issue 7, Art. No.: CD006937.

Rescher, N. (1980). *Scepticism: A critical reappraisal*. Oxford: Basil Blackwell.

Robinson, R. (1971). Arguing from ignorance. *The Philosophical Quarterly, 21*(83), 97–108.

Toulmin, S., Rieke, R., & Janik, A. (1984). *An introduction to reasoning*. New York: Macmillan.

Tsoumanis, A., Hens, N., & Kenyon, C. R. (2018). Is screening for chlamydia and gonorrhoea in men who have sex with men associated with reduction of the prevalence of these infections? A systematic review of observational studies. *Sexually Transmitted Diseases, 45*(9), 615–622.

Vogel, A. P., Keage, M. J., Johansson, K., & Schalling, E. (2015). Treatment for dysphagia (swallowing difficulties) in hereditary ataxia. *Cochrane Database of Systematic Reviews*, Issue 11, Art. No.: CD010169.

Walton, D. N. (1996). *Argumentation schemes for presumptive reasoning*. Mahwah, NJ: Erlbaum.

Slippery Slope Arguments

L. Cummings, *Fallacies in Medicine and Health*,
https://doi.org/10.1007/978-3-030-28513-5_3

3

LEARNING OBJECTIVES: Readers of this chapter will
- be able to distinguish between logical (argumentative) and non-logical (metaphorical) uses of slippery slope in a range of medical and health contexts.
- be able to distinguish slippery slope arguments from the argument from negative consequence.
- be able to identify the logical features of slippery slope arguments including the drivers and series of interlinked actions that take us down the slope.
- be able to recognise logical pitfalls in the use of slippery slope arguments including misrepresentation of the role of drivers in these arguments and a lack of evidential support for the actions on the slope.
- be able to determine when slippery slope arguments are more or less rationally warranted in certain contexts of use, and understand the reasons for the popular construal of these arguments as a scaremongering tactic.
- be able to characterize the way in which slippery slope arguments may serve as a cognitive heuristic during reasoning, and understand the cognitive gains that can derive from its use.

3.1 Introduction

Of any argument that we will examine in this book, the slippery slope argument has had a particularly bad press. This argument conjures up images of a complete loss of control over our decision-making and actions, as if we are being pulled by external forces along an ever more perilous path towards eventual destruction. No-one wants to be on a slippery slope any more than they would want to be behind the wheel of a car on a steep hillside without functioning brakes or on a ski slope without knowing how to stop. The question that concerns us in this chapter is whether these images of harm and loss of control are warranted, or whether they are a misrepresentation of a set of events that should not elicit fear or panic. After all, we can bring our car with no functioning brakes to a halt by steering it into a barrier on our descent down the hillside. We might still sustain some injury. But at least we would have averted total disaster by crashing at top speed into other vehicles and pedestrians at the bottom of the hillside. In the same way, we want to consider in this chapter if a **slippery slope argument**, once initiated, is not something that can be halted in a controlled way even as it is in progress. If this were possible, then some of the impending doom that this argument appears to arouse in us may lessen or even disappear altogether. At this point, we may be able to view the slippery slope argument in a new and altogether more positive light. But before we are in a position to consider the merits of this argument, we must say something more about the term 'slippery slope' and explain why this argument is so often associated with argumentation in medicine and health.

In ▶ Chapter 1, we described how terms like 'fallacy' and 'begging the question' may be used with a logical and non-logical sense or meaning. The same is true of the expression 'slippery slope'. In only some of the contexts in which this expression is used can we identify an arguer who may be said to advance claims that lead inexorably to an unwelcome or catastrophic conclusion. This logical use of the expression occurs in arguments about the legalization of abortion. When anti-abortionists argue that if we violate the sanctity of human life by permitting a woman to terminate a pregnancy on non-medical grounds, then it will not be long before we are seeking to terminate the lives of all other sorts of human beings whom we judge to be inconvenient—children with severe disabilities and elderly people who are no longer economically productive—a slippery slope is unfolding in the context of an **argument**. Anti-abortionists are using the legalization of abortion as the first dangerous step in a sequence of events that culminates in the morally repugnant practice of involuntary euthanasia of disabled and elderly people. It is this indefensible end point that is used to dissuade people from accepting the claim that abortion should be legalized. We will examine the logical structure of the slippery slope argument in more detail in ▶ Sect. 3.2. For the moment, suffice it to say that in the logical use of slippery slope, a disastrous scenario represented in the conclusion leads us to reject a premise that captures the first action or event in a sequence of increasingly negative events. But this logical use of slippery slope should not be confused with non-logical uses of the same expression. Consider the following extract from a journal article by Feig (2012). The author is describing the increased risk of diabetes in women who experience gestational diabetes:

> Women with a history of gestational diabetes clearly have an increased risk of diabetes. We have interventions that will help prevent them from sliding down this slippery slope including lifestyle modification, drugs (metformin) and breast feeding. By identifying women early in their course towards diabetes we have the opportunity to change this course. (319)

Like the logical use of slippery slope, this example describes a sequence of events that leads over time to an unwelcome state of affairs, namely, the development of diabetes. Also like the logical use, this outcome can be averted if appropriate action is taken—the woman with gestational diabetes can be encouraged to modify her lifestyle and comply with pharmacological interventions. So the slope in this example, like the slope in the abortion example, develops slowly over time and is certainly not inevitable. But there is no sense in which the author of the above extract is using the descent from gestational diabetes into late-onset diabetes in an argument. Feig is describing a sequence of physiological events that unfolds if left unchecked. This author is certainly not using the negative end point in the slope (the development of diabetes) as a reason not to accept a claim. In fact, it makes no sense to even use words like 'accept' and 'claim' to describe gestational diabetes, which is a complication of pregnancy for some women, and not a proposition that can be accepted or rejected. Feig is using 'slippery slope' as a **metaphor** to capture a sequence of events that terminates in a pathological condition. This non-logical use of the expression is certainly a vivid way in which to represent the decline into diabetes. But it is not in any way an argumentative sequence that unfolds through a series of premises and terminates in a conclusion.

The focus of this chapter will be the logical use of slippery slope argument. But the figurative or metaphorical use of slippery slope cannot simply be disregarded. This is because there are many processes in medicine and health that can best be characterized in terms of a slope of increasingly negative states or events. If we think of the neurodegenerative processes that accompany a condition like Alzheimer's disease, we can see that this is the case. Initially, an individual with Alzheimer's disease may experience impairments of memory and word-finding difficulty but have little or no functional limitation. As the disease progresses, more marked cognitive and language impairments become evident. At this point, an individual may struggle to understand aspects of conversation, may display confusion about the day of the week and the month of the year, and may struggle with daily activities like making a meal and managing finances. With further deterioration, an individual may lose the ability to speak, may become reliant on others for all aspects of self-care (e.g. toileting), and may display severe disorientation. Death, most often caused by pneumonia, eventually ensues. It cannot be denied that this pattern of deterioration is anything other than a sequence of increasingly negative states that terminates in the most catastrophic outcome of all, namely, a person's death. But the slope in this case is simply an effective way of representing a pathological process that, once started, continues unabated until the patient's body finally succumbs to disease. There is no argumentation in progress and the disastrous negative outcome of the patient's death is not used to dissuade us from taking an initial action. But the notion of a slippery slope is still doing important descriptive work.

Slippery slope argument is used extensively in medicine and health, particularly when ethical concerns are at issue and persuasion is required in order to secure public acceptance of a new technology or policy. Technological developments have forced us to consider how far human genetic engineering should be permitted to proceed. Strident opponents of this technology view it as unwelcome meddling in human genetics that will eventually result in the selection of traits that are judged to be desirable for social reasons, rather than the medical reasons for which the technology was originally adopted (viz., the elimination of serious genetic disorders). Even those who are not opposed to the use of genetic engineering for the treatment of serious genetic disorders are expressing concerns about the next slippery slope that new technological developments in the field have brought into focus. This is the proposal to use mitochondrial-replacement procedures to treat mitochondrial disease, a technique that would amount to a modification of the human germline. This is because mitochondria contain a small amount of DNA which, if modified or replaced, would effectively change the genetic features of future generations of children. Marcy Darnovsky, Executive Director of the Center for Genetics and Society in Berkeley, California, identifies the slippery slope that she believes supporters of this technology are about to head down. By implication, she is urging UK regulatory authorities not to take the initial action that would put this 'high-tech eugenic social dynamic into play':

> » "Mitochondrial-replacement procedures would constitute germline modification. Were the United Kingdom to grant a regulatory go-ahead, it would unilaterally cross a legal and ethical line on this issue that has been observed by the entire international community. This consensus holds that genetic-engineering tools may be applied, with appropriate care and safeguards, to treat an individual's medical condition, but should not be used to modify gametes or early embryos and so manipulate the characteristics of future children.

> Supporters argue that these concerns do not apply to modifications of mitochondrial DNA, which they characterize as an insignificant part of the human genome that does not affect a person's identity. This is scientifically dubious. The genes involved have pervasive effects on development and metabolism. And the permissive record of the UK regulatory authorities raises the prospect that inheritable mitochondrial changes would be used as a door-opening wedge towards full-out germline manipulation, putting a high-tech eugenic social dynamic into play." (Darnovsky 2013: 127)

Darnovsky is arguing that if the UK regulatory agencies take the first step of licensing mitochondrial-replacement procedures, it will unleash a sequence of events from which we will not be able to pull back. It will not be long before there is 'full-out germline manipulation' and with it the very real prospect that a policy of eugenics will be pressed into action. The latter can only be avoided by the UK continuing to operate within the ethical and legal line that has been observed by the entire international community to date.

Human genetic engineering involves a mix of competing factors. There are technological developments occurring on a continual basis which make it possible for us to manipulate the human genome in increasingly sophisticated ways. But just because we *can* perform these manipulations does not mean that we *should* perform them. Overlying technological developments are ethical considerations about how these techniques should be used to the benefit of people and society. It is in the tension between technological developments that extend the boundary of what it is possible to do in practical terms, and ethical concerns about how a new technology should be applied that slippery slope arguments can take root. Walton (2017) describes technological developments as drivers of the sequence of actions that take us along the slope. Another important driver of these actions is social acceptance. Acceptance often operates in tandem with technology. The introduction of a new technology may initially be greeted with some concern or alarm. There then follows a period of time during which the technology is demonstrated to have a beneficial purpose such as the treatment of human illness. These benefits win people over and social acceptance of the technology grows. Increasing acceptance permits further technological developments to take place, and so the process continues. There may be nothing but gains in this scenario for everyone involved, in which case there is no slippery slope at work. But the problem is that these mutually reinforcing moves between technological development and social acceptance can occur with such stealth that we often do not even recognise when we are on a slippery slope. This is one of the dangers of this type of argument. It can only be recognized through a sound appreciation of the logical features of slippery slope.

3.2 Logical Features of Slippery Slope Argument

The discussion so far has identified certain features of slippery slope argument. But no **argumentation scheme** for this argument has yet been advanced. Walton (2017) describes the slippery slope argument as a type of **argument from negative**

consequences. This is a single-premise argument that takes us directly from one or more negative consequences of an action to the conclusion that this action should be averted:

Premise: If action *A* is brought about, negative consequences will (or may) occur.
Conclusion: Therefore *A* should not be brought about (Walton 2017: 1513).

This argumentation scheme captures the central intuition in a slippery slope argument, that a highly undesirable consequence or outcome of an action should stand as grounds for rejecting the action that leads to this consequence or outcome. But slippery slope argument is altogether more specific than the argumentation scheme for the argument from negative consequences suggests. In 2015, an editorial in the journal *EBioMedicine* entitled 'Banning psychoactive substances: A slippery slope' presents a convincing argument in support of resisting a ban on new psychoactive substances. The argument unfolds as follows. A ban on new psychoactive substances has a deleterious effect on researchers who need to work with these substances in order to develop new drugs for the treatment of neuropsychiatric disorders. For this reason, a complete ban on these substances should be avoided. However, notwithstanding the title of this editorial, the argument that is advanced is an argument from consequence and *not* a slippery slope argument. So a slippery slope argument must have additional logical features beyond that captured by the argumentation scheme for the argument from consequence. For the moment, let us summarize the logical feature that the slippery slope argument shares with an argument from negative consequence:

Logical feature 1: Avoidance of negative consequence(s)

All slippery slope arguments involve an arguer who is reasoning from a negative consequence or set of negative consequences to the rejection of the action that brings these consequences into existence.

It will be instructive to return to the editorial in *EBioMedicine* to examine other logical features of slippery slope arguments that go beyond those of the argument from consequence. The reason that the argument advanced in this editorial qualified as an argument from consequence, and not as a slippery slope argument, is that there was no series of actions or events linking the ban on new psychoactive substances to the inability of researchers to develop the next generation of drugs that would be needed to treat neuropsychiatric disorders. A single step took us from the ban on new psychoactive substances to the failure of researchers to pursue much-needed drug development. There were no intermediate actions between these two events, with each action associated with further descent along the slope. Yet, this is a necessary feature of all slippery slope arguments (cf. Spielthenner [2010] who argues that a one-step slippery slope argument is possible). It is not simply that one action produces a negative consequence, but that a series of such actions lead to a negative consequence. We can formulate this second logical feature of slippery slope argument in the following terms (◘ Fig. 3.1):

Fig. 3.1 A single action to a negative consequence is a slippery step rather than a slippery slope (Courtesy of Nathan John Albury, Hong Kong, 2018)

***Logical feature 2*: Progression through interlinked actions**

All slippery slope arguments involve several premises that represent the series of interlinked actions through which a first action leads ultimately to a negative consequence. There is not a single action or step (or single premise) en route to the consequence.

In actual argumentation, it may not always be evident what the interlinked actions are that lead to the negative consequence. Considerable work may be required to make these actions explicit in the form of premises during **argument reconstruction**. For example, a popular argument against the legalization of cannabis is that taking a soft drug like cannabis leads to the taking of hard drugs like heroin. But this is not a simple argument from consequence in which we jump in a single leap from the taking of cannabis to the use of heroin. Rather, the argument progresses through a series of interrelated actions, each of which can be represented by a premise in a slippery slope argument. The legalization of cannabis may be expected to lead to an increase in the use of the drug. Imagine a person who decides to use the drug for the first time given its greater availability as a result of legalization. Cannabis can give this person pleasurable feelings and sensations that cannot be experienced under normal circumstances. The decision to use cannabis sets this person on a parallel course of desensitization and habituation-addiction. During desensitization, a person who has never previously used drugs becomes increasingly accustomed to the legal and health risks associated with drug-taking behaviour. During habituation-addiction, a person adjusts over time to the pleasurable sensations that a drug can offer (habituation), with the result that there is a desire to take more of a particular substance, or a person may develop a severe physical dependency where the taking of a drug becomes necessary (addiction). Habituation-addiction requires the user to increase the dose of a drug or change to other, harder drugs in order to satisfy their desire or physical dependency.

The action of cannabis use may be followed in time by a switch to cocaine which the user takes initially through nasal insufflation or snorting. The dual processes of desensitization and habituation-addiction continue to act as important drivers of the person's drug-taking behaviour. The desensitized user is unconcerned by the fact that he is taking greater and greater risks with his health and is increasing his likelihood of arrest as he attempts to source the illegal drugs that he requires. The addicted user who has developed a physical dependency on cocaine must take larger and larger amounts of the drug in order to avoid the unpleasant effects of withdrawal. Over time, the increasingly desensitized and addicted user starts to inject cocaine as a means of achieving faster delivery of the drug into his bloodstream and more rapid sensations of euphoria, increased energy and alertness. But even these pleasurable effects lessen over time as the individual's addiction to cocaine continues. The user's drug-taking behaviour is now as much about managing the unpleasant physical effects of withdrawal from cocaine, when the concentration of the drug in his bloodstream is low, as it is about deriving any pleasurable sensations from cocaine. Eventually, the user starts to inject heroin. He is now in the grip of a severe drug addiction that poses a very real and significant danger to his life. He has reached the bottom of the slope from which there appears to be no point of return. The most serious consequence of all—the drug user's death—can only be avoided at this late stage by prompt medical intervention.

We have gone to great lengths to show how an initial action (the legalization of cannabis) leads to a negative consequence (physical dependency on heroin) by means of a series of interrelated actions. Each action is a step in the descent down the slope. These actions are displayed below, along with the premises and conclusion in a slippery slope argument that are based on them:

Action 1: A cannabis legalization bill is signed into law.
Action 2: Legalization results in greater availability of cannabis.
Action 3: Greater availability results in an increase in the number of first-time users.
Action 4: First-time users smoke cannabis for the pleasurable sensations it provides.
Action 5: Cannabis users become desensitized to health risks and habituated to sensations.
Action 6: Cannabis is replaced by more addictive cocaine as the drug of choice of users.
Action 7: Users initially snort cocaine in relatively small and infrequent doses.
Action 8: The frequency of cocaine snorting increases over time as addiction takes hold.
Action 9: Users start to inject cocaine as a means of intensifying its effects.
Action 10: The frequency of cocaine injection increases to avoid symptoms of withdrawal.
Action 11: Users start to inject heroin as the 'positive' effects of cocaine start to diminish.

***'Cannabis' slippery slope argument*:**

Premise 1: There is a series of interlinked actions A_1 to A_{10} that results in a highly negative consequence represented by A_{11}.

Premise 2: The only way to avoid the negative consequence A_{11} is to not embark on the series of interlinked actions A_1 to A_{10}.

Premise 3: The only way to avoid the series of actions A_1 to A_{10} is to not take first action A_1.

Conclusion: Action A_1 should not be taken.

This argument draws heavily on inevitability in propelling us forward to the conclusion. In premise 1, heroin addiction is represented as an inevitable consequence of the actions in A_1 to A_{10} when we in fact know that someone could take each of these actions and still not end up with an addiction to heroin. In premise 3, the actions after A_1 in the sequence A_1 to A_{10} are represented as an inevitable consequence of the initial action A_1. But we also know that it is possible for cannabis to be legalized and for the subsequent actions in this sequence not to take place. For example, thirty states and the District of Columbia in the USA currently have laws broadly legalizing cannabis in some form. Yet, the entire populations of these states, or even significant proportions of them, have not deteriorated into dependency on hard drugs like cocaine. So what is the basis of this inevitability that propels us down the slope? What makes these actions appear to be so inevitable are a number of drivers of human behaviour. The driver that takes us from the legalization of cannabis in A_1 to the actions represented by A_2 to A_5 is social acceptance. As soon as a substance or activity is legalized, it acquires a level of social acceptance that it previously lacked. If cannabis use is legalized, people will no longer experience the social disapproval of others when they use the drug or have anxiety about the risk of arrest. Cannabis users will feel able to make use of the drug and purchase it in public places. Even the views of those who were formerly opposed to the legalization of cannabis may come to mellow over time as they are exposed to more people who are safely using the drug. There will be growing social acceptance of cannabis even among those who have no desire to make personal use of the drug. It is not difficult to see how social acceptance is a powerful driver of actions early in this particular slope.

When users replace the use of cannabis by the use of cocaine in A_6, social acceptance is no longer a significant driver of actions along the slope. This is because even in today's more permissive age, the vast majority of people are not supportive of the use of hard drugs like cocaine. Societal attitudes are still firmly opposed to the personal use of drugs like cocaine and no-one is seriously advocating that more dangerous drugs like cocaine should be legalized. A quite different and even more powerful driver of human behaviour takes over from social acceptance at this point in the slope. That driver is addiction in the form of physical dependency on cocaine and eventually heroin. To get some indication of the strength of this driver of behaviour, we need only consider the lengths that people go to in order to obtain drugs like cocaine. Users subordinate every responsibility and relationship in their lives in their desire to sustain their addiction. It is well known that users of cocaine and other narcotics will steal money from strangers and family members in order to buy drugs. They will risk criminal prosecutions, loss of employment, family breakdown, and even violence and injury at the hands of dealers and gangs in order to obtain the drugs they need. Addiction is such a strong driver of behaviour for drug addicts that many addicts would say that their immoral and illegal actions to obtain drugs at this stage of the slope are in every sense 'inevitable'—they are no longer able to exercise any form of self-control over their behaviour. Descent down the slope at this late stage is uncontrolled and proceeds at a more accelerated rate than at an early stage in the slope. Drivers like social acceptance and addiction are the basis of our third logical feature of slippery slope argument which can be summarized as follows:

Logical feature 3: Drivers propel series of actions

A range of drivers can propel us along the series of actions that take us down the slope. Examples of these drivers are social acceptance and technological developments and, in more extreme cases, dependency on drugs.

It is worth remarking that although the notion of a driver derives from Walton (2017), the above analysis of the 'cannabis' slippery slope argument differs from Walton's analysis in a number of significant respects. Walton believes that the social acceptance driver is in operation along the full length of the slope. However, I have claimed that social acceptance yields to the more powerful driver of addiction at a certain point in the slope. This reveals two different readings of what actually constitutes the slippery slope argument against the legalization of cannabis. For Walton, if cannabis is legalized, then society's attitudes towards drug use will change over time to such a degree that people will eventually advocate for the legalization of hard drugs such as cocaine and heroin. For my part, I believe that when opponents of the legalization of cannabis advance a slippery slope argument against legalization, they are basing their argument not only on concerns about where changing social acceptance of drugs might take us, but also on even greater concerns about the role of drug addiction in propelling us down the slope. Addiction provides a more plausible explanation of Walton's (correct) observation that there is always a point on the slope at which we lose control. For once dependency on drugs is established, there is complete loss of volitional action on the part of the user. The user is compelled to pursue a course of increasingly reckless and immoral actions in the service of his addiction. We were able to identify that point as A_6 in the sequence of interlinked actions. This is the point at which cocaine use replaces cannabis use. But while we can identify the stage at which loss of control occurs in this slope, Walton's observation that this is often not possible seems correct for the most part.

DISCUSSION POINT: Heading down the slippery slope

Commentators are divided on whether we can exercise control in a slippery slope argument and stop our descent down the slope. According to Walton (2017), control can be exercised at an early stage on the slope. However, we eventually enter a 'grey zone'. At some point in this zone, we lose control of our actions and our further descent down the slope cannot be stopped. In

an article in *The Guardian* on 2 April 2015 entitled 'Why we should avoid the "slippery slope"', Steven Poole takes a quite different view. He argues that "there is enough friction on the slope to enable us to stop wherever we choose. The invocation of a slippery slope is therefore almost always anti-rational fearmongering."

Which of these views of our descent down the slope do you consider to be most plausible? To answer this question, you will need to think about different types of drivers of actions along the slope. Are some of these drivers so powerful that they cannot be resisted and so we cannot choose to stop our descent down the slope? Or do you believe like Poole that we always have a choice not to continue our descent down the slope?

There is a fourth logical feature of the slippery slope argument. Because this argument concerns future events, it has a certain predictive nature. Boer (2003) states that "the force of any slippery slope argument, however, is by definition limited by its reference to future developments which cannot empirically be sustained" (p. 225). But any predictions about future events, particularly when they concern complex aspects of human behaviour such as the use of drugs, may be shown ultimately to be erroneous or false. We may surmise that the legalization of cannabis will result in an increase in its use only to discover that legalization results in no change in consumption of the drug. We may believe that cannabis users are more likely to turn to the use of cocaine than non-cannabis users. And yet this prediction may not be borne out by the actual behaviour of people. The predictive character of any slippery slope argument means that it can be defeated or overturned as new evidence emerges. This evidence may emerge at a later point in time, or it may arise from a similar or closely related case about which we may currently have some evidence. For example, evidence from countries and cities that have already moved to legalize certain cannabis products may be used to defeat the 'cannabis' slippery slope argument. It is because all slippery slope arguments, even those that have been carefully crafted and appear strongly warranted, can be overturned or defeated by the emergence of contrary evidence that we characterise these arguments as a type of defeasible or presumptive argument. This fourth and final logical feature of slippery slope argument can be summarized as follows:

Logical feature 4: Defeasible, presumptive argument

All slippery slope arguments are advanced on a tentative basis in the knowledge that they may be overturned or defeated by the emergence of contrary evidence. The defeasible, presumptive nature of these arguments is related to the fact that they all involve predictions about future events and behaviour.

It is now time for you to get practice at identifying the logical features of slippery slope argument by attempting Exercise 3.1.

EXERCISE 3.1: The 'euthanasia' slippery slope argument

Like the 'cannabis' slippery slope argument, the 'euthanasia' slippery slope argument sets out from an initial action that involves the legalization of a contentious practice. That practice is voluntary euthanasia or physician-assisted suicide. The 'euthanasia' argument is discussed below by Lerner and Caplan (2015). Examine what these authors say about this argument, and then answer the questions that follow:

> The slippery slope is an argument frequently invoked in the world of bioethics. It connotes the notion that a particular course of action will lead inevitably to undesirable and unintended consequences. Saying no to the original action, even if that act is moral in itself, may, in light of the slope that looms, be the ethical thing to do. Slippery slope arguments have been especially pervasive in discussions of euthanasia, in which physicians actively end patients' lives, and physician-assisted dying (or physician-assisted suicide), in which physicians supply medications to patients that enable them to end their own lives. The concern, fuelled by the German experience with racially motivated euthanasia in the last century, has been that approving either of these procedures for a few individuals will inevitably lead to overuse and abuse. (p. 1640)

Questions

(1) It was described above how in any slippery slope argument there must be progression through interlinked actions (logical feature 2) between an initial action and a negative consequence. Indicate what these interlinked actions might look like in the case of the 'euthanasia' slippery slope argument.

(2) Describe the type of economic factors that serve as a driver of actions along the slope.

(3) In their article, Lerner and Caplan (2015) reported a number of findings from two studies that examined the experience of euthanasia in the Netherlands and Belgium. The Dutch findings were based on data collected during a 1-year period from the End-of-Life Clinic, an organisation that was established in the Netherlands in 2012 to consider euthanasia and physician-assisted suicide requests from patients whose primary physicians had turned down a request. The Belgian findings are based on data collected from a nationwide postal questionnaire survey of physicians who certified a random sample of 6,871 deaths that occurred from 1 January to 30 June 2013 in Flanders. Examine these findings, and describe their significance in relation to the 'euthanasia' slippery slope argument:

The Netherlands:

6.8% of euthanasia requests accepted because person was 'tired of living'.

3.7% of successful requests reported only psychological suffering.

49.1% of successful requests characterized loneliness as part of their suffering.

1 in 30 people in the Netherlands died by euthanasia in 2012 (roughly triple that in 2002 when practice was first decriminalized).

Belgium:
1.9% of all deaths in Flanders were by euthanasia in 2007 (increased to 4.6% in 2013).
1 in 22 deaths in Belgium due to euthanasia.
55% of euthanasia requests approved in Flanders in 2007 (increased to 77% in 2013).
People allowed to use 'tiredness of life' as a reason for euthanasia in 2013 but not in 2007.

(4) As well as economic factors, it is clear that moral considerations can also serve as a significant driver of actions along the slope. Explain the role of moral considerations in this slippery slope argument.
(5) Clearly, it is possible to advance a rationally warranted slippery slope argument against the legalization of euthanasia without resorting to the use of racially motivated euthanasia by the Nazis in the twentieth century. Describe one risk of introducing this analogy into a slippery slope argument for the individual who is opposed to the legalization of euthanasia.

3.3 Evaluating Slippery Slope Arguments

We have already mentioned some of the ways in which slippery slope arguments may misfire or go awry. What appears to be a slope through a series of interlinked actions may actually only be a single step to a negative consequence. Also, a premise may appear to be rationally warranted only for its supporting grounds to be shown to be weak in some respect. There are many different pitfalls that can arise in a slippery slope argument despite the most honourable motivations on the part of the proponent of the argument. These pitfalls are even more pronounced when an arguer is using a slippery slope argument to deceive an opponent in a critical discussion. It is during the deceptive use of the argument that hyperbolical language may be employed, most often with a view to amplifying emotions such as fear. A fearful opponent is more easily persuaded of the need to reject an action that leads to a negative consequence, regardless of whether or not the supporting argument can withstand rational criticism. On such occasions, the slippery slope argument shares certain features of the **fear appeal** or *ad baculum* argument, another of the so-called informal fallacies (Cummings 2012). Alongside various fallacious uses of the slippery slope argument, there are other uses of this argument that are rationally warranted. If, as we saw in Exercise 3.1, the experience of euthanasia in other countries indicates that initially strict selection criteria are subsequently relaxed to the point where almost any ground whatsoever can be used to justify use of the procedure, then we would do well to listen to the arguer who develops a slippery slope argument along these lines. For this particular use of the argument is indeed empirically validated. In this section, fallacious and non-fallacious uses of the slippery slope argument will be examined.

There has been no shortage of authors over the years who have attempted to convey how a good slippery slope argument may be distinguished from a bad argument. According to Oakley and Cocking (2005), "[a] good slippery slope argument will give us strong reason to believe that […] significant morally worse future circumstances will come about as a result of our introducing or engaging in [a] practice here and now" (p. 232). This rather general formulation of what constitutes a good slippery slope argument is matched by an equally general account of how a slippery slope argument may be judged to be problematic. The *strong reason* to believe that a particular adverse consequence will come about in a good slippery slope argument is replaced by a lack of *compelling evidence* for the consequence in a weak argument:

> It is widely recognised that the standard problem with many slippery slope arguments is that they fail to provide us with the necessary compelling evidence that these significantly morally worse circumstances will actually come about as a result of our introducing or engaging in the practice in question. As such they seem rightly criticised as 'scare-mongering' through speculating impending doom without support or sufficient support from relevant empirical evidence. (p. 232)

A weak or bad slippery slope argument may indeed amount to little more than scaremongering. But in the absence of more specific formulations than *strong reason* and a lack of *compelling evidence*, it seems difficult to say if this is the case. Burgess (1993) is more specific about the shortcomings of proponents who advance weak slippery slope arguments. Such proponents "rarely if ever work it into a detailed slippery slope argument", preferring instead to shift the **burden of proof** onto an opponent who would deny any negative consequence of a reforming action:

> They rest content with the sketchiest of formulations, leaving the detailed work to their opponents: we've shown you (sketchily) that it might happen; now show us (in detail) that it couldn't. But this is a fraud. The mere presentation of a slope does nothing to show that the onus of proof is on the reformer to demonstrate that a proposed change will not lead to disaster. (pp. 169–170)

At the other extreme, Burgess acknowledges that there are those who regard slippery slope argument as "nothing more than a hollow rhetorical flourish", an attitude which he relates to "the prevalence of sketchy and implausible examples". However, this attitude must also be abandoned, he contends, as there are some modest slope arguments that are good arguments. What is needed, according to Burgess, is "some sound and (preferably) non-technical practical advice in sorting the good slippery slope arguments from the bad" (p. 170). It is the aim of this section to provide this advice.

In general, there are a number of circumstances under which a slippery slope argument may be deemed not to be rationally warranted. These circumstances tend to coalesce around the logical features of these arguments that were examined in ► Sect. 3.2. When a slippery slope argument does not observe these features, or these features are subverted in some respect, the argument can be said to be used fallaciously. Let us return to the first logical feature which we called the *avoidance of negative consequences*. Readers may wonder how this particular aspect of the argument can possibly go awry—after all, if a consequence of an action can be shown to cause harm or injury to an individual or group of people, then the action that brings this consequence about cannot possibly be defended. But for the argument to be used in a rationally warranted way, its proponent must succeed in demonstrating not only that an action leads to a negative consequence, but that this negative consequence is not outweighed by any of the benefits that might derive from the action in question. For most slippery slope arguments, there are benefits as well as negative consequences of the action that triggers our descent down the slope. For example, the legalization of voluntary euthanasia or physician-assisted suicide clearly terminates the suffering of many seriously ill people for whom there is no prospect of recovery. But for a slippery slope argument against the legalization of these practices to be advanced non-fallaciously, the proponent of the argument must succeed in demonstrating that the negative consequence at the bottom of the slope exceeds any benefits that derive from voluntary euthanasia. One or more negative consequences may not warrant the rejection of an initial action if significant benefits can also be shown to result from this action:

Logical pitfall 1: Failure to consider benefits of initial action

The proponent of a slippery slope argument must consider the benefits as well as the negative consequences of the action at the top of the slope. The argument is only used non-fallaciously if the negative consequences of an initial action can be shown to outweigh any benefits to be derived from the action.

Clearly, if the negative consequence at the bottom of the slope is the use of euthanasia in people who are unable to give informed consent to the procedure (e.g. individuals with cognitive impairment or other disabilities), then such a consequence is so morally unacceptable for most people that they would be inclined to argue that the termination of suffering of terminally ill people does not justify this consequence. But imagine that a proponent argues that euthanasia should not be legalized because it will lead to people requesting the procedure on the grounds that they are 'tired of living', as we saw in Exercise 3.1. This particular consequence of the procedure may not be considered to be sufficiently negative to warrant denying people with terminal illnesses access to the procedure. After all, people who are 'tired of living' can still give informed consent to euthanasia. In this case, there may be grounds for arguing that the proponent has made fallacious use of the slippery slope argument because the so-called negative consequence has not been adequately evaluated against the benefits that are derived from the procedure by people with interminable suffering on account of terminal illness.

DISCUSSION POINT: Evaluating consequences in slippery slope arguments

Spielthenner (2010) argues that slippery slope arguments are logically fallacious. He enlarges on his grounds for this viewpoint by discussing a prominent issue in medical ethics, the use of therapeutic and reproductive cloning. In therapeutic cloning, nuclear material isolated from a somatic (body) cell is transferred into an enucleated oocyte (egg cell) with the goal of deriving embryonic cell lines with the same genome as the nuclear donor. However, these cells are not implanted into a female uterus and do not develop into a person or animal. In reproductive cloning, implantation does occur. This is how Spielthenner develops his objection to the 'cloning' slippery slope argument:

> **The main reason, I suspect, why authors have often regarded this type of reasoning as valid is that they have ignored the simple fact that drawing a conclusion from a slippery slope argument requires comparing the values of available alternatives and not only considering the bad outcome of a certain act or policy [...] The putative fact that allowing therapeutic cloning will inevitably lead to reproductive cloning does not entail the conclusion that we must not allow therapeutic cloning. This is so for the simple reason that *not* allowing therapeutic cloning might have consequences that are even worse. (2010: 152)**

How do you think the consequences of a policy or action should be evaluated in a slippery slope argument? To help you discuss this issue in a group, you might want to undertake some background reading in the area of cloning. You can read the chapter 'Cloning: Definitions and Applications' at the following address: ▶ https://www.ncbi.nlm.nih.gov/books/NBK223960/.

In ▶ Sect. 3.2, we discussed how in any slippery slope argument, there must be progression through a series of interlinked actions between the initial action at the top of the slope and the negative consequence at the bottom of the slope. Problems can arise, however, when there is little or no evidence to support these actions, or the purported relationships between them appear weak or implausible. Given that many slippery slope arguments concern events that have yet to unfold, the evidence base to support these interlinked actions can often be quite limited. If the proponent of a slippery slope argument acknowledges the limited or tentative nature of the evidence in an area, and uses proportionate language to represent the interlinked actions along the slope as a result, then a slippery slope argument may indeed be rationally warranted. Use of a statement or premise during argumentation such as 'A_1 *will definitely lead to* A_2' rather than 'A_1 *may possibly lead to* A_2' conveys through its use of the modal auxiliary verb (*will*) and adverb (*definitely*) a better developed evidence base relating to the argument than may actually be the case. The uncertainty expressed by the modal auxiliary verb (*may*) and adverb (*possibly*) in the second statement is more appropriate given the defeasible nature of all slippery slope reasoning. If the proponent of a slippery slope argument exaggerates the strength of the evidence or warrant for actions along the slope, then the charge that a **fallacy** has been committed is certainly warranted. Such a proponent seeks to force acceptance of the conclusion of the argument—that a particular negative consequence necessitates rejection of the initial action on the slope—by overstating the strength of evidence that supports the series of interlinked actions. This is the basis of the second logical pitfall in the use of slippery slope argument:

Logical pitfall 2: Interlinked actions are weakly warranted

There is little evidence to support the series of interlinked actions that takes us along the slope. However, the proponent of the argument overstates this evidence with a view to forcing the opponent's acceptance of the conclusion.

In illustration of this flaw in the use of slippery slope argument, consider the following statements from two newspaper articles in *The Washington Post*. These articles are discussing the positive and negative implications of a new gene editing technology called CRISPR-Cas9. The technology in question allows scientists to target specific stretches of genetic code and to edit DNA at precise locations. Through this technology, it will be possible to correct mutations at precise locations in the human genome in order to treat genetic causes of disease. However, non-medical uses of the technology are also possible and, as these journalists acknowledge, are a cause of concern:

> It's certain that we will quickly move past questions of "fixing" disease to enhancing human capability more generally. ('If we're going to play God with gene editing, we've got to ask some moral questions', Christine Emba, 20 February 2017, *The Washington Post*)
>
> Some therapies that can be used to treat a disease could potentially be used for purely cosmetic or competitive purposes. For example, gene therapy developed as a treatment for muscular dystrophy could potentially be exploited to make a healthy person more muscular. ('Ethicists advise caution in applying CRISPR gene editing to humans', Joel Achenbach, 14 February 2017, *The Washington Post*)

The context of these statements is a discussion of the potential for this new gene editing technology to lead us down the slippery slope towards full-scale manipulation of the human genome for non-medical purposes. But while the first of these statements represents the actions that will take us down the slope as 'certain', the second statement characterizes these actions in more tentative terms through the use of the modal auxiliary verb (*could*) and the adverb (*potentially*). It is unclear how the force of the first statement can be warranted when the journalist who wrote the article does not present any evidence to support the transition between use of the new technology for the treatment of human disease and its use in achieving socially desirable genetic enhancements. This lack of evidence becomes apparent as soon as we ask: *What are the grounds for your certainty that we will move from* $Action_1$ *to* $Action_2$ *in this case?* If Christine Emba has such grounds, she does not present them in her article. Such unsubstantiated claims are a problem when her aim is to argue that we should be wary of the slope that this new technology could take us down. To the extent that she is advancing a slippery slope argument, it is clearly a weakly warranted one.

Quite different considerations come into play in the second statement above. The journalist, Joel Achenbach, is also aware of where this new gene editing technology could take us. As well as preventing congenital diseases, he states that the new technology "could also be used for cosmetic enhancements and lead to permanent, heritable changes in the human species". But unlike Emba, who represented the transition between disease intervention and non-medical uses of the technology as certain, Achenbach presents a more considered analysis of actions along the slope. Gene editing for the treatment of disease *could potentially* lead to the use of this technology to achieve socially desirable manipulations of the human genome. But there is also the very real possibility that this negative scenario will *not* come about. Indeed, Achenbach describes in his article a number of the 'checks and balances' that serve as a bulwark against an inevitable or certain descent down the slope. The human germline modifications that would have to occur in order for heritable genetic changes to come about are tightly regulated, as this extract from Achenbach's article indicates:

> The list of criteria for going down that road is a long one, said Alta Charo, a professor of law and bioethics at the University of Wisconsin, speaking at a news conference Tuesday in Washington. For example: The intervention would have to replace the defective, disease-causing gene with a gene already common in the human species. There would also have to be no simpler alternative for parents wishing to have a healthy child. And first and foremost, there needs to be more research to show that such modifications are safe and target well-understood genes, she said. "We are not even close to the amount of research that we need before you can move forward," Charo said.

Like Emba, Achenbach is making readers aware of the slope that this new gene editing technology might take us down. But unlike Emba, he is at pains to point out that the actions on the slope are not certain or inevitable and that they may not actually come about. In fact, based on current evidence in the form of regulations and criteria that this new technology must satisfy, it is highly likely that we will *not* plummet down the slope. In rehearsing the concerns of many that this new technology sets us on a slippery slope, Achenbach is more concerned than Emba to reflect the probabilistic nature of actions on the slope and the uncertainty of the evidence that supports those actions.

DISCUSSION POINT: Evaluating actions on the slope

We described above two very different approaches to the series of interlinked actions that carry us along the slope towards gene editing for non-medical purposes. Emba characterized the transition between these actions as certain, although no evidence was presented to support this stance. Achenbach characterised this same series of actions in more probabilistic terms as events that 'could potentially' occur, but which were not in any sense certain or guaranteed to occur. The basis for this more tentative stance towards the likelihood of these actions occurring was a number of restrictions on the use of gene editing technology. These restrictions had been recommended in a report that was written by 22 experts worldwide and published by the National Academy of Sciences and the National Academy of Medicine in the US. This is how one commentator, Eric Lander, characterized the guidelines in the report. Lander is president of the Broad Institute of MIT and Harvard. He was not involved in the writing of the report:

> It's a very careful, conservative position that's just a little bit beyond an absolute bar. And I think that's the right place to go for now. … They say you cannot do this unless you put double-stick tape on the slippery slope so that nothing can slip. That's a pretty strong set of restrictions. ('Ethicists advise caution in applying CRISPR gene editing to humans', Joel Achenbach, 14 February 2017, *The Washington Post*)

Emba describes Lander's characterization of the restrictions as a double-stick tape on the slippery slope so that nothing can slip as "an un-reassuring metaphor if there ever was one". To what extent do you think Emba's certainty that we will plummet to the bottom of the slope can be justified by a belief on her part that these restrictions are inadequate to the task for which they were designed?

Alongside minimal rational warrant for individual actions on the slope and the relationships between these actions, there may also be little or no evidence that factors such as social acceptance and technological developments can serve as drivers of these actions. To illustrate this point, just think about how many slippery slope arguments trade on social acceptance as a driver of actions along the slope. Proponents of slippery slope arguments against the legalization of euthanasia argue that if this procedure is legalized, then attitudes to voluntary euthanasia and physician-assisted suicide will change to such an extent that it will only be a matter of time before we are performing involuntary euthanasia of people with disabilities and addictions. Attitude change is also presumed to drive movement down the slope in arguments about the legalization of cannabis, human genetic engineering, and non-invasive prenatal testing. This raises the question of the extent to which each of these uses of social acceptance as a driver of actions along the slope is warranted. Certainly in some of these slippery slope arguments, social acceptance is a genuine driver of actions. When Ian Birrell argues in the *Daily Mail* that the introduction of non-invasive prenatal testing will take us down a slope 'into a new age of eugenics' (see [3] in end-of-chapter questions), it is growing social acceptance of abortion of foetuses with conditions like Down's syndrome which he believes is propelling us down the slope:

> "Even government advisers accept that when the new test is offered on the National Health Service, almost 100 more babies with Down's syndrome are likely to be discarded before birth every year after the condition is identified.
>
> In Denmark, which terminates more Down's children than Britain (about 98 per cent of these babies are aborted), it is predicted the disorder will soon all but disappear. Polls show most people see this as a good thing.
>
> 'When you can discover almost all foetuses with Down's, then we are approaching a situation in which almost all of them will be aborted,' said Lillian Bondo, head of the Danish Midwives Association, two years ago." ('I fear this new Down's test is a slippery slope to eugenics', Ian Birrell, 1 March 2017, *Daily Mail*).

However, there is little or no evidence that women who are prepared to abort a foetus with Down's syndrome would also be prepared to abort a foetus on grounds such as gender, eye and hair colour, or intellectual attributes, the conditions that would need to obtain in order for us to descend into full-scale eugenics. In short, in only some of the slippery slope arguments that we encounter can social acceptance be unequivocally credited with driving our movement down the slope. And even in these cases, it is only responsible for our movement along part of the slope.

Social acceptance is a somewhat intangible driver of actions along the slope. Short of opinion polls, many of which are limited in various respects, it is very difficult indeed to identify in a reliable way the extent to which social acceptance may be driving actions along a slope. This allows the proponents of many slippery slope arguments to misrepresent the influence of this particular driver on these actions. More often than not, this misrepresentation involves exaggeration of the part played by social acceptance in propelling actions along the slope. There is no evidence, for example, that attitudes to people with disabilities have deteriorated to the point where the majority of people would regard involuntary euthanasia of these individuals to be an acceptable practice. Indeed, there are now protections for people with disabilities enshrined in law that would suggest a general improvement in our attitudes towards these individuals and their right to participate as full and equal members of society. Slippery slope arguments that would have us believe that attitudes towards people with disabilities have declined so significantly that we no longer recognize the right to life of these people serve only to misrepresent the more positive attitudes that many people have towards individuals with disabilities in today's society, and to exaggerate the negative attitudes to disability that undeniably still exist in some quarters. The failure to accord drivers of actions along the slope the weight and influence that they warrant is the basis of the third logical pitfall in slippery slope arguments:

Logical pitfall 3: Misrepresenting drivers of actions on the slope

The proponent of a slippery slope argument may misrepresent the influence of one or more drivers of actions along the slope. A common error is to exaggerate the extent to which attitudes in society deteriorate over time, and then to use that deterioration to claim that people are increasingly willing to accept grossly immoral actions.

While social acceptance is difficult to represent in evidential terms, another driver of actions along the slope is more readily verifiable. That driver is technological developments. Technological developments in areas such as human genetic engineering and reproductive medicine have made once unimaginable activities a practical reality. However, along with each new achievement, challenging ethical questions are raised about how far technological developments should be allowed to determine what constitutes human life itself. In the following extract, Gunning (2008) describes the technological developments that have made preimplantation genetic diagnosis possible. This is the diagnosis of genetic disorders in embryos during IVF treatment with a view to rejecting those embryos for implantation in which disorders are identified. The procedure differs from non-invasive prenatal testing, which is the identification of genetic and other anomalies during a pregnancy:

> The invention of the polymerase chain reaction (PCR) for the amplification of DNA led to the use of the technology for the genetic analysis of DNA from a single cell and to the development of preimplantation genetic diagnosis (PGD). The focus of this new technology was on the detection of autosomal single gene disorders such as cystic fibrosis and X-linked disorders such as Duchenne muscular dystrophy. In 1993 the application of fluorescent in situ hybridisation (FISH) in the preimplantation diagnosis of chromosomal abnormalities was reported and heralded the introduction of preimplantation genetic screening (PGS) for a number of common aneuploidies. This was followed by the use of PGD to detect chromosomal translocations, and the use of preimplantation human leukocyte antigen (HLA) typing to obtain sibling stem cell donors. (p. 29)

Key developments such as polymerase chain reaction and fluorescent in situ hybridisation have resulted in significant diagnostic achievements that would not have been possible in the absence of these technologies. Moreover, the presence of these technologies and the advances that they have allowed scientists to make are both concrete and verifiable. However, what technological developments gain over a driver like social acceptance in terms of verifiability and evidential status, they can lose in other respects. It is still possible for the proponent of a slippery slope argument to misrepresent these developments and overstate the ways in which they may be misused with a view to forcing acceptance of the conclusion of an argument. Preimplantation genetic diagnosis may be used to perform sex selection of embryos for social rather than medical reasons, for example. Misrepresentation of this particular driver may be facilitated by the expertise and technical competence that are required to understand these procedures and their applications to genetic diagnosis. A lay person who is required to evaluate a slippery slope argument that makes extensive use of a technological driver may be unable to detect when the proponent of this argument is misrepresenting this particular driver.

EXERCISE 3.2: Evaluating drivers of actions on the slope

In an article in the *Los Angeles Times* in December 2009 entitled 'The slippery slope of marijuana regulation', Tim Rutten describes some of the difficulties that lawmakers and enforcement authorities have had in maintaining a consistent position on the legalization of marijuana. For example, although lawmakers voted to cap the number of marijuana dispensaries at 70, 186 establishments that registered with the city after a poorly drafted moratorium on new dispensaries was ruled illegal have been allowed to operate. Rutten's article analyses the source of this disarray in the city's approach to the legalization of marijuana. Read this extract from the article carefully, and then answer the questions that follow:

> "The real reason the City Council is having such a hellish time coming to grips with this issue is that this is one of those areas where social attitudes and thinking simply have moved beyond conventional legal thinking or, for that matter, the permissible language of politics. Medical marijuana was, from the start, a back door to legalization, and now it's swung wide open. If we really believed cannabis was a normative medical remedy, it would be sold in pharmacies like everything else your doctor prescribes. Instead, the council is trying to regulate it in just the way we control bars or liquor stores or any other vendor of recreational intoxicants, while paying lip service to the really rather limited medicinal necessities.
>
> A recent Field Poll found that 60% of Los Angeles County voters and 56% statewide favour legalizing and taxing marijuana. As The Times reported Tuesday, a proposition to do both those things already has qualified for next year's ballot."

Questions

(1) In the typical slippery slope argument around the legalization of marijuana, an arguer claims that legalization will lead to an increase in the use of so-called hard drugs like cocaine and heroin, with all of the problems that this entails.

These problems are sufficiently costly to individuals and to society to necessitate our rejection of attempts to legalize marijuana. Rutten develops a different argument around the legalization of marijuana. What is his argument, and how does it differ from the typical argument?

(2) What driver does Rutten think is particularly influential in propelling us along the slope to the point where we will permit the legalization of marijuana?

(3) What evidence does Rutten present to support his view that the driver identified in response to (2) is particularly significant?

(4) Rutten argues that '[i]f we really believed cannabis was a normative medical remedy, it would be sold in pharmacies like everything else your doctor prescribes.' What conclusion does Rutten invite readers to draw from this conditional statement? Reconstruct the argument that takes us to this conclusion.

(5) Aside from social attitudes, Rutten identifies another factor that has served as a driver of actions along the slope towards full legalization of marijuana. What is that factor? Does it appear to have any legitimacy according to Rutten?

The final way in which the proponent of a slippery slope argument may commit a logical error involves the arousal of emotion. The purpose of any act of reasoning is to bring forward good reasons or grounds in support of a claim. However, when a proponent is unable to advance such reasons or grounds, often because they do not exist, he may resort to the use of emotions such as fear to achieve acceptance of a conclusion. When the content of an argument concerns issues such as when someone should be allowed to die or terminate a foetus during pregnancy, emotions can run very deep indeed and distort any logical reflection that we may attempt to undertake. Affective states such as fear are often aroused by slippery slope arguments, many of which address highly contentious and emotive issues. This is why these arguments have often been described, not unfairly, as scaremongering. In ▶ Chapter 4, it will be seen that not all uses of emotion in argument are fallacious. However, when emotions are used to bypass logical argumentation, or to make an audience receptive to a weak argument, then a proponent is making fallacious use of reasoning (if we can even call it 'reasoning'). To illustrate this point, consider the following extract which appears in an article about euthanasia in the *Belfast Telegraph*:

> "When we study the barbarous history of the Nazis, we can see that the origin of their extermination programme was in 1939 and started off with the euthanasia of mental patients and disabled children.
>
> Rightly, the world condemned them for their gross atrocities, but what the Nazis started out with in 1939, some countries are now carrying out for themselves under the cloak of legality.
>
> Clearly it was not right for the Nazis, so why then should it be regarded as right now for others?
>
> Euthanasia not only corrupts medical ethics but also erodes respect for human life, which is the very foundation for human rights in the world.

> Where all this will lead in the future is the question.
> But, sadly, once opened, this Pandora's Box of deathly measures could lead anywhere."
> ('The Nazis were condemned for their policy of euthanasia from 1939 to 1945, so what is different now?', Alban Maginness, 28 March 2018, *Belfast Telegraph*)

There can be little doubt that the author of this article is exploiting the fear and horror aroused by Nazi genocide to make us reject any place for euthanasia in today's society. Early in the extract, we are encouraged to think about the 'gross atrocities' of mental patients and disabled children undergoing involuntary euthanasia. The fear engendered by these atrocities is compounded by the fear of the unknown, in that we do not know where euthanasia, even if initially well regulated, will lead us in the future. Once 'Pandora's box of deathly measures' is opened we could be led along a path of increasingly amoral acts, each one more depraved than the one which preceded it. The question that concerns us is whether this arousal of emotion is legitimate and warranted, or whether it is intended to replace careful, reasoned argument. The weakness in this author's argument is that it is simply assumed that the euthanasia that campaigners and others wish to see legalized and that is already practiced by 'some countries' *is* the very same extermination programme that the Nazis implemented. The author explicitly states, for example, that what the Nazis started out with in 1939 is now being carried out by some countries 'under the cloak of legality'. No grounds are advanced for such a strong claim. In fact, the author appears to treat this statement as so self-evidently true that no evidence in support of it need even be brought forward. The author is not undertaking the argumentative work that is required to support this viewpoint, and is relying instead on the arousal of fear to encourage readers to reject the legalization of euthanasia. This use of slippery slope argument as a scaremongering tactic is the basis of the fourth logical pitfall in the use of the argument:

Logical pitfall 4: Illegitimate use of emotion in argument

The proponent of a slippery slope argument makes fallacious use of this argument when he uses emotions like fear to force acceptance of his conclusion. In this case, emotions are used to subvert the requirement to advance evidence or grounds in support of the conclusion.

You will get further practice in identifying the use of emotion in slippery slope arguments in the questions at the end of the chapter. In the meantime, you should attempt Exercise 3.3.

EXERCISE 3.3: Emotions and the slippery slope argument

In an article in *The Spectator*, Carol Sarler argues that many beneficial medical therapies and other advances are stifled by the use of slippery slope arguments. These arguments, she claims, plant sufficient fear and alarm in the minds of people that legislation relating to issues such as the legalization of cannabis and euthanasia is invariably blocked, even when there is considerable public support for it. This is an extract from Sarler's article. Read the extract carefully and then answer the questions that follow:

» "Assisted dying bit the dust not because anybody seriously wishes to prolong agony among the terminally ill but because, in the dark minds of scattergun alarmists and conspiracy theorists, to allow it would be a slippery slope towards truckloads of septuagenarians being hurled, still kicking, into the gaping mouths of crematoria.

Lightening up the law on cannabis may be opposed for several reasons, good and bad, worthy of consideration and far-fetched [...] But when it returns to debate next month, the move will fail not by dint of the reasoned arguments. It will fail because, as always, the ignorant cling to the belief that the use of cannabis is a slippery slope towards the use of, say, heroin [...]

Taken simply as a tool of argument, the slippery slope demonstrates a paucity of intellectual rigour: it is one thing to oppose what is being proposed and another altogether to oppose what is not. The first requires knowledge, study and fact; the second needs neither evidence nor proof and is validated as a warning by nothing more than its own utterance."

('Why I'm sick of slippery-slope arguments', Carol Sarler, 19 September 2015, *The Spectator*)

Questions

(1) Proponents of slippery slope arguments often use emotive language to persuade audiences to accept the conclusions of their arguments. In the above extract, Carol Sarler also makes use of emotive language but with the purpose of opposing those who would advance slippery slope arguments. Give *one* example of the use of this language.

(2) At points in her article, Sarler uses abusive *ad hominem* reasoning to characterize the position of proponents of slippery slope arguments. Give *two* examples of where this occurs.

(3) Sarler argues that slippery slope argument demonstrates a "paucity of intellectual rigour". What does Sarler believe is the logical flaw at the heart of this lack of intellectual rigour?

(4) Sarler also states that those who use slippery slope argument do not consider themselves bound by any requirement to produce evidence or proof of their position. Instead, they appear to believe that their position "is validated as a warning by nothing more than its own utterance". Where else in our discussion of logical pitfalls in slippery slope arguments have we seen an author who does not consider himself bound by a requirement to produce evidence?

(5) How would you characterize the position that Sarler takes on slippery slope argument? Do you think she views the argument as inherently fallacious, or as more or less rationally warranted in different contexts of use? Provide evidence to support your answer.

3.4 Slippery Slope Reasoning as a Cognitive Heuristic

It will not have escaped the attention of readers that most of the discussion in this chapter has been concerned with ways in which slippery slope arguments fail certain standards of rational argument, or may be used to deceive an audience into acceptance of a conclusion. However, the widely held view that this argument is inherently defective or is little more than a scaremongering tactic is as unwarranted as the claim that these arguments always embody the most exacting standards of **logic** and **rationality**. At least this much is assumed in the pragmatic approach to argument evaluation that is conducted throughout this book. According to this approach, some slippery slope arguments are rationally warranted within certain contexts of use. The aim of this volume is to equip readers with the logical skills that are required to determine when this is the case. On at least some of the occasions when slippery slope arguments are employed in a rationally warranted way, it is contended that these arguments can be shown to fulfil an important function as a cognitive heuristic within our practical deliberations. As a heuristic, this argument provides cognitive agents with a quick, effective shortcut in reasoning by means of which practical decisions can be made with minimal expenditure of cognitive effort. This heuristic function has previously been described in relation to a number of the so-called informal fallacies, including **argument from expert opinion** (or *argumentum ad verecundiam*) and the argument from ignorance (Cummings 2014, 2015; Walton 2010). However, this is the first attempt to characterise slippery slope argument in these terms within a wider analysis of fallacies-as-heuristics.

To help us understand what a 'slippery slope' heuristic might look like, consider the following scenario. Many readers will have had the experience of trying to decide if they are safe to drive a vehicle when they have consumed alcohol or when they have taken prescribed or illicit drugs. For most people, good sense prevails and we decide not to take the risk of having an accident, and opt to hire a taxi or take the bus instead of driving. In such a case, a simple argument from consequence guides our decision-making:

Premise: If I engage in drink driving or drug driving, a (possibly fatal) accident may occur.
Conclusion: Therefore I should not engage in drink driving or drug driving.

However, a slippery slope argument may also steer our decision-making in the direction of leaving the car at home and taking a taxi for our journey. Each premise in this argument is strongly warranted given what we know about the legal actions that will be taken against us if we are arrested by the police for drink or drug driving, and the actions that will be taken by employers and others if we are banned from driving for breaking the law. These actions are represented below, along with the 'driving' slippery slope argument that is based on them:

Action 1: I decide to drive my car after a party where I have consumed considerable alcohol.
Action 2: Alcohol in my bloodstream impairs my judgement and reactions behind the wheel.

Action 3: I drive erratically on my way home and do not observe the police car behind me.
Action 4: The two police officers in the car use their siren to pull me over to the roadside.
Action 5: They ask me questions and get me to blow into their breathalyser device.
Action 6: The reading on the device is twice the legal limit and the police arrest me.
Action 7: I appear in court a week later and am fined for my actions and given a year's ban.
Action 8: My employer learns of the ban and decides to terminate my employment.
Action 9: I have no income and no means of earning money while I am banned from driving.
Action 10: I cannot financially support my family and my spouse and children leave me.
Action 11: I have lost my family and employment and have nothing of value left.

'Driving' slippery slope argument:
Premise 1: There is a series of interlinked actions A_1 to A_{10} that results in a highly negative consequence represented by A_{11}.
Premise 2: The only way to avoid the negative consequence A_{11} is to not embark on the series of interlinked actions A_1 to A_{10}.
Premise 3: The only way to avoid the series of actions A_1 to A_{10} is to not take first action A_1.
Conclusion: Action A_1 should not be taken.

Although we may not be aware of it, this reasonable slippery slope argument has prevented many people from engaging in drink driving. It could also be legitimately argued that it is a failure to engage in exactly this type of reasoning that leads people to make the unwise decision to drink and drive. This argument observes all the logical features of slippery slope arguments. There is a negative consequence—the loss of everything that someone might value—that the proponent of the argument wishes to avoid at all costs. There is a series of interlinked actions that carries us down the slope, with each action inching us closer to the negative consequence that we wish to avoid. There are also forceful drivers of these actions. The intoxication caused by alcohol consumption is a powerful driver of actions in the early part of the slope. This is followed by legal procedures and employment practices which take us further down the slope. In the final part of the slope, it is the human distress and hardship that these procedures cause which guarantee our descent to the very bottom of the slope. The final logical feature of slippery slope argument, its defeasibility, is also satisfied by this example. My lawyer may successfully argue in court that there were mitigating circumstances and that a fine and driving ban are not warranted on this occasion. In this case, I may be able to retain my employment and there is no further descent down the slope. If a ban is imposed and I am not able to drive for employment, I may still be able to retrieve the situation by travelling on public transport. Even at this late stage in the slope, I may avoid the loss of everything valuable in my life by means of a range of factors that apply brakes to my descent down the slope (Fig. 3.2).

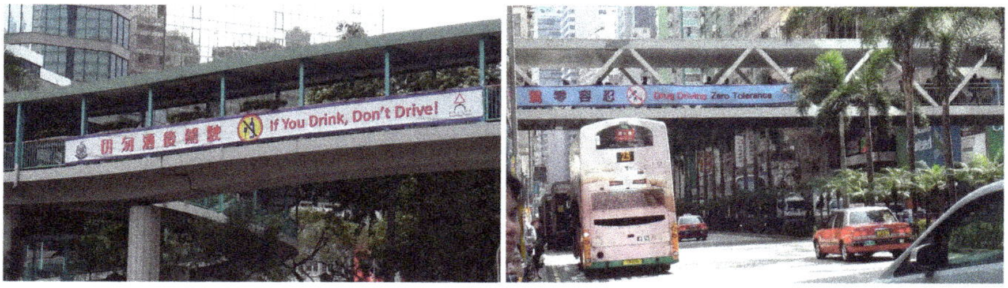

Fig. 3.2 Campaigns to warn the public about the dangers of drink driving and drug driving are a common feature in many cities around the world (Reproduced courtesy of the Road Safety Council of Hong Kong; photographs by Nathan John Albury, Hong Kong, 2018)

So there are clear grounds for treating the 'driving' slippery slope argument as a reasonable form of argument in the context of a practical deliberation. But there is still some way to go before we can claim that this argument is serving as a cognitive heuristic in our decision-making about drink driving. For the latter to be achieved, it must be possible to demonstrate that this argument confers some cognitive gains on those who employ it during reasoning. Gains include increased speed of processing as well as reduced expenditure of mental resources such as memory. These gains can be illustrated by the 'driving' slippery slope argument, but only when we conceive of it in terms of a 'condensed' argument. The explicit mental representation of all the actions in this argument not only places considerable demands on our memory, but also slows processing as we evaluate each action. If these actions can be collapsed or condensed, in the sense of existing as implicit premises in the argument, then it is possible to achieve the cognitive efficiencies that we so keenly desire. In a condensed slippery slope argument, memory that would otherwise be required to store each action (or premise) can be given over to other information. Also, time that would otherwise be devoted to the processing of all the actions in this argument can be used for other cognitive operations. With its individual premises collapsed or implicit, it may be argued that a condensed slippery slope argument has all the appearance of an argument from negative consequence. That appearance is certainly true. But where a condensed slippery slope argument can have its implicit premises unpacked and opened to scrutiny, there are no such premises to make explicit in an argument from negative consequence. This latter argument is truly a one-premise argument.

The 'driving' slippery slope argument is not unique, either on account of its status as a rationally warranted argument or on account of its role as a cognitive heuristic during reasoning. There are many such arguments in medicine and health. An individual's decision to decline the use of cannabis when offered the drug at a party, for example, may be guided by a condensed slippery slope argument. The context is one of a practical deliberation that precludes the use of time- and resource-intensive systematic reasoning. A quick and accurate shortcut through this reasoning is required. This is provided by a condensed slippery slope argument. When unpacked, the premises of this argument are similar to those examined in the 'cannabis' slippery slope argument in ▶ Sect. 3.2. The condensed slippery slope argument also functions as a heuristic in medical decision-making. Doctors use this type of reasoning when they are trying to decide which course of treatment to pursue in a particular case. Imagine a scenario where a drug causes side-effects which must then be treated with other drugs, and that these drugs also cause unpleasant symptoms which must be treated in turn. The administration of no single one of these drugs is a risk to the patient's life. However, when each newly administered drug causes physical symptoms that must be treated with further drugs, the cumulative toxicity of these various drugs may lead to the patient's death. The series of interlinked actions in this case involves several iterations of drug prescription followed by the development of side-effects, with each action down the slope an almost inevitable consequence of the one that precedes it. A condensed slippery slope argument may help doctors decide in this case that the initial act of drug prescription is best avoided.

Chapter Summary

Key points

- Slippery slope arguments are used extensively in medicine and health, particularly where ethical issues intersect with decisions about medical interventions and the termination of life. These arguments are commonly found in public and medical discourses about euthanasia, human genetic engineering, and reproductive medicine. In these contexts, slippery slope arguments are most often used to persuade an audience not to undertake an action which, it is argued, will lead ultimately to a disastrous consequence.
- There are logical and non-logical uses of slippery slopes. In the logical use, the slope is represented by a series of premises which may or may not provide support for a conclusion. The purpose is one of argumentation. In the non-logical use, the slope is used as a metaphor to capture the downward descent in many naturally-occurring processes (e.g. disease progression). There is no attempt to support a conclusion with premises in the non-logical use.
- Slippery slope arguments are a type of argument from negative consequence. However, they differ from this argument in an important respect. An argument from consequence is a single-premise argument. This is because a single action takes us directly to the negative consequence that is to be avoided. The slippery slope argument is a multi-premise argument in which each of the actions that takes us down the slope is represented.
- An argument must satisfy certain logical features in order to be a slippery slope argument. It must contain a conclusion that describes a negative (usually disastrous) consequence that is to be avoided. It must capture in its premises a series of interlinked actions that take us down the slope. It must have identifiable drivers that propel us forward along the actions on the slope. It must exhibit defeasibility in that any of its premises and the conclusion can be overturned or defeated by the emergence of contrary evidence.

- There are a number of logical pitfalls that we can fall into when we use slippery slope arguments. We may only consider the negative consequence of an action and not the benefits of an action. If the negative consequence is allowed to dominate and an initial action is rejected, we may be denied the benefits of an initial action. There may be little or no evidence to support the interlinked actions along the slope. Drivers of actions along the slope can be misrepresented or exaggerated. Emotion may be used to force the audience to accept the conclusion of a slippery slope argument.
- The slippery slope argument is not inherently fallacious. It may be more or less rationally warranted in certain contexts of use. On at least some of the occasions when it is rationally warranted, it may assume the function of a cognitive heuristic. A condensed slippery slope argument is just such a heuristic. It can facilitate decision-making in medicine and health.

Suggestions for Further Reading

(1) Walton, D. (2015). The basic slippery slope argument. *Informal Logic, 35*(3), 273–311.

In this article, Walton presents a basic argumentation scheme for slippery slope argument. Using this scheme, Walton demonstrates that slippery slope argument can be a reasonable argument in some instances. Some of the issues addressed in this chapter are also examined by Walton. This includes drug use, mitochondrial-replacement procedures, and euthanasia.

(2) Den Hartogh, G. (2009). The slippery slope argument. In H. Kuhse & P. Singer (Eds.), *A companion to bioethics* (2nd ed., pp. 321–332). Oxford: Wiley-Blackwell.

This chapter has examined how slippery slope arguments are used extensively in bioethics. Issues such as euthanasia, genetic engineering, and reproductive medicine forcefully bring these arguments into contact with some of the most difficult medical and ethical problems that we face. In this chapter, Govert den Hartogh examines how slippery slope argument is used to navigate these complex problems, on some occasions more adequately than others.

(3) Jefferson, A. (2014). Slippery slope arguments. *Philosophy Compass, 9*(10), 672–680.

In this article, Jefferson examines different variants of slippery slope arguments, their argumentative strength and the interrelations between them. She discusses the factors that affect the likelihood of slippage on the slope in the most common variant of the argument, the empirical slippery slope argument, as well as examines the relation between the strength of the prediction and the justificatory power of the argument.

Questions

(1) We discussed in this chapter how the expression 'slippery slope' can have a logical use and meaning and a non-logical use and meaning. Each of the following extracts mentions a slippery slope. For each extract, identify if the slope in question is part of an argument (logical use) or is used as a type of metaphorical or figurative language (non-logical use):

(A)

Title	A slippery slope: On the origin, role and physiology of mucus
Source	Academic article, *Advanced Drug Delivery Reviews*, volume 124, 16–33

The aims of this article are to elucidate the different physiological, biochemical and physical properties of bodily mucus, a keen appreciation of which will help circumvent the slippery slope of challenges faced in achieving effective mucosal drug and gene delivery.

(B)

Title	The slippery slope of legalization of physician-assisted suicide
Source	Academic article, *Annals of Internal Medicine*, volume 167, issue 8, 595–596

The "slippery-slope" objection to medical suicide and euthanasia may be dismissed as alarmist, but it is not easily refuted. Euthanasia was legalized in the Netherlands in 2002, with multiple safeguards against abuse. However, in 2015, the Dutch government reported that hundreds of persons were put to death without their express consent or because of psychiatric illness, dementia, or just "old age". In addition, the Groningen protocol has legalized infanticide in the Netherlands. In view of these developments, it is laudable that Oregon, Canada, and other jurisdictions have built safeguards into their end-of-life legislation. However, a slope still exists, and it may be fairly steep.

(C)

Title	The slippery slope: Prediction of successful weight maintenance in anorexia nervosa
Source	Academic article, *Psychological Medicine*, volume 39, issue 6, 1037–1045

The current study provides evidence for an anecdotally recognized clinical phenomenon, that early weight loss following acute treatment and weight restoration among patients with anorexia nervosa is a slippery slope and a worrisome early marker of poor long-term outcome.

(2) In ► Sect. 3.2, we saw how increasing addiction to illicit drugs was a powerful driver of actions along a slippery slope that might terminate in the death of a drug user. It is also possible to develop a tolerance for, or dependency on, medications that are prescribed by medical professionals. Burgess (1993) refers to this tolerance in the following slippery slope argument. Examine this use of the argument and then answer the questions that follow:

> Many slippery-slope arguments in applied ethics are simple in structure, highly specific in scope and modest in the practical counsel they offer us. A good example involves the question whether to prescribe drug A or drug B to a

patient. For the condition concerned, A might score best on almost all relevant criteria whilst B does adequately on all, if less well on some. Suppose, further, that there is no realistic possibility of switching drugs in mid-treatment. Now, if A leads to tolerance, eventually needing to be administered in a lethal dose, a simple and sound slippery-slope argument leads to the conclusion that drug B is to be preferred. (Burgess 1993: 169)

Questions

(a) When the 'cannabis' slippery slope argument is used, it is with the purpose of influencing decision-making in areas like politics and law. How is the slippery slope argument described by Burgess being employed?

(b) A key reason why physical dependency on illicit drugs is such a powerful driver down the slope is that there are few, if any, factors that might intervene on this decline to bring it to a halt. These factors might include the actions of friends and family members, many of whom may have abandoned the drug user by this stage in his or her addiction. What factors might halt the decline down the slope of someone with a physical dependency on prescribed medications?

(c) The decision to opt for drug B over drug A prioritises the avoidance of a negative consequence—the administration of a lethal drug dose—over the effectiveness of a particular treatment (recall that drug A scores best on almost all relevant criteria, while drug B does adequately on all and less well on some). What does this weighing of different factors tell us about the type of reasoning at work in a slippery slope argument?

(d) Burgess states that many slippery slope arguments in applied ethics are 'highly specific in scope'. Describe *three* ways in which the slippery slope argument presented above is specific in scope.

(e) The slippery slope argument examined above does not counsel against the legalization of an activity or practice. Name *two* slippery slope arguments in applied ethics where matters relating to legalization are raised.

(3) In the following extract from the *Daily Mail*, writer Ian Birrell discusses how he believes the introduction of non-invasive prenatal testing will take us down a slippery slope 'into a new age of eugenics'. The technique can be used to test for conditions like Down syndrome, a chromosomal disorder that it has only been possible to detect to date through the use of amniocentesis (a procedure that carries the risk of miscarriage). Birrell is opposed to the use of prenatal testing, and had a daughter 24 years ago with a genetic disorder called CDKL5. Examine the extract in detail and then answer the questions that follow:

'I fear this new Down's test is a slippery slope to eugenics', Ian Birrell, *Daily Mail*, 1 March 2017.

» "A new technique — Non-Invasive Prenatal Testing — is set to be rolled out across the National Health Service (NHS) from next year after winning backing from ministers four months ago. […]

In a report published yesterday, the Nuffield Council on Bioethics warns that if it is made widely available, this test is likely to lead to a large increase in the number of babies being aborted on the basis of disability.

What it also points out is that the test, which can identify a foetus's gender as early as nine weeks into pregnancy, could lead to a rise in abortions based on gender among various communities where there is a preference for male children.

These disturbing findings suggest we are hurtling towards a world that once sounded like science fiction; one in which imperfections are eliminated, disabilities eroded and parents enabled to pick idealised children from a medical production line.

Already some scientists [...] talk brazenly about the 'immorality' of producing children with disabilities.

Some senior doctors have suggested the NHS should work out whether caring for children with Down's syndrome during their entire lives was 'cost effective'.

The Royal College of Obstetricians and Gynaecologists, no less, even suggested that the cost of the new test could be justified on the basis that the NHS would be spared the cost of a lifetime of care of babies aborted as a result.

Surely, there needs to be more discussion about moves that raise deep philosophical questions for medicine, politicians and society."

Questions

(a) Identify the initial action that Birrell believes will initiate a descent down the slope. Has that action been taken?

(b) What is the negative consequence that Birrell is arguing non-invasive prenatal testing will lead to?

(c) To what extent are social factors serving as a driver of actions along the slope?

(d) To what extent are economic factors serving as a driver of actions along the slope?

(e) What role is expertise playing in the slippery slope argument that Birrell is advancing?

(4) The field of genetic engineering is a rich source of slippery slope arguments. This chapter has examined a number of the technologies used in this field, including preimplantation genetic diagnosis, gene editing, reproductive cloning, and mitochondrial-replacement procedures. Media outlets have used a range of terms in their reporting of these technologies to the general public. Terms include 'designer babies', 'three-parent babies', 'genetically modified babies', and 'cloned babies'. Relate each of these terms to one or more of the technologies used in genetic engineering. How do these terms affect slippery slope arguments about the use of these technologies?

Answers

Exercise 3.1

(1) Interlinked actions in the 'euthanasia' slippery slope argument:

Action 1: A euthanasia legalization bill is signed into law.
Action 2: Physicians and clinics that offer euthanasia services become available to the public.
Action 3: Significant numbers of people with terminal illnesses begin to access these clinics.
Action 4: Regulatory bodies extend the criteria for patient selection to include conditions other than terminal illnesses such as severe depression and addiction (e.g. alcoholism).
Action 5: There are calls for individuals with severe brain injuries, dementia and a range of other conditions that affect the ability to give informed consent to have access to euthanasia services.
Action 6: The criteria for patient selection are changed again to permit euthanasia of people who are unable to give informed consent to the procedure as well as people who are not economically active (e.g. the elderly and disabled).

(2) As the health systems of countries come under increasing financial burdens, there may be growing reluctance by governments to continue to fund expensive medical treatment of individuals with conditions that will never improve to the point where they can participate economically in society. The families of individuals with these conditions may also become increasingly reluctant to sustain the economic challenges posed by caring for a disabled or ill relative when they are unable to undertake employment on account of their caring duties. It is not difficult to imagine how the combination of these economic factors may lead to a relaxation of the criteria for patient selection for euthanasia and drive us further down the slope towards involuntary euthanasia.

(3) These figures from the Netherlands and Belgium show that the 'euthanasia' slippery slope argument may not be irrational scaremongering after all. Rather, they appear to confirm the series of interlinked actions that take us down the slope. First, there has been an expansion in the criteria used for patient selection. Patients in both countries are now able to use 'tiredness of living' as a reason for euthanasia, so that the procedure is no longer restricted to patients who have terminal illnesses. Second, as patient criteria have been relaxed, there has been a substantial increase in the number of people seeking euthanasia. Euthanasia is now a significant cause of death in both countries.

(4) Particularly in the early part of the slope, a moral duty to alleviate and terminate human suffering is a significant driver of actions. For patients with terminal illnesses such as cancer than involve significant pain, or with severe disabilities that compromise functioning, there may be very poor quality of life. A moral duty on physicians and society as a whole to address that suffering may lead to the

legalization of euthanasia initially. However, this moral driver of early actions on the slope may come to be replaced by an economic driver in which our duty of care to others is subordinated to economic considerations such as the costs of extending the lives of terminally ill people. It is this economic driver that may propel us forward on the slope to extend the practice of euthanasia to groups of people who are considered to be expendable.

(5) The risk that attends the use of the Nazi analogy in a slippery slope argument against the legalization of euthanasia is that it will be perceived as a scare tactic. An otherwise rationally warranted slippery slope argument may lose any legitimacy if the proponent of the argument is perceived to be using emotional factors such as fear rather than 'good reasons' to achieve persuasion.

Exercise 3.2

(1) In the typical argument, the legalization of marijuana or cannabis is the initial action on the slope which, if taken, leads ultimately to the disastrous consequence of hard drug use. In Rutten's argument, full legalization of marijuana is not the initial action on the slope, but the end point that we are inching towards when we permit concessions such as legalization for medicinal purposes to guide law making.

(2) The driver that Rutten believes has been most influential in propelling us along the slope towards full legalization of marijuana is changing social attitudes towards use of the drug. This driver has been so powerful, Rutten argues, that it has exceeded the moderating influences of both 'conventional legal thinking' and 'the permissible language of politics' in relation to marijuana.

(3) Rutten uses the results of polls to support his view that social attitudes are a significant driver of actions towards the legalization of marijuana. He reports that a recent poll found that 60% of Los Angeles County voters and 56% of voters statewide now support the legalization and taxation of marijuana.

(4) Rutten invites readers to draw the conclusion that cannabis is *not* a normative medical remedy. The premises (P) that take us to this conclusion (C) can be reconstructed as the following argument:

P1: If cannabis were a normative medical remedy, then it would be sold in pharmacies.

P2: Cannabis is not sold in pharmacies.

C: Cannabis is *not* a normative medical remedy.

This is a deductively valid *modus tollens* inference.

(5) The other driver of actions along the slope towards the legalization of marijuana is the medicinal use of cannabis to alleviate the suffering of people with terminal illnesses and serious disease. The medical use of marijuana to alleviate human suffering is, in Rutten's view, not well supported. He describes the medicinal necessities of the drug as 'really rather limited'.

Exercise 3.3

(1) Sarler uses emotive language when she characterizes the position of those who oppose euthanasia in the following terms: "to allow it [euthanasia] would be a

slippery slope towards *truckloads of septuagenarians being hurled, still kicking, into the gaping mouths of crematoria*".

(2) Sarler uses abusive *ad hominem* reasoning to characterise proponents of slippery slope arguments when she describes them as "scattergun alarmists and conspiracy theorists" and she states that "the *ignorant* cling to the belief that the use of cannabis is a slippery slope towards the use of, say, heroin".

(3) The logical flaw that is made by proponents of slippery slope arguments is the decision to oppose what is not even being proposed by those who would wish to see the legalization of euthanasia or cannabis.

(4) Alban Maginness does not consider himself bound by a requirement to produce evidence for the claim that euthanasia as practiced in a number of countries is none other than the extermination programme of the Nazis. This claim appears to have self-evident status, in his view.

(5) Sarler views slippery slope arguments as inherently fallacious. Her characterization of these arguments is invariably negative. Slippery slope arguments are what come about when 'reasoned arguments' are suspended. Also, they represent a 'paucity of intellectual rigour'.

End-of-chapter questions

(1)

(a) non-logical use;

(b) logical use;

(c) non-logical use

(2)

(a) This slippery slope argument is being used to guide the decision-making of a medical professional or pharmacist who is attempting to decide between one of two drugs for the treatment of an individual's medical condition.

(b) For the patient who has a physical dependency on prescribed medication, there is a greater likelihood that effective medical intervention may be available and may halt the descent down the slope. It is, after all, within the context of medical treatment that these drugs are being administered to the patient. So although the illicit drug user and the person taking prescribed medication may both have a physical dependency on drugs, it is less likely that factors will intervene to prevent the descent down the slope in the former case than in the latter case.

(c) The reasoning in a slippery slope argument is a type of practical reasoning in which an agent weighs up the costs and benefits of different courses of action. A course of action that incurs severe costs to an agent (in this case, death resulting from a lethal drug dose) may force us to consider an alternative course of action where the benefits are less significant but severe costs are avoided.

(d) This slippery slope argument is specific in scope in the following three ways: (1) the argument concerns the treatment of a specific patient; (2) the argument concerns the treatment of a specific medical condition; and (3) the argument concerns two specific drugs.

(e) Two slippery slope arguments in applied ethics: (1) argument against the legalization of euthanasia and (2) argument against the legalization of abortion.

(3)

(a) According to Birrell, the initial action that starts our descent down the slope is the introduction of non-invasive prenatal testing. There are two parts to this action. First, there is parliamentary approval which has been obtained (the technique received backing from ministers four months ago). Second, the procedure needs to be implemented by the National Health Service. We are told in the article that this new procedure is due to be rolled out by the NHS from 2018. So at the time Birrell was writing, the first part of the action had been completed, while the second part had yet to be completed.
(b) Birrell is arguing that non-invasive prenatal testing will lead to a form of eugenics (negative consequence) as parents opt to abort foetuses where disabilities are identified, or where a foetus is not the desired gender in a particular community.
(c) Social factors are a powerful driver of actions along the slope. These factors are of two kinds. First, parents are opting not to have babies with severe disabilities. Their support of procedures which make this possible ensures that non-invasive prenatal testing will be widely adopted. Second, many cultures and communities continue to prefer babies of male gender over babies of female gender. Parents in these cultures and communities will also support the use of non-invasive prenatal testing.
(d) Economic factors are an equally powerful driver of actions along the slope. Babies who are born with severe disabilities require medical, educational, and social support for the rest of their lives. Health systems like the NHS are increasingly asking if the costs of this support can continue to be absorbed when the demand for health services outstrips the available resources.
(e) The Royal College of Obstetricians and Gynaecologists is a recognised expert body. However, the expertise of this body is used to support the case for prenatal testing. So they are one of the key actors who, according to Birrell, are driving us down the slope towards the widespread practice of eugenics.

(4) The terms 'three-parent babies' and 'cloned babies' are associated with mitochondrial-replacement procedures and reproductive cloning, respectively. The terms 'designer babies' and 'genetically modified babies' are both associated with gene editing, while 'designer babies' is associated with preimplantation genetic diagnosis. The terms 'designer babies' and 'three-parent babies' are negatively emotionally loaded in the slippery slope arguments in which they appear. The former implies the commodification of human beings in the same way that someone can own a designer handbag or item of clothing. The latter implies an aberration of nature like Frankenstein ('three-parent babies' have often been characterised as Frankenstein science by the media). In slippery slope arguments the use of these terms serves to arouse fear and encourage rejection of the various technologies that lead to them.

References

Boer, T. A. (2003). After the slippery slope: Dutch experiences on regulating active euthanasia. *Journal of the Society of Christian Ethics, 23*(2), 225–242.
Burgess, J. A. (1993). The great slippery-slope argument. *Journal of Medical Ethics, 19*(3), 169–174.
Cummings, L. (2012). Scaring the public: Fear appeal arguments in public health reasoning. *Informal Logic, 32*(1), 25–50.
Cummings, L. (2014). Informal fallacies as cognitive heuristics in public health reasoning. *Informal Logic, 34*(1), 1–37.
Cummings, L. (2015). *Reasoning and public health: New ways of coping with uncertainty*. Cham, Switzerland: Springer.
Darnovsky, M. (2013). A slippery slope to human germline modification. *Nature, 499,* 127.
Feig, D. S. (2012). Avoiding the slippery slope: Preventing the development of diabetes in women with a history of gestational diabetes. *Diabetes/Metabolism Research and Reviews, 28,* 317–320.
Gunning, J. (2008). The broadening impact of preimplantation genetic diagnosis: A slide down the slippery slope or meeting market demand. *Human Reproduction & Genetic Ethics, 14*(1), 29–37.
Lerner, B. H., & Caplan, A. L. (2015). Euthanasia in Belgium and the Netherlands: On a slippery slope? *JAMA Internal Medicine, 175*(10), 1640–1641.
Oakley, J., & Cocking, D. (2005). Consequentialism, complacency, and slippery slope arguments. *Theoretical Medicine and Bioethics, 26*(3), 227–239.
Spielthenner, G. (2010). A logical analysis of slippery slope arguments. *Health Care Analysis, 18*(2), 148–163.
Walton, D. N. (2010). Why fallacies appear to be better arguments than they are. *Informal Logic, 30*(2), 159–184.
Walton, D. (2017). The slippery slope argument in the ethical debate on genetic engineering of humans. *Science and Engineering Ethics, 23*(6), 1507–1528.

Fear Appeal Arguments

L. Cummings, *Fallacies in Medicine and Health*,
https://doi.org/10.1007/978-3-030-28513-5_4

LEARNING OBJECTIVES: Readers of this chapter will

- be able to distinguish fear appeal argument from non-argumentative uses of fear in discourse, and identify different contexts in which fear-based language is used.
- be able to describe the logical structure of fear appeal argument as a special type of argument from negative consequence, and understand that a negative consequence is not necessarily a fearful consequence.
- be able to appreciate the difference between fear appeal and threat appeal in argument, particularly as these arguments relate to health.
- be able to describe the different ways in which fear appeal may be misused in argument, and understand that most logical pitfalls arise when the argument is pursued too forcefully against a respondent.
- be able to discuss some of the key empirical findings about fear appeal argument in the social scientific literature.
- be able to explain how fear can constitute an effective heuristic during reasoning about health issues, and characterize the nature of a fear appeal heuristic.

4.1 Introduction

In ► Chapter 3, we saw how even a weakly warranted slippery slope argument could persuade an opponent or audience to accept a conclusion if fear was aroused by advancing the argument. In this chapter, we will see how the appeal to fear can be an argument in its own right. Fear appeal has received something of a bad press in logic and critical thinking where it is often viewed as the antithesis of rational argumentation. Indeed, logicians and some argumentation theorists routinely contend that the person who appeals to fear in order to persuade an opponent to accept a claim in argument has resorted to the use of a scare tactic. This chapter will examine the extent to which this is true, and whether a strategy to use fear to achieve the rational persuasion of an audience can be warranted under certain circumstances. A difficulty for any argument analyst is that fear is not an easily delineated concept. In some cases, fear can be conceived in terms of affective states such as horror or disgust. I may experience these states, for example, when I see images of diseased bodies and organs in public health campaigns about alcohol consumption and smoking (see ◘ Fig. 4.1). In other cases, fear may take the form of anxiety such as the anxiety I may have about my own health when I receive a letter inviting me for a mammogram. In still other cases, fear can overlap with emotions such as vanity and psychological states like self-esteem. It is exactly these mental phenomena that public health agencies are attempting to arouse when they use male concerns about sexual performance and female concerns about aging in campaigns on smoking cessation (see ◘ Fig. 4.1). Each of these different ways of defining fear will be illustrated by the examples of fear appeal argument that will be used throughout this chapter.

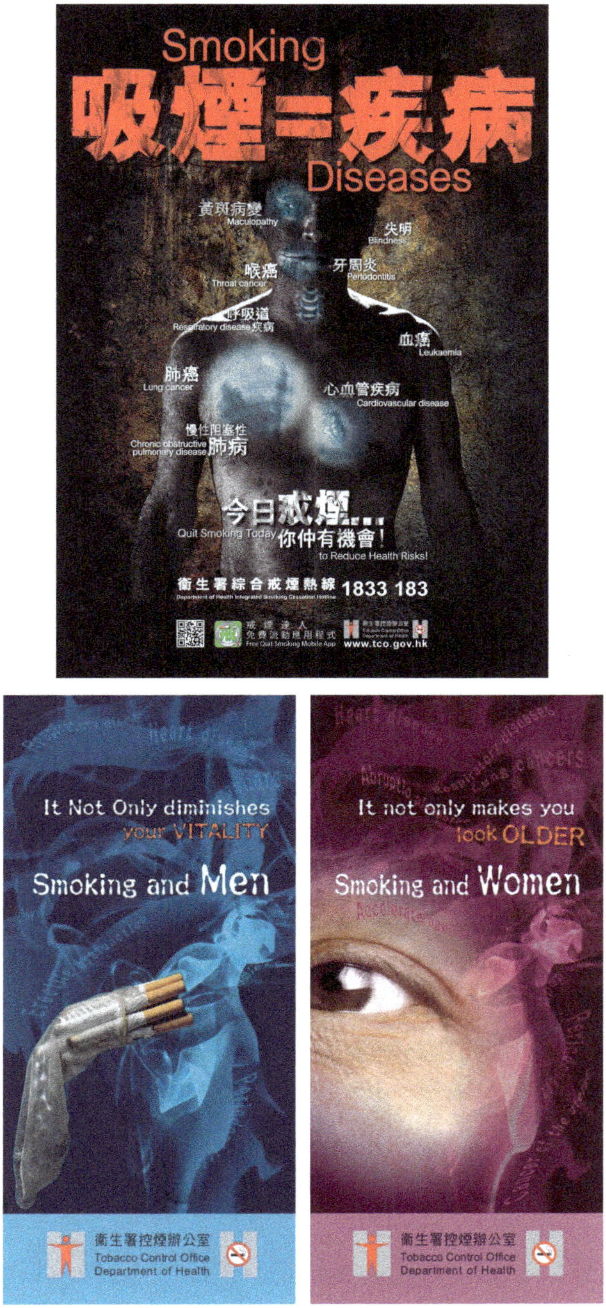

Fig. 4.1 Fear and related emotions are often aroused in campaigns about smoking cessation (Reproduced courtesy of the Department of Health, The Government of the Hong Kong Special Administrative Region)

The sections in this chapter will unfold as follows. In ▶ Sect. 4.2, it will be argued that fear-based language is used in fear appeal argument but can also be used in **speech acts** other than argumentation (e.g. warnings). Distinguishing the argumentative use of such language from these other uses is challenging, and may in some cases involve a balance of probabilities. In ▶ Sect. 4.3, the logical features of fear appeal arguments will be considered. We have already seen how these arguments can overlap with slippery slope arguments. This is by virtue of the fact that they are both types of argument from negative consequence. However, fear appeal argument is a special type of argument from negative consequence—not every negative consequence can arouse fear, after all. The conditions under which fear appeal arguments are more or less rationally warranted are addressed in ▶ Sect. 4.4. It is undeniable that these arguments are pressed into use quite often by politicians, advertisers and others, particularly when they want to achieve 'quick and easy' acceptance of their viewpoint by the public or purchase of a commercial product. But these fallacious uses of the argument should not overshadow those occasions when rationally warranted appeals to fear are made during argument. Fear appeal argument is almost unique among the informal fallacies in that it has also been the focus of considerable social scientific research. In ▶ Sect. 4.5, some of the findings of this research are examined. Finally, in at least some of the instances when fear appeal argument is used non-fallaciously, it can be construed in terms of a fear heuristic that confers certain cognitive gains on the reasoning in which it participates. The chapter concludes in ▶ Sect. 4.6 with an examination of this heuristic.

4.2 Logical and Non-logical Uses of Fear

Like ignorance and slippery slopes, fear appeal has both logical and non-logical uses in **discourse**. It is not always easy to tease these uses apart as fear-based language may be employed in a range of discourse processes that are unrelated to argumentation as such. Fear-based language may be used to warn or threaten a person not to undertake a certain action, or to suggest that one course of action may be preferable over another course of action. Warnings, threats, and suggestions are not arguments and need not involve arguments. By way of illustration, consider the following extract from an article about use of the drug crystal meth (crystal methamphetamine) in the British tabloid newspaper *The Daily Star*. The article is describing the severe and often rapid transformation of one's physical appearance that results from use of the drug. There are several photographs of addicts throughout the story that illustrate this transformation in a very graphic way. These photographs are not reproduced here:

> **REVEALED: The horror of crystal meth—Most shocking EVER before and after pictures**
>
> THESE disturbing mugshots look like characters from a zombie horror flick.
> [Photos]
>
> SCARY: These meth-heads look more like the cast of a terrifying horror film.

But they reveal the devastating impact on people hooked on crystal meth. The deadly substance, made world famous by telly hit Breaking Bad, is now one of the most dangerous drugs in the world.

Shocking before and after pictures show how rapidly meth can erode people's appearances—and destroy their lives.
[Photos]

SHOCKING: These pictures show how meth erodes users' appearances.
[Photos]

NOW: The dramatic changes to the woman after just five years.

And many of the images are taken just two years apart, demonstrating the speed which addiction can take hold.

Users often develop acne and "obsessive skin-picking" can result in their faces becoming riddled with sores and scars.
[Photos]

ZOMBIE: This guy has been transformed in just two years.

This is commonly caused by hallucinations of BUGS crawling under their skin. Meth also suppresses the appetite, leading addicts to typically have "hollowed-out", gaunt faces.

Eventually the body starts to eat ITSELF to stay alive, consuming muscle tissue and facial fat.
[Photos]

DISTURBING: These pictures show how meth ravages the body.
[Photos]

AFTER: Two years on and this woman is a shadow of her former self.

One of the most common features is "meth mouth"—which sees teeth and gums DISSOLVED by the harsh chemicals in the drugs.

Addicts often neglect their dental hygiene and grind their teeth at night, causing further damage.

The overall result leads to users appearing DECADES older.
[Photos]

DEVASTATING: The impact of crystal meth addiction.
[Photos]

RAVAGED: In just five years this woman has destroyed her looks.

The drug, a form of methamphetamine, is extremely addictive, producing a powerful high followed by a severe comedown.

The pictures were put together by online drug recovery directory, ► Rehabs.com.

Meth is one of the most serious drug problems in many Mid-west states in America, according to the site.

"No one is immune to the frightening long-term impact of hard drug abuse"

Rehabs.com

Revealing the horrors of meth abuse, ▶ Rehabs.com said: "Addiction touches nearly every family, ravaging physical and mental health, relationships, and personal finances".

"Mothers, fathers, brothers, sisters, daughters and sons".

"No one is immune to the frightening long-term impact of hard drug abuse".

"What follows is a sobering depiction of REAL individuals who've fallen victim to the temptation of drug use - in this case, Methamphetamine - whose devastating effects are all too apparent."

The startling photographs of drug abuse come as the *Daily Star Online* reveal that ISIS killers are pumped up on speed-like drugs so they can carry out atrocities in Syria without a second thought.
[Photos]

ADDICT: This woman has aged dramatically since taking meth.
(Siba Jackson, 29 January 2016, *The Daily Star*)

Reproduced courtesy of Express Newspapers.

This article is littered with fear-inducing language. Noun phrases such as *horror, victim, zombie horror flick*, and *cast of a terrifying horror film* arouse the type of fear that is experienced when one watches horror movies. This fear is compounded by frequent use of adjectives like *shocking, devastating, disturbing*, and *frightening*, many of which are capitalised for emphasis. The author employs graphic descriptions similar to those that may be used to capture the effects of a deadly infectious disease on the body. They include: *body starts to eat itself, ravages the body*, and *teeth and gums dissolved*. In case there is any doubt that the author is attempting to instil fear in readers, the article concludes by drawing an analogy between crystal meth and speed-like drugs that are used by ISIS killers to commit atrocities in Syria.

There can be no doubt that the language used in this article is intended to arouse fear in readers. But the question that we need to address is whether the author is using this language in a fear appeal argument, or whether the article is serving only to describe the effects of crystal meth on the body and warn readers against use of the drug. The simple answer is that we cannot say for certain in this case. It is true that this article will have the effect of deterring people from embarking on meth use. The website referred to in the article, ▶ Rehabs.com, conducted an online survey to determine what, if any, effect graphic images of the type featured in the article have on peoples' attitudes towards drugs and drug addicts. A total of 1598 respondents answered the question 'Does seeing the physical effects of severe drug addiction make you less likely to abuse drugs?', to which 89.3% responded 'yes' and 10.7% responded 'no'. However, a warning about meth use that succeeds in deterring people from using the drug is not a fear appeal *argument* about meth use. It is also true that this article lacks any of the linguistic markers of argument. There are no **logical connectors** like *so* and *therefore* that indicate the author is drawing a conclusion based on certain premises. If a fear appeal argument is advanced by this author, it is difficult to identify it, and distinguish it from other speech acts such as a warning.

The author of the above article is clearly intent on making readers aware of the devastating effects of meth use on the body, albeit in a rather sensationalist way. On learning about these effects, if readers decide not to use this drug, then we can certainly say that any warning in the article has been acted upon. However, the author has still not produced an argument to the effect that a particular action—in this case, meth consumption—has fearful consequences that can only be avoided by not embarking on the use of this drug. This can be explained by the fact that the author is a journalist for a newspaper and, as such, has an aim to inform (or terrify) readers without advising them to modify their behaviour or pursue a certain course of action. The same is not true of a public health agency like the Centers for Disease Control and Prevention (CDC) in the United States, where positive behaviour modification is very much part of the message to be communicated. This can be seen in the *Rx Awareness* campaign that was launched by the CDC in 2015 to address the large number of deaths related to prescription opioid overdoses in the United States. According to the CDC (2016), more than 183,000 people in the United States died from overdoses related to prescription opioids between 1999 and 2015. This large number of deaths demanded an effective public health campaign that warned of the dangers of opioids with a view to discouraging widespread use of these drugs. The CDC's campaign was directed at adults aged 25–54 years who had taken opioids at least once for medical or nonmedical (recreational) use. The main poster and message used in this campaign are displayed in Fig. 4.2.

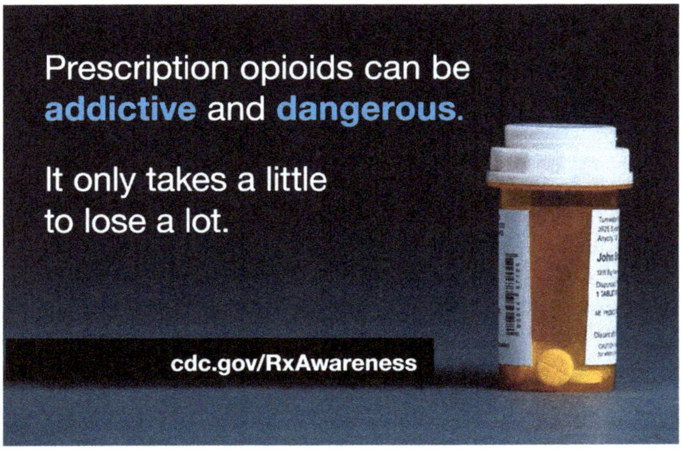

Fig. 4.2 The *Rx Awareness* campaign by the CDC was in response to the escalating number of deaths in the US related to prescription opioid overdoses (Reproduced courtesy of the Centers for Disease Control and Prevention)

Even in the absence of the fear-arousing language of the article in *The Daily Star*, the reader is left in no doubt about what can be lost as a result of taking prescription opioids—one's life is the ultimate price of these drugs. By any standard, death and addiction are fearful consequences that most (or all) of us would wish to avoid. But the poster and its message take us beyond a warning about these fearful consequences to the only course of action that can avert these consequences—the avoidance of prescription opioids. The implied directive to avoid the use of opioids is the conclusion in a fear appeal argument. It is the recommended behaviour modification that is implicit in this message from the CDC that sets this fear appeal argument about opioids apart from the newspaper's warning about meth. It is only in the former case that we can be said to act on the logical consequences of one or more premises that express a fearful scenario.

These two examples illustrate a number of points about fear appeal argument that have general relevance to this chapter. First, language can be used to arouse fear without conveying a fear appeal argument, as was the case in the article in *The Daily Star*. The aim to arouse fear and even terrify readers may be an end in itself, especially when this is done in a sensational way. A fearful readership may be all that a journalist intended to achieve by means of writing an article. Second, the logical use of fear in argument does not treat fear as an end in itself but as the first step towards behaviour modification. When public health agencies like the CDC create a fearful scenario in the mind of readers, it is with a view to recommending a course of action that will allow us to avoid or diminish the fear-arousing situation. We will see in the next section that the scenario which generates fear is expressed in the premises of a fear appeal argument while the protective action to be taken is expressed in the conclusion. Third, a fear appeal argument is seldom expressed in a fully explicit way. Typically, one of the premises or the conclusion remains implicit in the argument and must be made explicit at the stage of argument reconstruction. In the *Rx Awareness* campaign poster in ◘ Fig. 4.2, we are in little doubt that the CDC intends readers to conclude that prescription opioids should be avoided altogether or their use restricted at least. But the campaign poster *implies* this conclusion rather than *states* it. Fourth, visual images can play an important role in fear arousal, both on their own and alongside language. Images can contribute to fear arousal as an end in itself (non-logical use) and as a premise in a fear appeal argument (logical use). We will return to each of these points in the following sections.

EXERCISE 4.1: Opioid use on US college campuses

The following poster is produced by the San Francisco Department of Health. It contains a warning to college students about the use of oxycodone, an opioid that is a prescribed medication but is also often used as a recreational drug. Along with other opioid drugs, including hydrocodone (a prescription opioid), fentanyl (a synthetic opioid), and heroin (an illegal opioid), it is responsible for an escalating number of adult accidental deaths in the United States. Naloxone is a medication that can rapidly reverse opioid overdose, and is administered by medical personnel, police officers, and non-emergency first responders. Examine the poster in ◘ Fig. 4.3, and then answer the questions that follow it.

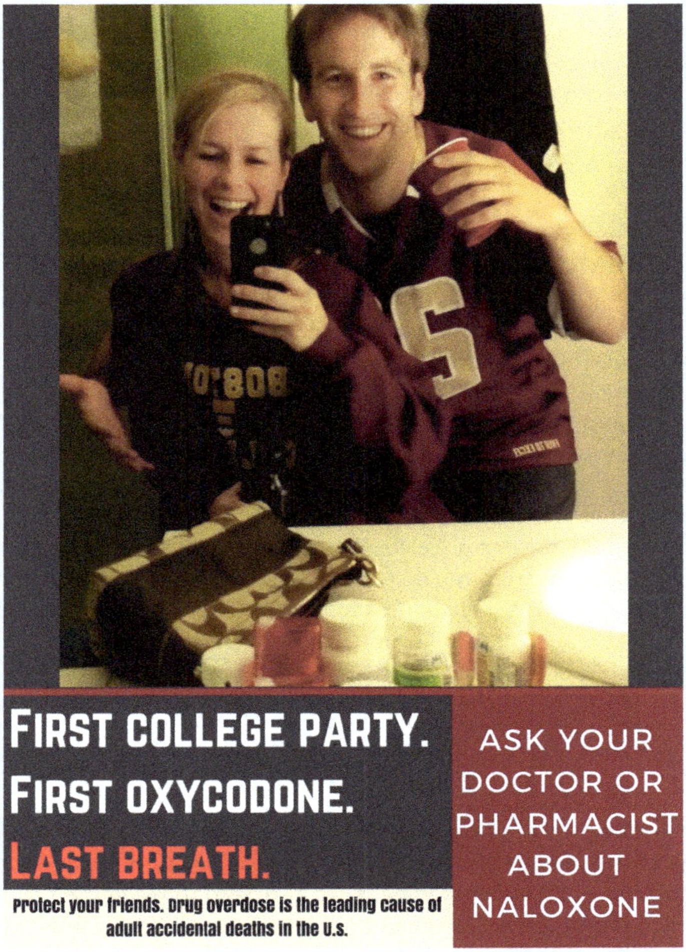
FIRST COLLEGE PARTY.
FIRST OXYCODONE.
LAST BREATH.
Protect your friends. Drug overdose is the leading cause of adult accidental deaths in the U.S.
ASK YOUR DOCTOR OR PHARMACIST ABOUT NALOXONE

Fig. 4.3 A poster warning college students about the dangers of the opioid drug oxycodone (Reproduced courtesy of the San Francisco Department of Health)

Questions

(1) What are (a) the *fearful consequence* identified in the poster, and (b) the *action* that gives rise to this consequence? Are the responses you have given to (a) and (b) the same as or different from those that were identified in the CDC poster examined previously?

(2) What information in the poster suggests that the action identified in response to (1b) has an increased likelihood of resulting in the consequence that was identified in response to (1a)?

(3) In the CDC poster, a protective action was strongly implied in response to the fearful consequence. Is the same protective action suggested in this case?

(4) In the CDC poster, the agent of the *initial action* (the action that causes the fearful consequence) is the same as the agent of the *protective action* (the action that avoids or diminishes the fearful consequence). Is that also the case in this poster?
(5) Is this poster advancing a fear appeal argument? Provide a justification of your response.

4.3 Logical Features of Fear Appeal Argument

We have already had cause to examine some of the logical features of fear appeal arguments. These arguments set out from premises that describe an action that is undertaken by the recipient of the argument, and a consequence of this action. The premises further express that the consequence of this action is particularly negative for the recipient. In fact, the consequence is so serious (maybe even disastrous or catastrophic) for the recipient that it induces fear. The conclusion states that the only way to avert this negative consequence and the state of fear that it arouses is to avoid taking the action that brought it about in the first place. Readers will no doubt have recognised the logical structure of an argument from negative consequence in what has just been described. Indeed, this is exactly how Walton (2000: 140) characterizes fear appeal argument:

If you (the respondent) bring about *A*, then *B* will occur.
B is a very bad outcome, from your (the respondent's) point of view (or interests).
Therefore, you (the respondent) should not bring about *A*.

The logic of this argument is incontestable. What rational agent would not want to avoid taking an action that placed its safety and wellbeing in grave danger? But in acknowledging the logic of this argument, we also need to recognize that fear appeal argument is not simply the argument from negative consequence that is set out above. Fear appeal argument demands an additional premise beyond the two that occur in the argument from negative consequence. That premise makes explicit the role of fear in the argument. It can be stated as follows:

B arouses considerable fear in you (the respondent).

The introduction of a 'fear' premise into an argument will leave many traditional logicians feeling uneasy. They argue that such a premise gives a logical status to fear, and that no emotion should be afforded logical standing in argument. This is essentially the challenge to fear appeal argument by logicians who characterize this argument as a fallacy. But not all uses of fear in argument are unwarranted. Fear may indeed be rationally warranted if there is evidence to support it. We will address this issue further when we come to an evaluation of fear appeal argument in ▶ Sect. 4.4. In the meantime, we can say that fear appeal argument is an argument from negative consequence that is modified to include a premise which explicitly articulates the fear of the respondent. Fear assumes a logical role as a ground or reason for the acceptance of the conclusion in an argument from negative consequence:

P1: If you (the respondent) bring about *A*, then *B* will occur.
P2: *B* is a very bad outcome, from your (the respondent's) point of view (or interests).
P3: *B* arouses considerable fear in you (the respondent).
C: Therefore, you (the respondent) should not bring about *A*.

The representation of fear in *P3* is doing more than placing fear on a logical footing. It is also allowing fear to be rationally assessed in the same way that we would wish to rationally evaluate any premise in argument. The structure of a typical or standard argument from negative consequence seems to miss the central intuition about an appeal to fear in argument. That intuition is that it is often rational to avoid a certain action exactly because that action arouses fear and not because it leads to a bad outcome. If I do not undertake revision for an exam, and I fail the exam as a result, the failure would amount to a bad outcome for me, according to most observers. But this bad outcome may have no logical weight whatsoever in my decision to comply with the recommended action in the conclusion of a fear appeal argument. That action—the requirement to undertake extensive revision—may only be rationally warranted when I consider the fearful situation that I will experience when my parents are informed of my exam failure. In this case, fear is doing logical work that the bad outcome of exam failure is not able to do. A bad outcome per se may not be a 'good reason' to undertake a recommended action if that outcome has no affective (specifically, fearful) consequences for me. The first logical feature of fear appeal argument can be stated as follows:

Logical feature 1: A modified argument from consequence

Fear appeal argument is a modified argument from negative consequence. In addition to the standard structure of an argument from negative consequence, there must be an additional premise that captures the fear that is aroused in the recipient of the argument by the outcome of an action.

It could be objected that fear arousal is a psychological phenomenon that has no place in the logical structure of an argument. The charge is one of **psychologism** in logic, the idea (mistaken in the view of many philosophers) that logical principles should be based on psychological laws. However, as the discussion of drivers in slippery slope argument in ▸ Chapter 3 illustrated, psychological, social, and other factors routinely undertake logical work in argument with no loss of the normative force of logic. A fear appeal argument will fail in its purpose of rational persuasion of an audience if its premises merely state the bad outcome of an action. The extra logical step of fear must be taken to relate this outcome to the protective action that will be able to avert it. An anti-smoking campaign that tells the public that smoking causes lung cancer is certainly describing a bad outcome (lung cancer) of an action (smoking) from the recipient's point of view. But this bad outcome has almost no logical force for smokers, almost all of whom already knew of this consequence before they started smoking. However, what does have logical weight for smokers in the decision to stop smoking is the thought of a protracted, painful death, and the distress and hardship that are caused to loved ones when a smoker dies prematurely from smoking-related disease. It is the fear associated with each of these scenarios that provides the logical link between the bad outcome of an action and compliance with the recommended protective action in the conclusion of a fear appeal argument. Fear is as much a component of rational persuasion in this argument as are these other logical features (Fig. 4.4).

4

The other premises in a fear appeal argument also require some discussion. The wording of *P1* strongly suggests that the action which leads to a bad outcome is under

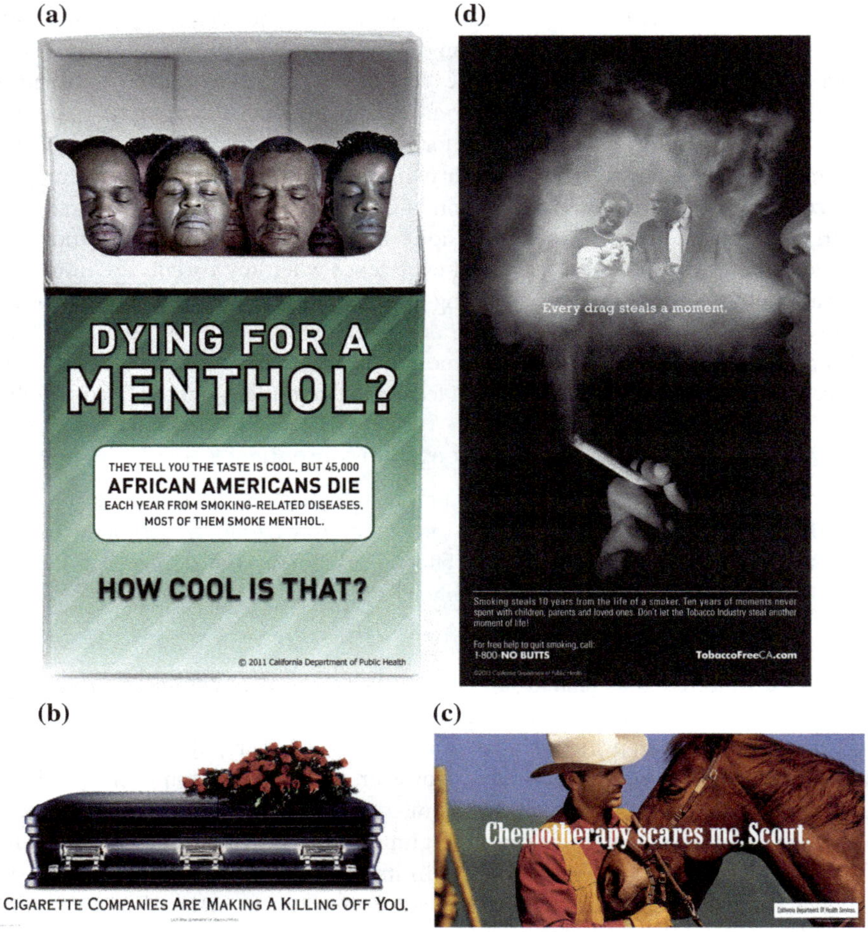

Fig. 4.4 All anti-smoking campaigns provide warnings about the adverse consequences of smoking. But only some of these campaigns arouse fear by confronting people with their own mortality (a and b), the need for medical treatment (c), and the loss of precious family experiences (d) (Reproduced courtesy of the California Department of Public Health)

the volitional control of an agent. This agent—the recipient or respondent of the argument—'brings about' an action. For many fear appeal arguments, this is an accurate characterization of the action that leads to a bad outcome for the recipient of the argument. If I decide to use illicit drugs, smoke tobacco, or drink alcohol to excess, then the adverse outcomes that I will very likely experience have resulted from actions that are under my volitional control, at least initially. But there are many events that lead to adverse outcomes and that may be used in fear appeal arguments, but which it may seem cannot be characterized in these terms. If I contract influenza or develop a vector-borne disease like Zika virus infection and dengue fever (both of which are transmitted by mosquitoes), it may be argued that I have not acted under my volitional control in these circumstances. I cannot be said to have willed either of these situations upon myself, or intended that either of them should come about. To all intents and purposes, it may appear that these events are completely outside of my volitional control.

To some extent, this characterization of these events is true—I did not purposely set out to contract influenza or develop a mosquito-borne infectious disease. But there is another important respect in which I am still able to exercise some control over these situations. Indeed, a fear appeal argument cannot work unless we can assume that this is the case. This is because the recommended protective action in the conclusion of the argument requires that some degree of volitional control must be possible. Otherwise, and somewhat illogically, this conclusion would encourage the recipient of the argument to undertake actions that cannot in any way influence the initial event that leads to a bad outcome. So I can get a flu vaccination that will in most cases protect me against influenza. I can also use insect repellent and take other precautionary measures to protect myself against mosquito bites (see ◘ Fig. 4.5). Despite my best efforts, these actions may not be successful in preventing me from contracting flu or developing a mosquito-borne infectious disease. But they still allow me to exercise some degree of control over events that might initially appear to lie outside of my control. These considerations give rise to a second logical feature of fear appeal argument:

Logical feature 2: Volitional control of initial action

The action that leads to a bad outcome must be under *some* degree of volitional control, even in those cases where it appears that an event or action 'just happens'. The recommended protective action in the conclusion of a fear appeal argument only makes sense to the extent that some degree of volitional control can be assumed.

The wording of *P2* also requires some elaboration. This premise states that an action must have a 'very bad outcome' from the respondent's point of view or interests. Some restriction of the evaluative adjective 'bad' is required as actions can have a range of very bad outcomes, only some of which arouse fear. If I lose my house in payment of a gambling debt, this is clearly a very bad outcome for me that resulted from my decision to engage in gambling. Yet, this outcome is much more likely to give rise to emotions like anger and despair than it is to arouse fear. Even in the context of medicine and health, there can be very bad

4

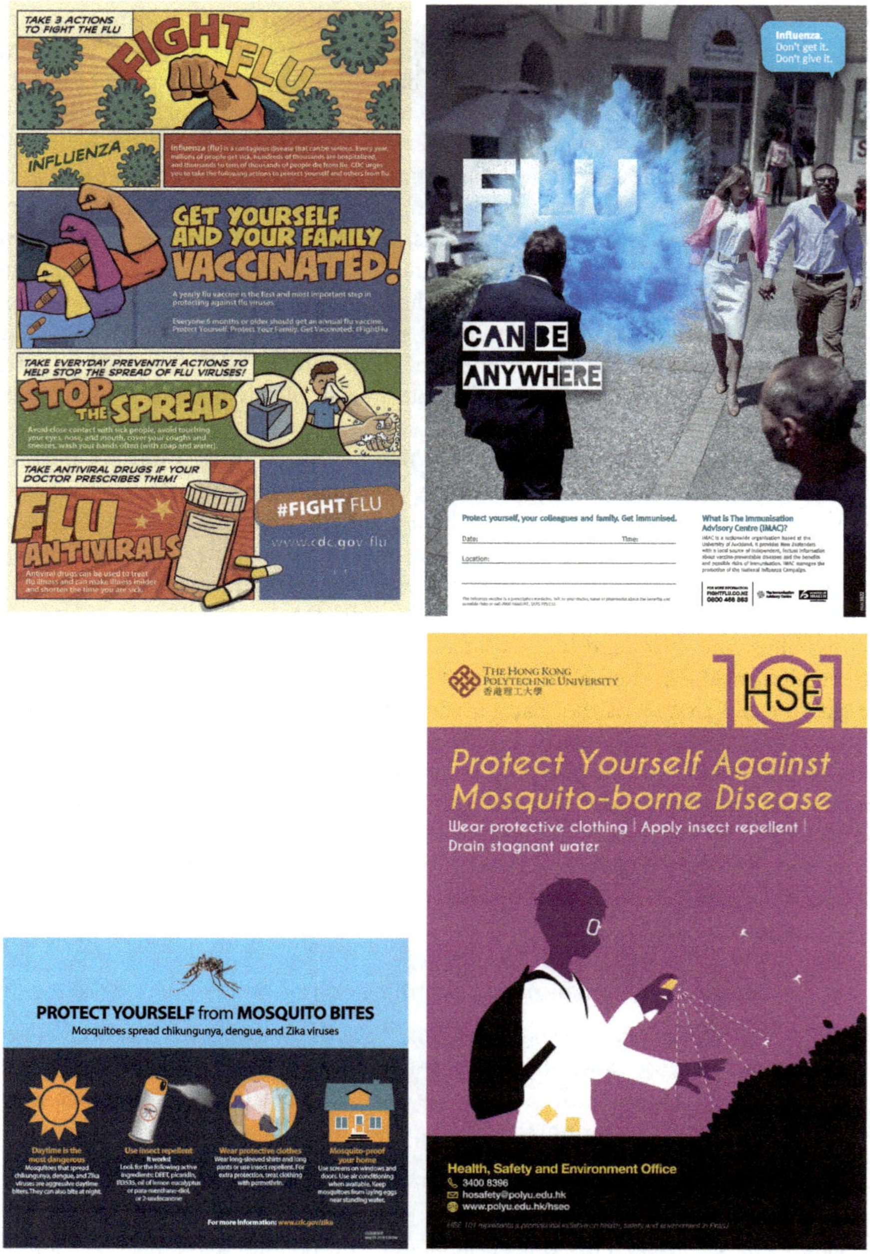

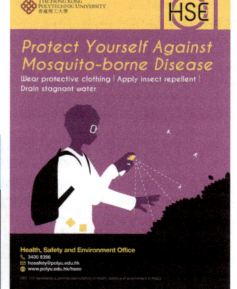

Fig. 4.5 The recipient of a fear appeal argument must be able to exert some control over the initial action, even when this involves contracting infectious diseases like influenza and mosquito-borne infections such as Zika virus (Reproduced courtesy of the Centers for Disease Control and Prevention in the United States, the Ministry of Health of the New Zealand Government, and the Health, Safety and Environment Office at The Hong Kong Polytechnic University)

outcomes of actions that I have initiated that do not in any way lead me to experience fear. I may have smoked 60 cigarettes a day for 30 years and developed lung cancer as a result. Yet, my overriding emotional state may be one of regret about my earlier actions and not fear about the treatment that lies ahead or even my premature death. What scenarios like these demonstrate is that the negative evaluation of the outcome of an action in *P2* of a fear appeal argument is necessary, but not sufficient, for that action to arouse fear. An additional conceptual and psychological step must be taken between negative evaluation on the one hand and fear arousal on the other hand. If this step cannot be taken because an emotion other than fear intervenes (e.g. anger, regret), then there are grounds for saying that whatever other type of argument we may be dealing with, it is *not* a fear appeal argument. But if the transition between negative evaluation and fear arousal is uncomplicated by the presence of other affective states, then we may be said to be appealing to fear in argument. These considerations give rise to the third logical feature of fear appeal argument:

Logical feature 3: Negative evaluation and fear arousal

A negatively evaluated outcome of an action is necessary, but not sufficient, for fear arousal. In a fear appeal argument, the relationship between negative evaluation and fear arousal must not be mediated by any other affective state.

There is a second feature of premise *P2* that requires examination. In fear appeal argument, the outcome of an action is judged to be 'very bad' from the respondent's *point of view or interests*. This allows for the possibility that there are fear appeal arguments where the negatively evaluated outcome of an action does not involve direct injury or harm to the recipient of the argument. And yet the recipient is motivated to undertake the protective action recommended in the conclusion of the argument because it is in his interests to do so. To illustrate this point, consider the type of fear appeal argument that is used by public health agencies to persuade parents not to expose their children to the harmful effects of second hand smoke. The argument may describe the increased risk of asthma and other respiratory illnesses in children who are exposed to tobacco smoke. These harmful consequences, the argument continues, can only be averted if parents stop smoking in the presence of their children. It should be noted in this case that, quite unlike other fear appeal arguments that we have examined in this chapter, it is not the recipient of the argument who experiences the 'very bad outcome' of smoking (although the adult who smokes will, of course, experience adverse health effects as well). Rather, it is the children of the recipient who are placed at an increased risk of developing respiratory illnesses like asthma. The key point, however, is that it is in the *interests* of the recipient to prevent exposure of his or her children to tobacco smoke, at least on the assumption that the recipient is concerned about their safety and well-being. It is with a view to advancing these interests that the recipient is motivated to undertake the protective action recommended in the conclusion of a fear appeal argument (Fig. 4.6). The final logical feature of fear appeal argument can be formulated as follows:

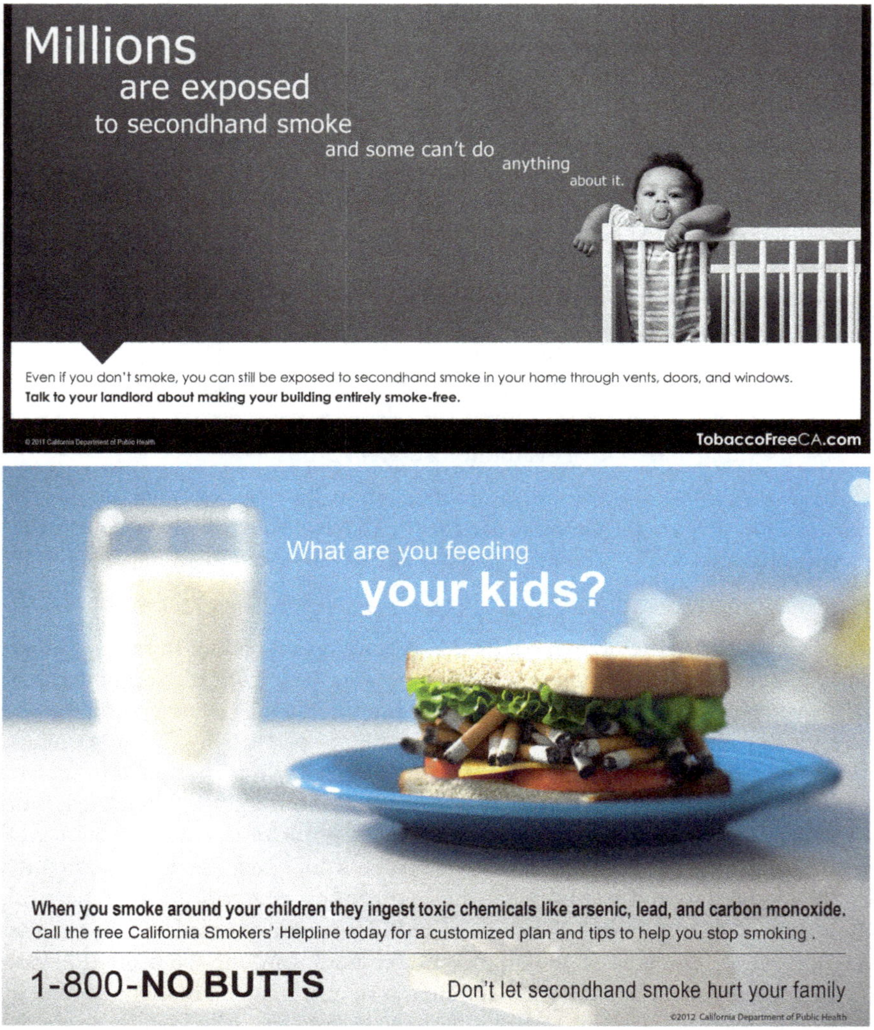

Millions
are exposed
to secondhand smoke
and some can't do
anything
about it.
Even if you don't smoke, you can still be exposed to secondhand smoke in your home through vents, doors, and windows.
Talk to your landlord about making your building entirely smoke-free.
TobaccoFreeCA.com
What are you feeding
your kids?
When you smoke around your children they ingest toxic chemicals like arsenic, lead, and carbon monoxide.
Call the free California Smokers' Helpline today for a customized plan and tips to help you stop smoking .
1-800-NO BUTTS
Don't let secondhand smoke hurt your family
©2012 California Department of Public Health

Fig. 4.6 Parental smoking damages children who are not the recipients of fear appeal arguments (Reproduced courtesy of the California Department of Public Health)

Logical feature 4: Negative outcomes and their harm

The person who sustains the harmful effects of an action need not be the recipient of a fear appeal argument. However, it must nonetheless be in the *interests* of the recipient to avoid any harm to this person by carrying out the protective action recommended in the conclusion of a fear appeal argument.

You should now get practice at identifying the logical features of fear appeal argument by attempting Exercise 4.2.

EXERCISE 4.2: Lead poisoning in children

Lead poisoning is a significant public health problem in the United States. A reference level of 5 micrograms per decilitre (μg/dL) is used to identify children with blood lead levels that are much higher than most children's levels. In California, the annual number of children under 6 years of age with blood lead levels ≥ 10 μg/dL is estimated at over 1000 cases. This increases to 10,000 cases when blood lead levels between 4.5 and 9.5 μg/dL are included (Handley et al. 2017). Sources of lead poisoning include paints, toys and toy jewellery, imported candies and traditional home remedies, and some water pipes. Exposure to lead can damage the brain and nervous system, slow growth and development, cause learning and behaviour problems, and lead to hearing and speech impairments.

Health agencies in the US such as the Centers for Disease Control and Prevention undertake a range of activities to raise public awareness about lead poisoning in children. One such activity is the National Lead Poisoning Prevention Week that is held every year. The poster below was used to publicise this event in 2009. It refers to lead-based paints which were banned in 1978. Currently, some 24 million homes in the US contain deteriorated lead-based paint and elevated levels of lead-contaminated house dust (Centers for Disease Control and Prevention 2017). Examine the poster in detail, and then answer the following questions (Fig. 4.7):

Questions

(1) This poster contains the elements of a fear appeal argument, even if they are not arranged as such. Identify (a) the action that leads to a negative consequence or bad outcome, (b) the individuals who are most likely to sustain this negative consequence, and (c) the protective action that must be taken to avoid this consequence.

(2) Are the intended recipients of this fear appeal argument the people who are most likely to sustain damage from lead-based paints? If not, what logical feature of a fear appeal argument ensures that the recipients of the argument are nevertheless motivated to undertake protective actions?

(3) This poster describes 'damage' or harm to the reader's children. This is a significant source of fear arousal for the reader. What other feature of the poster contributes to fear arousal?

(4) This poster differs in a significant way from the posters displayed in Fig. 4.6. What is this significant difference? Which aspect of the logical structure of a fear appeal argument is most likely to be affected by this difference between the posters?

(5) The ambiguity of a particular expression is vital to the message that is conveyed by this poster. Identify the expression in question, and state the ambiguity that it generates.

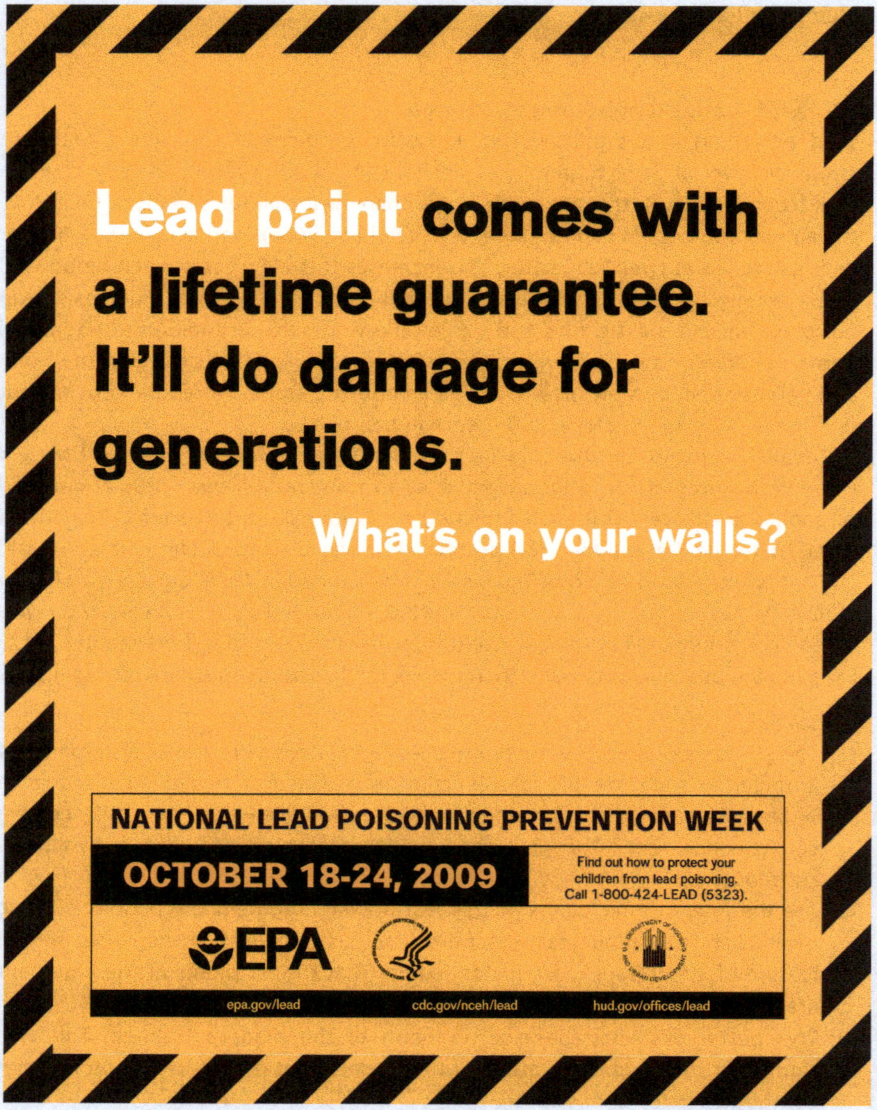

Fig. 4.7 Childhood lead poisoning is a significant public health problem. The National Lead Poisoning Prevention Week in the US attempts to raise awareness of this problem (Reproduced courtesy of the Centers for Disease Control and Prevention)

SPECIAL TOPIC: Children and fear appeal argument

So far, we have characterized adults in the roles of both the proponent and respondent of fear appeal arguments. When we have mentioned children, they have always been viewed as sustaining the negative outcome of an action, which it is then the responsibility of adults, namely their parents, to avoid or rectify. However, there is evidence that children, even pre-teenage children, are adept at constructing fear appeal arguments. This is amply demonstrated by a radon poster contest that is held each year by the New York State Department of Health. The contest is for children aged 9–14 years. The goals are to raise awareness about the harmful effects

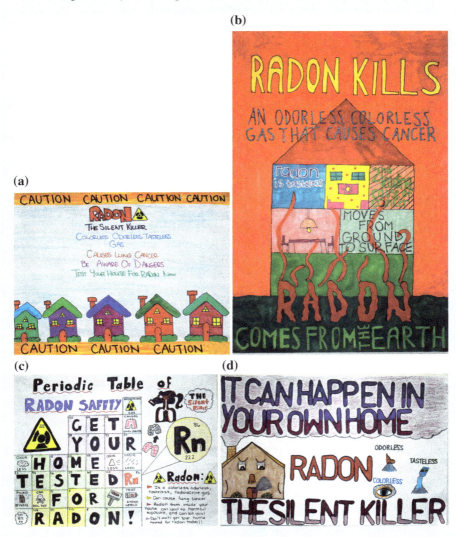

Fig. 4.8 Winning entries in the annual radon poster contest that is held by the New York State Department of Health (Reprinted with permission of the New York State Department of Health)

of elevated levels of indoor radon gas and to increase the number of homes that are tested. The posters in Fig. 4.8 were among the winning entries in recent years.

These posters convey effective fear appeal arguments about the health risks of radon gas. Each poster identifies exposure to radon as the event that leads to a negative and fearful consequence. All the posters tell readers what radon is—a colourless, odourless, tasteless gas that they cannot detect by means of their normal senses of sight, smell, and taste. The negative consequences of exposure are also clearly expressed. All the posters state that radon kills or is a silent killer. With the exception of poster (d), they all state that radon causes lung cancer or is the second leading cause of cancer. Posters (a) and (c) successfully communicate the only protective action that is available to readers—they must get their homes tested for radon gas.

Clearly, the children who designed these posters have a sound appreciation of the key elements in fear appeal arguments. But where they really excel is in their ability to arouse fear in order to achieve the compliance of readers with the recommended protective action of the argument. The threat of death is forcefully conveyed through the use of a gas mask, skull and crossbones, and diseased lungs in poster (c). The international symbol for ionizing radiation is used in posters (a) and (c). This symbol alerts us to danger and harm wherever it is used. It also reflects the fact that radon is an important way in which we are exposed to ionizing radiation. Further fear arousal is achieved in poster (d) with noxious radon fumes bellowing from the chimney and front door of a house. Poster (b) shows radon fumes rising from the earth and permeating a house. The red fumes and vivid red background of the images are evocative of flames from hell. These deathly images complete the fear appeal argument by securing the reader's compliance with the recommended protective action of the argument.

4.4 Evaluating Fear Appeal Argument

Fear appeal arguments are frequently misused and abused. I may realize that my argument is weak and that I have little prospect of rationally persuading you to accept its conclusion. And so I resort to the use of fear to achieve your acceptance of my claim. On another occasion, I may think that my argument is quite strong, but I know that you are resolutely opposed to its conclusion. So an appeal to fear may be made to give me additional leverage in winning you over to my point of view. I may stand to gain financially from your acceptance of the conclusion of a fear appeal argument. For example, I may be selling a product or service that I am claiming is the best or only way of protecting you and your family from the adverse outcome of an action or event (e.g. indoor radon testing). With this personal gain in mind, I may set out to induce in you an overwhelming level of fear that cannot possibly be supported by the available evidence. On still other occasions, I might use fear to distract an opponent from interrogating benefits that might also derive from an action, an action that I have chosen to characterize in wholly negative terms. What these scenarios demonstrate is that deceptive uses of fear in argument certainly abound. It is the task of argument evaluation to establish when fear appeals are used illegitimately and when other instances of these arguments are rationally warranted.

This task is not as straightforward as it may at first seem. This is because logical pitfalls in the use of fear appeal arguments are many and varied, depending on the contexts in which these arguments are advanced. In this section, we identify some of the most common logical flaws in the use of fear appeal arguments. We also consider some of the contexts in which these arguments may be used in a rationally warranted way.

Logical flaws arise in the use of fear appeal argument when the relations expressed within premises, and between the premises and conclusion of the argument, are characterized in terms of deductive certainties rather than probabilities. Consider the first premise in a fear appeal argument:

P1: If you (the respondent) bring about *A*, then *B* will occur.

This premise refers to future events that may or may not occur. I may take considerable risks with my sexual health by not practicing safe sex, and yet I may never contract a sexually transmitted infection (STI). I may drink alcohol to excess for most of my adult life and never develop cirrhosis of my liver. When fear appeal argument is used appropriately, the probabilistic nature of *P1* is made evident. The respondent to whom the argument is directed must know that contracting STIs and developing liver cirrhosis are not deductively certain or inevitable consequences of a failure to practice safe sex and engage in responsible drinking, respectively. When the proponent of a fear appeal argument uses this argument fallaciously, the probabilistic or uncertain nature of the relation between an action and its consequence(s) in *P1* is never made apparent. In fact, the probabilistic nature of this relation is effectively transformed into deductive certainty. A fear appeal argument where actions have inevitable, certain consequences upon which no external factors can intervene to achieve an alteration of outcome is unlikely to work as a tool of rational persuasion. A heavy smoker who believes that his smoking behaviour will at some future point in time result in adverse health effects, each of which is inevitable and certain, will never be persuaded to stop smoking, no matter how aggressively a fear appeal argument is pursued against him. The misrepresentation of probabilistic or uncertain relations between actions and consequences within the premises of fear appeal arguments, and also between the premises and conclusions of these arguments, gives rise to the first logical pitfall in the use of fear appeal argument:

Logical pitfall 1: Relations misrepresented as deductive consequence

Probabilistic relations between actions and future consequences are misrepresented as deductive certainties that are inevitable and immutable. A fear appeal argument that misrepresents probabilistic relations in terms of deductive consequences distorts the probative standards of the practical deliberations in which fear appeal argument operates.

It is not difficult to see how this logical flaw might come about. If you are conducting a public health campaign, and it is your aim to get people to stop smoking, to practice safe sex, and to drink alcohol responsibly, then it serves your purpose to present the adverse health outcomes of these lifestyle choices as certain, inevitable events. You are no doubt motivated in doing so by the belief that people will be more likely to comply with recommended protective actions in the conclusion of a fear appeal argument if they believe that it is certain, and not just likely, that they will experience an adverse health outcome of an action. But this concern to present probable outcomes as certain outcomes creates a paradox for the proponent of fear appeal argument in a public health campaign. This is because for any fear appeal argument to work, the public must believe that they can positively influence the outcome of an action. So, smokers must believe that although they have smoked heavily for years that they can avoid developing lung cancer if they stop smoking now. However, this latter belief is only warranted to the extent that lung cancer is a probable and not an inevitable consequence of smoking. If we construe the relation between smoking and lung cancer in terms of certainties rather than probabilities, the smoker may simply reason that serious illness is a certain outcome of his smoking behaviour and that efforts to influence this outcome in a positive way are entirely futile. There is only one solution to the paradox that the proponent of a deductively inflated fear appeal argument has created. That solution is for the proponent of this argument to represent truly probable events in terms of probabilistic relations and not as deductive consequences.

So, a fear appeal argument may be advanced too forcefully, with the result that probable consequences are misrepresented as deductively certain consequences. Another flaw that arises when there is aggressive use of fear appeal argument against a respondent is that a single negative consequence of an action is allowed to outweigh one or more benefits that might also derive from the action. Clearly, when the action is as harmful an activity as smoking, it is difficult to imagine what those benefits might be—although many smokers would argue that the relaxation and pleasure that they derive from tobacco smoking outweighs even the risk of developing serious smoking-related illnesses. However, if we think about alcohol consumption, most of us are aware that there are cardiovascular protective effects of moderate alcohol consumption (Xi et al. 2017). Cannabis use also appears to have some benefits in that it can deliver effective pain relief to people who do not respond to other pain medications (Haroutounian et al. 2016). When fear appeal argument is forcefully advanced against a respondent, it can seem that negative consequences are the only outcomes that should fall within our purview. However, a fear appeal argument is only properly rationally warranted when the negative outcome of an action outweighs any of the benefits that might derive from an action. In order for this latter assessment to be made, the respondent of a fear appeal argument must be given sufficient argumentative space in which to weigh up negative *and* positive consequences of an action. The premature closure of that space so that only the negative consequences are evaluated is the basis of the second logical pitfall in the use of fear appeal argument:

Logical pitfall 2: Failure to consider positive consequences of action

A proponent can overstate the negative consequences of an action and disregard positive consequences, with the result that the respondent is unduly coerced into accepting the recommended protective action in the conclusion of a fear appeal argument.

To illustrate this logical error, consider the fear appeal argument that gained momentum in the UK following media reports that questioned the safety of the measles, mumps, and rubella (MMR) vaccine. Concerns about the safety of MMR vaccine were first raised by Dr Andrew Wakefield and his colleagues in an article that appeared in *The Lancet* (Wakefield et al. 1998). These investigators examined a consecutive series of 12 children with chronic enterocolitis and pervasive developmental disorder (or autism). It was claimed by Wakefield and his colleagues that the onset of the behavioural symptoms of autism in 8 of the 12 children was associated with the MMR vaccination. At a press conference subsequent to the publication of the article, Dr Wakefield set out the course of action that he believed should be taken:

> For the vast majority of children the MMR vaccine is fine, but I believe there are sufficient anxieties for a case to be made to administer the three vaccinations separately. I do not think that the long-term safety trials of MMR are sufficient for giving the three vaccines together. ('Andrew Wakefield—The Man Behind the MMR Controversy', Rebecca Smith, *The Telegraph*, 29 January 2010).

Parents of children who were due to receive the MMR vaccination read Dr Wakefield's comments about the lack of MMR safety as a recommendation to avoid the combined vaccine. As a result, there was a sharp reduction in the number of parents who consented to the vaccination of their children. This sequence of events has all the hallmarks of a fear appeal argument. An initial action, administration of the MMR vaccination, purportedly resulted in a negative and fearful consequence, namely, the development of autism in children. (It should be emphasized that the purported link between MMR vaccine and autism has now been entirely discredited.) The protective action that Dr Wakefield recommended to avert this negative consequence was the avoidance of the combined MMR vaccination. However, the emphasis that was placed by Wakefield and others on the negative consequence in this case entirely overlooked the significant health benefits that derive from the vaccination of children against these three infectious diseases, each of which can cause death and serious complications. These benefits were to be clearly demonstrated some years later when an unprotected population of 10–16 year-olds, who had missed out on vaccination in the late 1990s and 2000s, contracted measles in significant numbers during outbreaks of the disease in the UK. The increase in measles cases, which totalled 587 cases in the first three months of 2013, prompted Public Health England, NHS England and the Department of Health to announce a national catch-up programme on 25 April 2013. The aim of this programme was to increase MMR vaccination uptake in children and teenagers who had been left susceptible to infection as a result of the crisis in MMR safety that had been prompted by Dr Wakefield (see Fig. 4.9).

The negative consequence in this case, even one as devastating as the development of autism in children, did not outweigh the benefits of MMR vaccination, namely, the protection afforded to children by means of the vaccine to three serious infectious diseases. In the absence of any evaluation of the positive consequences of vaccination, and a failure to balance these consequences against the negative consequence identified by Dr Wakefield and his colleagues, the fear appeal argument at the centre of the MMR crisis was logically flawed.

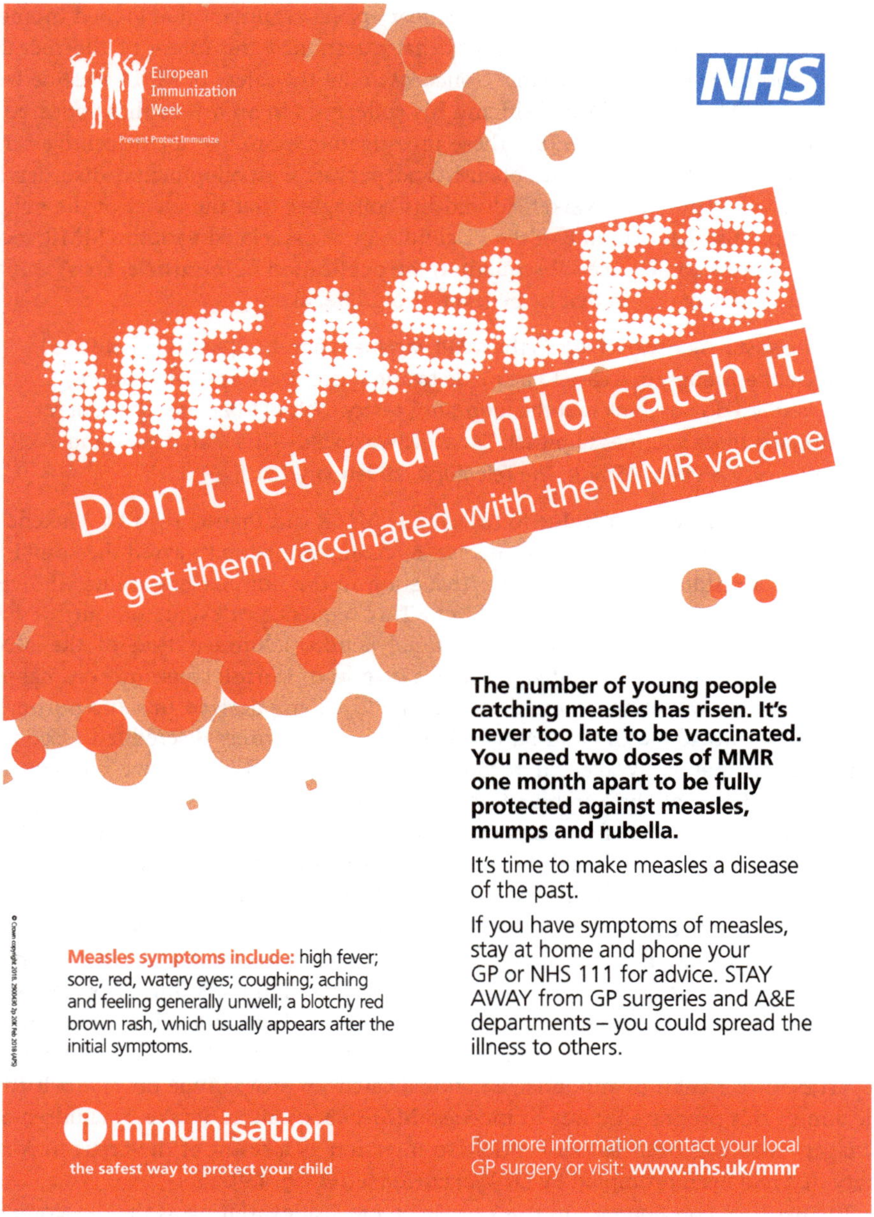

Fig. 4.9 A campaign to encourage uptake of MMR vaccinations in children was launched in 2013 in response to the growing number of measles cases in the UK (Contains public sector information licensed under the Open Government Licence v3.0. ▸ http://www.nationalarchives.gov.uk/doc/open-government-licence/version/3/)

Another common logical error in the use of fear appeal argument is the inclusion of a fear premise which has little or no evidential support. In ▶ Sect. 4.3, the fear premise was represented as follows:

P3: *B* arouses considerable fear in you (the respondent).

In ▶ Sect. 4.3, it was argued that a negative consequence, denoted by *B*, is not necessarily a fearful consequence and that only certain negative consequences can arouse fear in the respondent of an argument. Even a particularly negative consequence need not arouse fear if certain other conditions do not hold. A health campaign may emphasize serious illness and premature death as a means of encouraging people to stop smoking. Yet, even the contemplation of severe disease and loss of years of life may arouse no fear in the smokers who are the target of this campaign if family relationships are fractured, rewarding activities do not exist, and purposeful life goals are absent. In order for a negative consequence to arouse fear, there must be some evidence that it threatens relationships, livelihoods and assets, and people in whom the recipient of a fear appeal argument places some value. If the latter cannot be established, then a consequence may be very negative indeed without arousing fear. In such a case, *P3* would be weakly warranted, if warranted at all. Alternatively, the proponent of a fear appeal argument may aggressively advance a fear premise, but the fear arousal contained in the premise is excessive to the rather limited evidence that can be advanced in support of it. These considerations lead to the third logical pitfall in the use of fear appeal argument:

Logical pitfall 3: A fear premise lacks evidential support

The proponent of a fear appeal argument advances a fear premise that cannot be supported by the available evidence. The proponent may falsely assume that a negative consequence *is* a fearful consequence and offer no independent grounds for the fear premise. Alternatively, the fear premise may be advanced too forcefully given the rather limited grounds that can be advanced in its support.

To illustrate this logical error, let us consider the standard way in which anti-smoking health campaigns are conducted. All these campaigns effectively state the negative consequences of smoking. These consequences may take the form of the number of premature deaths that are related to smoking (see [a] in Fig. 4.10), or the adverse health outcomes of smoking such as the increased risk of developing a range of cancers (see Fig. 4.1). However, one of the reasons why some anti-smoking campaigns may not be particularly effective in reducing rates of smoking[1] is that although they clearly state the negative consequences of smoking, they do not give people *reasons* to fear those consequences. One such reason may be the loss of the opportunity to fulfil a parenting role to a young child (see [b] in Fig. 4.10). If we begin to conceive of a fear appeal argument as an argument with a fear premise, rather than as an argument from negative consequence which may be influenced by fear, then we come to realize that we must advance grounds or reasons for fear in exactly the same way that we must advance grounds or reasons for the other premises in the argument. If grounds cannot

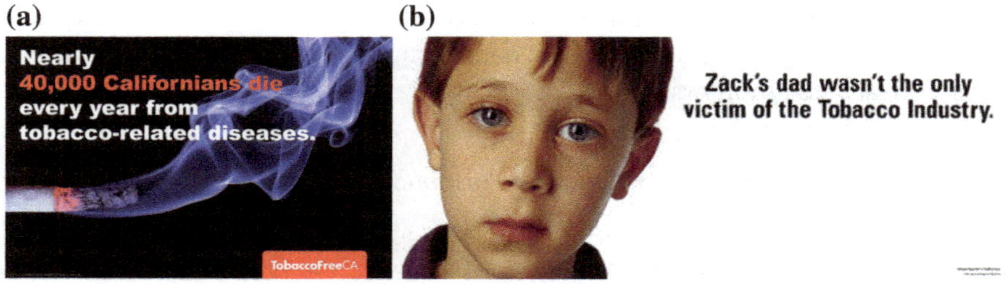

Fig. 4.10 Fear appeal arguments in anti-smoking campaigns should go beyond stating a negative consequence (**a**) to giving reasons for fearing that consequence (**b**) (Reproduced courtesy of the California Department of Public Health)

be advanced in support of a fear premise because they do not exist, or if such evidence as does exist cannot support the weight of the fear premise, then a fear appeal argument contains a logical weakness and the argument is used fallaciously. But if plausible grounds can be brought forward in support of a fear premise, the fear in a fear appeal argument may be as rationally warranted as any other premise.

The final logical flaw that can occur in the use of fear appeal argument concerns the recommended protective action in the conclusion of the argument. If this action is executed in full by the respondent of the argument, it must be possible to avert the negative consequence of an action and the fear that this consequence generates. However, a respondent can only comply with a recommended protective action if the action is expressed in a comprehensible way, and if the respondent has the cognitive, technical, and other skills that are necessary to bring about its implementation. Although these requirements appear straightforward, they are not always present in fear appeal arguments. For example, a fear appeal argument that urges parents to vaccinate their children against infectious disease is counter-productive if parents cannot afford to pay for vaccination or if the only health facility in an area that offers vaccination is some 50 miles away. In this case, financial difficulties and transport problems mean that compliance with the recommended protective action is either not possible or is difficult to achieve, and the respondent is left in a state of fear that cannot be dissipated through action. On other occasions, compliance may not be possible because a recommended protective action requires physical abilities and a commitment of time that are not available to most adults. Fear-based health warnings about coronary heart disease that recommend an hour of intense cardiovascular exercise each day are likely to result in low levels of compliance. In this case, the protective action involves conditions that are not readily satisfied, even by adults who possess high levels of motivation to comply with them.

Logical pitfall 4: Compliance with the recommended protective action

The proponent of a fear appeal argument falsely assumes that the respondent possesses certain abilities and resources. In the absence of these skills and resources, the recommended protective action in the conclusion of the argument cannot be implemented.

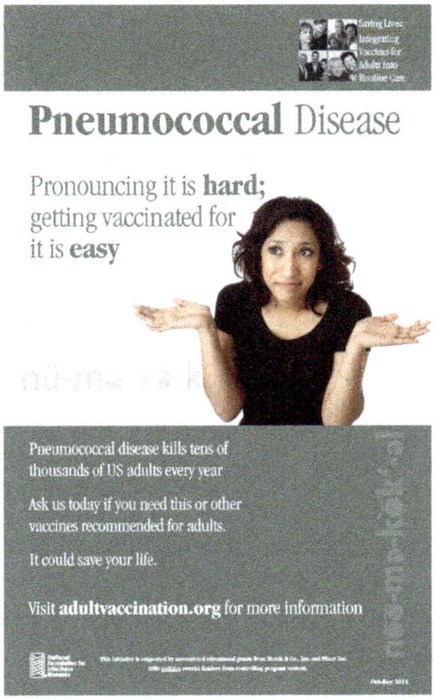
Pneumococcal Disease
Pronouncing it is hard; getting vaccinated for it is easy
Pneumococcal disease kills tens of thousands of US adults every year
Ask us today if you need this or other vaccines recommended for adults.
It could save your life.
Visit adultvaccination.org for more information
October 2014

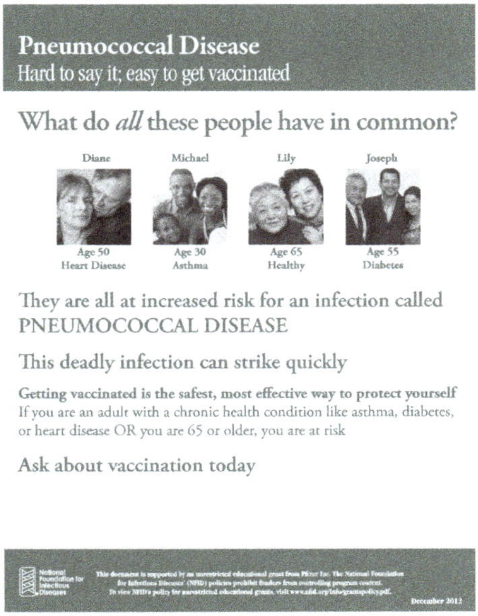

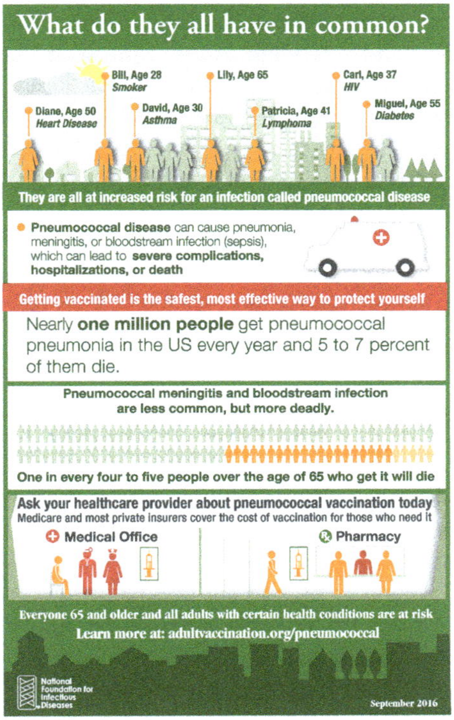

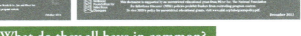

Fig. 4.11 Posters and an infographic promoting vaccination against pneumococcal disease among high-risk adults in the United States (Reproduced courtesy of the National Foundation for Infectious Diseases, ▶ www.nfid.org)

Health campaigns that achieve high levels of compliance recommend protective actions that can be reasonably implemented by respondents. People who are aged 65 years or older or who have chronic health conditions such as asthma and diabetes are at increased risk of developing pneumococcal infection. Pneumococcal infection is caused by the bacterium *Streptococcus pneumonia* (pneumococcus). This bacterium can cause a wide range of diseases, including middle ear infection (acute otitis media) and chest infection (pneumonia). Invasive pneumococcal diseases such as infection of the brain membranes (meningitis) and bloodstream (bacteraemia and sepsis) can be serious or even life-threatening. In the United States, adults aged 65 years or older or who have one or more chronic health conditions are urged to get vaccinated. Two posters for public display and an infographic that are produced by the National Foundation for Infectious Diseases and that advise adults at high risk to get vaccinated are shown in ◘ Fig. 4.11.

A distinctive feature of this campaign material is the emphasis that is placed on the *ease* with which the recommended protective action, namely vaccination, can be taken. The slogan of the campaign—pneumococcal disease is HARD to say, but it is EASY to get vaccinated—makes clear to high risk adults that there are no barriers to complying with vaccination. The accompanying infographic goes a step further in letting these adults know where they can be vaccinated (at medical offices and pharmacies), and that the cost of vaccination is covered by Medicare, the federal health insurance program in the US, and most private insurers. High risk adults from all socioeconomic groups thus have equal access to vaccination. The combination of these factors ensures that poor patient compliance with the recommended protective action (namely, vaccination) does not limit the effectiveness of this important public health campaign.

You should now get practice at identifying logical pitfalls in the use of fear appeal argument by attempting Exercise 4.3.

EXERCISE 4.3: Antibiotic resistance

A growing number of bacteria, viruses, parasites, and fungi are becoming resistant to the drugs that are used to control them. The World Health Organization (WHO) estimates that in 2016, 490,000 people developed multi-drug resistant tuberculosis globally. Drug resistance is also starting to complicate the fight against HIV and malaria. This has prompted WHO and public health agencies worldwide to launch campaigns warning about the diminishing effectiveness of many of the drugs that are used to treat infectious diseases. The misuse of antibiotics is a particular problem, with patients often seeking these drugs from doctors for the treatment of minor ailments such as colds. This has resulted in antibiotic resistance for many bacterial infections that were once effectively treated with antibiotics.

The following posters are produced by the Public Health Agency of Canada. Posters (a) and (b) warn readers about the dangers posed by antibiotic resistance. Poster (c) informs readers that antibiotics should not be used to treat illnesses such as colds and flu. The poster in (b) is targeted at First Nations and Inuit, two groups of peoples who are the traditional inhabitants of Canada. Examine the posters in detail, and then answer the questions below (◘ Fig. 4.12):

(a) © All rights reserved. *When you really need them, will antibiotics work?* Public Health Agency of Canada. Adapted and reproduced with permission from the Minister of Health, 2018.

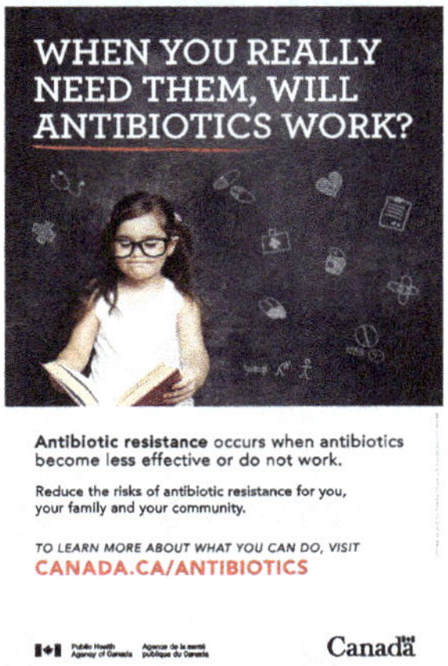

(b) © All rights reserved. *When you really need them, will antibiotics work? – for First Nations and Inuit.* Health Canada. Adapted and reproduced with permission from the Minister of Health, 2018.

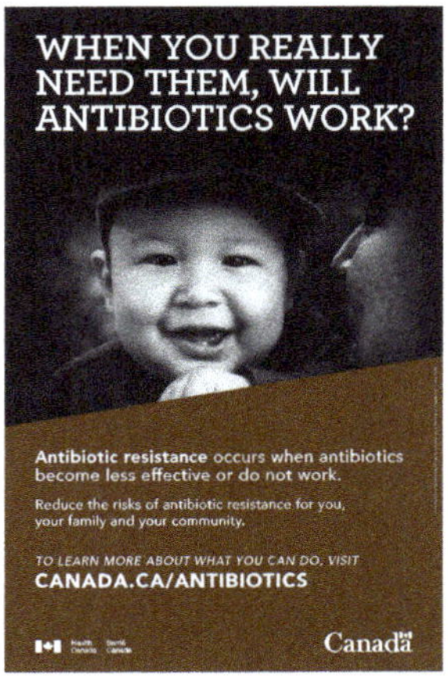

(c) © All rights reserved. *Use Antibiotics Wisely: Not All Bugs Need Drugs.* Public Health Agency of Canada. Adapted and reproduced with permission from the Minister of Health, 2018.

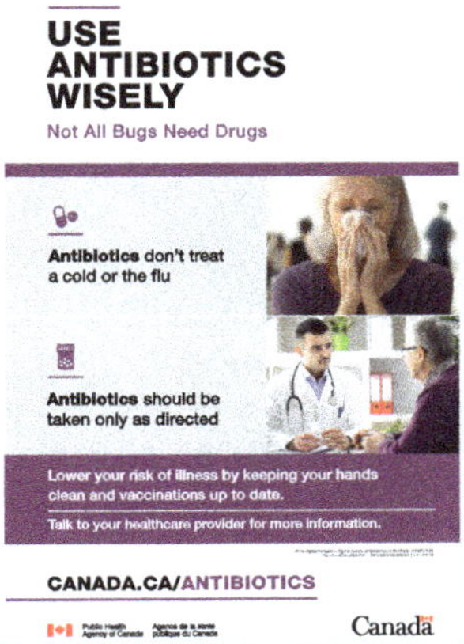

Fig. 4.12 Public health campaigns are addressing the global health threat posed by antibiotic resistance

Questions:

(1) The elements of a fear appeal argument can be found across all three posters, but not in any single poster. Those elements are an *initial action* that leads to a particularly *negative consequence*. This consequence *arouses fear* that is only diminished by carrying out a recommended *protective action*. Identify each of these elements in the fear appeal argument that is generated by the above posters.

(2) What elements in a fear appeal argument are conveyed through posters (a) and (b) but not through poster (c)?

(3) What elements in a fear appeal argument are conveyed through poster (c) but not through posters (a) and (b)?

(4) How likely do you think it is that the fear aroused by posters (a) and (b) will lead to the type of behaviour modification needed to address antibiotic resistance? Provide a justification of your response.

(5) How would you rationally evaluate the campaign adopted by the Public Health Agency of Canada to warn people about antibiotic resistance?

SPECIAL TOPIC: Fear appeal, threat appeal, and *ad baculum* argument

Douglas Walton (2000) describes the logical journey that has been taken by fear appeal argument to the present day. What we now regard as fear appeal argument started out as *argumentum ad baculum* (literally, "argument to the stick"). Until the late 1940s, *ad baculum* was consistently defined as an appeal to force. At that point in time, the notion of threat began to be used alongside force (Walton 2000: 34). In 1956, *ad baculum* came to be defined for the first time as an appeal to fear in argument, as opposed to an appeal to force (Walton 2000: 38).

Historical transitions in the definition of *ad baculum* would have little more than etymological significance were it not for the fact that terminological changes can represent different conceptions of argument. The terms *ad baculum*, *fear appeal* and *threat appeal* are widely used today in logic and beyond. While social scientists tend to use *threat appeal* and *fear appeal* synonymously, logicians recognize a conceptual distinction between these forms of argument. The negative consequence *B* in a fear appeal argument occurs without any agency by the proponent of the argument. However, in a threat appeal argument an agent, the proponent, gives an explicit commitment to bring about the negative consequence of an action *A*. As Walton (2000) remarks, in a fear appeal argument "whether B comes about is up to nature – or at least there is no stipulation that any persistent agent stands ready to see to it personally that B will occur" (p. 141). The logical form of fear appeal argument displayed in ▶ Sect. 4.3 contained the following conditional premise: If you (the respondent) bring about *A*, then *B* will occur. Some embellishment of this premise is required if it is to convey that an agent undertakes a commitment to carry out *B*. The first premise in what Walton (2000: 140) calls a conditional baculum threat argument is just such a premise:

I (the proponent) undertake to see to it that B will occur if you (the respondent) bring about A.
B is a very bad outcome, from your (the respondent's) point of view (or interests).
Therefore, you (the respondent) should not bring about A.

Walton's conditional baculum threat argument may appear to have limited relevance to health. After all, the adverse consequences of actions in the health arguments we are examining imply no agency on the part of the proponents of these arguments. If I develop serious complications from influenza or suffer respiratory depression from taking a prescription opioid, there is no sense in which the proponent of an argument that is warning me of these consequences has acted to bring them about. However, there is a type of argument that is increasingly used in healthcare that does have the structure of Walton's conditional baculum threat argument. As funding for healthcare comes under growing pressure, elective surgery and other forms of treatment are increasingly being rationed. In an article in *The Guardian* on 3 September 2016, Kevin Rawlinson and Chris Johnston reported on the decision of the Vale of York clinical commissioning group to postpone elective surgery in certain groups of patients. The patients were adult smokers and people with a body mass index (BMI) of 30 or more:

» The Vale of York group said: "The local system is under severe pressure. This work will help to ensure that we get the very best value from the National Health Service (NHS) and not exceed our resources or risk the ability of the NHS being there when people really need it."
Policy documents produced by bosses in the North Yorkshire authority make clear that adult smokers will have elective surgery postponed "for six months or until they've stopped smoking for eight weeks".
And, for people whose BMI is 30 or more – who are defined as obese – such treatment will be put back a year "or until 10% of weight loss is achieved, whichever is the sooner." ('Decision to deny surgery to obese patients is like "racial discrimination"', *The Guardian*, 3 September 2016)

The Vale of York clinical commissioning group is clearly signalling its intention to deny elective surgery (the negative consequence) to patients who do not stop smoking and who fail to lose weight. The intention to put a negative consequence into effect is what characterizes the actions of the clinical commissioning group as an appeal to threat in argument, and distinguishes the actions of this group from the type of fear appeals we have examined elsewhere in this chapter.

4.5 Fear Appeal in the Social Sciences

Of all the informal fallacies, fear appeal argument is in the rather unique position of being the focus of extensive empirical investigation. Health psychologists, public health scientists, politicians, and practitioners in marketing and advertising all have a professional interest in fear appeal argument. Through this interest these individuals share a common aim—to understand how fear appeal may be used to best effect in health campaigning, political rhetoric, commercials, and other forms of public discourse. To achieve this aim, investigators need to establish the features of fear appeal argument that are effective in persuading an audience to comply with a recommended protective action—equally, the features that are *not* effective. Features such as **emotionality**, thematic content, and **message frame**, for example, are known to play a significant role in audience persuasion. Investigators must also have a sound understanding of the cognitive and affective processes by means of which appeals to fear are interpreted and are acted upon, assessed and rejected, or quite simply ignored. In health and medical matters, the study of both these main dimensions of fear appeal argument has resulted in a burgeoning literature. A comprehensive discussion of this literature is beyond the scope of the present chapter—readers are referred to Ruiter et al. (2014) for an excellent overview. What can be achieved in this section is an examination of some of the main factors that are known to influence the processing of fear appeals and that can affect audience compliance with these arguments. We begin with two key concepts, self-efficacy and response efficacy, that have been discussed extensively in relation to fear appeal.

In ► Sect. 4.4, it was described how the proponent of a fear appeal argument might falsely assume that the recipient of the argument has the abilities and resources to carry out the recommended protective actions. A public health campaign that recommends adults to engage in cardiovascular exercise for two hours a day in communities with no sports facilities is unlikely to be greeted with high levels of compliance for the simple reason that people do not believe they can undertake this recommended action. What was characterized as a logical pitfall in the use of fear appeal argument is referred to as **self-efficacy** in the social scientific literature. This is how self-efficacy is typically defined:

> Self-efficacy refers to the individual's capacity to produce desired effects. Correspondingly, self-efficacy beliefs are the beliefs about what means lead to what goals and about possessing the personal capacity to use these means. (Flammer 2001: 13812)

There is extensive evidence that people are more likely to comply with protective health actions when they perceive that their 'personal capacity' to comply with those actions is high. Studies have shown that participation in Pap smear screening, breast cancer screening, and screening for colorectal cancer is greatest in individuls with high self-efficacy (Fernández et al. 2009; Melvin et al. 2016; Orbell et al. 2017). Huang et al. (2018) reported that medication self-efficacy is positively associated with diabetes medication adherence in subjects aged 20 years and above and diagnosed with type 2 diabetes. Medication self-efficacy was expressed as subjects' level of confidence about taking medications correctly under a number of different circumstances.

Even significant fear arousal in a fear appeal argument may produce minimal compliance with protective actions if the recipient of the argument exhibits low self-efficacy. Guignard et al. (2018: 1) state that smokers exposed to fear appeals "may resist the message by minimising the threat, denying the risk, rejecting the problem, or avoiding the message, particularly when they feel unable to stop smoking (low self-efficacy) or when they do not feel concerned by the risk (low perceived susceptibility)".

Guignard et al. studied 3000 smokers before, immediately after, and at 6 months after a French national highly emotional anti-smoking campaign. The campaign consisted of two TV ads (two 30-second videos) and radio messages (two 30-second messages). In a voice-over, a woman is heard saying goodbye to her two daughters, and a man to his wife. A video accompanying the voice-over showed hospital employees cleaning the room where the smoker had just died. It was found that campaign recall at 6 months was not significantly associated with a change in self-efficacy in smokers with low self-efficacy at the start of the study. These smokers had higher levels of dependency on smoking than the rest of the study population, leading Guignard et al. to conclude that "referral to a cessation help programme at the end of the ads might not have been strong enough to persuade low self-efficacy and highly addicted smokers of their ability to quit."

Response efficacy is another key concept in the social scientific literature on fear appeal argument. While self-efficacy describes individuals' perception of their ability or capacity to carry out a recommended action, response efficacy describes their perception of the likely effectiveness of the recommended action in averting a threat. Witte et al. (2001) state that "[i]f individuals perceive a recommended response to be effective in averting, stopping, diminishing, or avoiding a threat, then they are said to have high-response efficacy" (p. 21). Response efficacy has been examined across a range of health issues in different study populations. Choi et al. (2013) examined efficacy in the context of adolescent substance use in 2129 seventh-grade students in 39 rural Pennsylvania and Ohio schools in the fall of 2009. In this context, response efficacy was defined as refusal response efficacy. Refusal response efficacy was measured by means of four items: that simply saying no, offering an explanation, avoiding the situation, and leaving would be effective ways to resist alcohol and other drug use. These investigators found that refusal response efficacy was negatively related to alcohol and marijuana use—high refusal response efficacy was associated with low alcohol and marijuana use. Refusal response efficacy was also found to moderate the relationship between alcohol-resistance self-efficacy and alcohol use, and between marijuana-resistance self-efficacy and marijuana use.

A fear appeal argument may arouse considerable fear in an audience. But it is only when recommended actions are perceived to be successful in addressing a threat that a fear appeal argument can be an effective tool of persuasion. Roskos-Ewoldsen et al. (2004) examined the role of efficacy on attitude accessibility in fear appeal messages concerning breast cancer. A composite measure of efficacy was obtained by averaging responses to four scales used to measure response efficacy and four scales used to measure self-efficacy. One of the scales used to measure response efficacy asked subjects to rate their agreement with the statement "If I examine my breasts regularly myself, my chances of detecting cancer are extremely high". It was found that fear appeal messages that advocated the efficacy of breast self-examinations increased the accessibility of attitudes towards the adaptive behaviour which in turn predicted behavioural intentions to perform breast self-examinations. Carcioppolo et al. (2013) reported that response efficacy significantly mediated the relationship between message framing and prevention intentions in women who were exposed to prevention messages about human papilloma virus, the virus known to cause cervical cancer. Factors that influence response efficacy in fear appeal arguments have also been examined. For example, response efficacy has been found to increase significantly following repeated exposure to a fear appeal message about preventing melanoma (Shi and Smith 2016). In a study of fear appeals in HIV-prevention messages to young people in Tanzania, Bastien (2011) found that information-based posters were rated high in inducing response efficacy.

Other aspects of fear appeal arguments have also been investigated. When individuals with low efficacy perceive a significant threat in fear appeals, they may use a range of avoidance strategies to help them cope with the threat (a process called fear control). Carcioppolo et al. (2018) found that joking about colorectal cancer was a significant avoidance strategy in 209 older adults who were recruited from eight different worksites. Men were more likely to joke about colorectal cancer than women, particularly if they had low self-efficacy and perceived a significant threat. This study shows that fear appeals may be ineffective or even counter-productive in certain circumstances, a finding that is confirmed by Lee (2018) who examined the responses of college students to anti-alcohol abuse media messages. These messages were designed to appeal to either fear or humour. College binge drinkers who watched fear appeals reported that they were less likely to change their drinking behaviour than those who watched humour appeals. The opposite pattern was reported in college non-binge drinkers. The authors concluded that use of conventional fear appeal to scare college binge drinkers into changing their drinking behaviour may be an ineffective strategy. Demographic characteristics of the audience do not appear to influence how fear appeals are processed (Witte and Allen 2000). Rhodes and Wolitski (1990) reported that age, gender, ethnicity, and group membership did not, in general, influence rated effectiveness of fear appeals in AIDS education posters. There is evidence that the cultural orientation of respondents (namely, individualist versus collectivist orientation) is a significant factor in the processing of fear appeals (Murray-Johnson et al. 2001).

DISCUSSION POINT: Fear appeal in the social sciences

In the Introduction to his book *Scare Tactics*, Walton (2000) makes the following remarks:

> [G]overnments now use fear appeal ads on a wide scale, to try to get teenagers to stop smoking, to try and discourage drinking and driving, to warn of the dangers of AIDS, and for other purposes of promoting public health and safety […] Experimental findings are mixed, but the perception at present is that fear appeal ads can be successfully used to change behaviour and attitudes of the groups to whom they have been specially addressed. (p. xiv)

In discussion with other students, you should address the following question: To what extent are Walton's comments supported by recent social scientific research into fear appeal argument?

4.6 Fear Appeal Argument as a Cognitive Heuristic

Throughout this book, we have taken the view that the so-called informal fallacies are not so fallacious after all when viewed against the contexts in which these arguments are used. Fear appeal argument is no exception in this regard. This argument was shown to be rationally warranted when the proponent of the argument was able to bring forward grounds in support of the fear premise, *P3*. The question that we want to conclude this chapter by asking is whether rationally warranted fear appeal arguments, or some subset thereof, might not assume a heuristic function in our reasoning, similar to that already seen in the argument from ignorance and slippery slope argument. As a heuristic, fear appeal argument might be expected to confer certain efficiencies on reasoning in terms of increased processing speed and reduced cognitive effort over more systematic processes of reasoning. These gains, however, must not be achieved at the expense of the accuracy of the decisions and judgements that are licenced by means of fear appeal argument, such as the decision to pursue a recommended action as a means of averting a negative and fearful consequence.

As we begin to explore what a fear heuristic might look like and whether it can achieve these cognitive efficiencies, we might start by asking what form the arguments in this chapter would have had to take if we could not have appealed to fear to persuade the audience to comply with the recommended action in each case. Let us take as our example the use of fear appeal argument in the *Rx Awareness* campaign of the Centers for Disease Control and Prevention in the US. This campaign makes effective use of testimonials and other publicity materials to make people aware of the ease and speed with which someone can become dependent on prescription opioids. It also emphasizes the devastating consequences of these drugs in terms of deaths caused by accidental overdoses. The slogan of the campaign, “It only takes a little to lose a lot”, leaves little doubt that life itself is placed at risk from these prescribed medications. This is how one woman, Ann Marie, describes the loss of her 22-year-old son from a prescription opioid overdose:

> » My son, Christopher Perrotto, was 20 years old when he was prescribed opioids. It took him five days to get addicted. I'm not supposed to be the one to go get his suit and tie and pick which sneakers that I'm going to bury him in.

This powerful testimonial must surely strike terror into the heart of every person who hears it. The fear arousal generated by this brief statement must be particularly intense for parents whose children are the same age as Ann Marie's son. But let us imagine for a moment that the CDC opted for a different campaign strategy to warn people about the dangers of prescription opioids. This alternative strategy avoids the use of fear to achieve persuasion, and instead embarks on a systematic process of reasoning to caution people about the use of these drugs. Such a campaign may present extensive evidence of the risks associated with prescription opioid use. These risks may be characterized in terms of probabilities. For example, a campaign may include information such as the probability that someone will experience respiratory depression and death from taking a prescription opioid. Populations at particular risk of these adverse events may also be identified. This might include people who consume alcohol while taking prescription opioids, and older adults who have multiple prescriptions and chronic diseases, and are at an increased risk of drug-drug and drug-disease interactions. The increased risk to each of these populations may also be presented in terms of probabilities in our alternative campaign strategy. Aside from information about the risks associated with prescription opioid use, the alternative campaign strategy may also present evidence about the nature and impact of opioid dependency on those who become addicted to these drugs. This might include the damaging effect of these drugs on behaviour and decision-making in the workplace and home environment, and the detrimental consequences of dependency for familial and social relationships.

What we have outlined here is a prescription opioid campaign strategy based on **systematic reasoning**. In this campaign, extensive evidence and information are provided, much of it expressed in terms of probabilities. But what this campaign gains in terms of the quantity and quality of evidence that it provides, it loses in increased processing times and expenditure of cognitive effort. This is because we must use considerable cognitive resources in order to attend to and decode the evidence that is provided in this alternative campaign strategy, and to assess its implications for any recommended protective actions. Each of these resource-intensive cognitive activities takes time to complete. Accordingly, this alternative campaign strategy based on systematic reasoning results in slower processing speed relative to the CDC's campaign strategy based on fear appeal argument. Also, as discussed in Cummings (2012), evidence from the landmark experiments of Amos Tversky and Daniel Kahneman in the 1970s to the present day, indicates that people make a number of systematic errors when they engage in probabilistic reasoning. One such error is known as the gambler's fallacy, the belief that random processes self-correct: "if [a random] sequence has strayed from the population proportion, a corrective bias in the other direction is expected" (Tversky and Kahneman 2004: 193). Added to these errors in probabilistic reasoning are a number of other cognitive biases in our thinking such as the optimistic bias. This is the belief that an individual's risk from a certain agent or behaviour is less than that of the rest of the population (Weinstein 1980, 1984). Applied to prescription opioids, the optimistic bias may lead a person to believe that they are at less risk of accidental overdose than other people who also take these drugs.

So our alternative campaign strategy based on systematic reasoning is not without considerable problems. It makes significant cognitive demands of its audience, demands that are likely to exceed the cognitive capacities of many of those whom it is intended to persuade to modify their behaviour. The strategy also increases the likelihood that errors related to probabilistic reasoning will arise as well as cognitive biases such as the optimistic bias. In none of these scenarios is the critical safety message about prescription opioids likely to be successfully communicated to its intended audience. Another approach is clearly needed. That approach can be found in the use of a fear-based campaign strategy. Fear appeal argument effectively circumvents the need to engage in protracted systematic reasoning of the type that requires us to assess probabilistic information and that increases the opportunity for error and bias to arise. Fear appeal is a mental shortcut that serves us well in our practical deliberations even if, like any other cognitive procedure, it can sometimes lead us into error. A fear appeal heuristic takes us in a single leap from a fearful scenario to the action or actions that will diminish our fear. No extended deliberation is required during which evidence is weighed up, and different courses of action are considered. The simplicity of fear appeal's operation is what confers considerable cognitive gains on this heuristic, and reduces the opportunity for error and bias to afflict reasoning. In pressing fear into action in its *Rx Awareness* campaign, the CDC was encouraging maximally effective **heuristic reasoning** or processing of its opioid safety message, and avoiding the many logical challenges posed by systematic reasoning.

Note

1. The adult smoking prevalence has undoubtedly decreased in many countries. In the United States, for example, it has decreased from 42% in 1965 to 15% in 2015 (Drope et al. 2018). However, this decrease in smoking prevalence is not fully attributable to anti-smoking campaigns, only some of which are effective (Pechmann and Reibling 2000; Davis et al. 2018).

Chapter Summary

Key points

- Fear appeal argument is the use of fear to achieve audience acceptance of a conclusion in argument. Throughout the long history of logic, the appeal to any type of emotion in argument has generally been characterized as a fallacy. This is also true of the emotion of fear. However, there are many contexts in which an appeal to fear in argument is rationally warranted. These contexts include medicine and health.
- Fear appeal argument is a special type of argument from negative consequence. A proponent argues that an action *A* leads to a negative consequence *C* that arouses fear. However, *C* can be averted if the respondent undertakes a recommended protective action.
- It was argued in this chapter that in a fear appeal argument, the basic logical structure of an argument from negative consequence needs to be supplemented by the inclusion of a fear premise (*P3*). This premise explicitly states that *C* arouses fear in the respondent. This premise is necessary because a negative consequence, even a particularly serious negative consequence, need not arouse fear in a respondent.
- There are many logical pitfalls that can occur in the use of fear appeal argument. The proponent of the argument may misrepresent the consequence of the initial action as a deductive consequence when its standing is probabilistic in nature. Someone can smoke heavily for many years, for example, and *not* develop lung cancer. The proponent may also recommend protective actions that cannot avert the initial action and its consequence.
- Fear appeal argument is also studied in the social sciences. Concepts such as self-efficacy (a person's belief that he or she can carry out the recommended action) and response efficacy (a person's belief that the recommended action will be successful in averting a negative and fearful consequence) have been found to influence the effectiveness of fear appeal argument in a range of experimental populations.
- At least some rationally warranted uses of fear appeal argument can function as cognitive heuristics. A fear appeal heuristic is a quick and effective mental shortcut through systematic reasoning which is costly in cognitive terms and can be a source of logical errors and biases. Many effective health campaigns encourage heuristic processing of their critical safety messages to the public.

Suggestions for Further Reading

(1) Walton, D. (2000). *Scare Tactics: Arguments That Appeal to Fear and Threats.* Dordrecht, The Netherlands.

This is the only book-length treatment of fear appeal argument in informal logic. In seven chapters, Walton examines the logical structure of the argument, the relationship of fear to threat appeals, the evaluation of fear appeals, and the contribution of social science to an understanding of the argument. There are many everyday cases of fear appeal argument examined, including some that relate to health (e.g. anti-smoking ads).

(2) Tannenbaum, M. B., Zimmerman, R. S., Hepler, J., Saul, L., Jacobs, S., Wilson, K., & Albarracín, D. (2015). Appealing to Fear: A Meta-Analysis of Fear Appeal Effectiveness and Theories. *Psychological Bulletin, 141*(6), 1178–1204.

The aim of these authors was to compile the largest available meta-analytic database of empirical fear appeal research. A total of 127 articles yielding 248 independent samples from diverse populations were reviewed. The authors found that fear appeals are effective at positively influencing attitude, intentions, and behaviour, and that there are no identified circumstances under which they backfire or lead to undesirable outcomes.

(3) Kok, G. (ed.). (2014). The Effectiveness of Fear Appeals in Health Promotion. *International Journal of Psychology, 49*(2), 61–139.

This Special Section in an issue of the *International Journal of Psychology* contains five papers that address the use of fear appeals in health promotion. These papers discuss issues other than the logic of the argument, including the ethics of using distressing health promotion advertising, and neuroscientific evidence for defensive avoidance of fear appeals.

Questions

(1) For most people, flu is an infectious disease that causes unpleasant symptoms but is usually self-limiting after a few days. However, for some people serious complications can arise. These complications include pneumonia, myocarditis (inflammation of the heart), encephalitis (inflammation of the brain), and sepsis. Each of these conditions requires hospitalization of the patient and can result in death. For people with pre-existing conditions such as HIV, asthma and diabetes, the risk of developing serious complications is increased. The Centers for Disease Control and Prevention (CDC) in the US attempts to protect these high risk groups through targeted health campaigns. The poster in ◘ Fig. 4.13 warns individuals with asthma about their risk of developing serious complications of flu. Examine this poster in detail, and think about its content. Then answer the questions below.

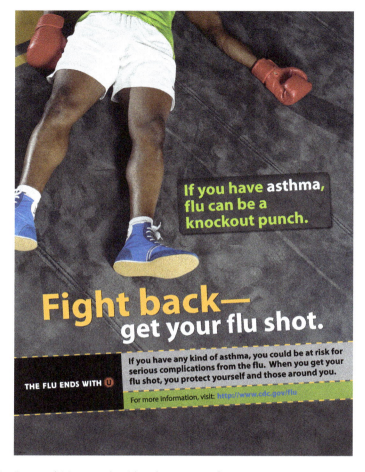

Fig. 4.13 Poster advising people with asthma to get a flu vaccination (Reproduced courtesy of the Centers for Disease Control and Prevention in the United States)

Questions

(a) This poster is intended to convey a fear appeal argument to people with asthma. Reconstruct the premises and conclusion of this argument.
(b) In most fear appeal arguments that we have encountered in this chapter, the initial action is an activity that is under the volitional control of an agent. So, an individual may use a prescribed or illegal drug, or engage in an activity like smoking. Does the initial action in this case differ from these earlier examples?
(c) What role is the boxer and boxing in general playing in this health message from the CDC?
(d) What is the logical function of the feature that you have identified in your response to (b)?

(e) Social scientists have found that fear appeal arguments are most effective when the actions that can prevent an undesirable consequence from arising display *self-efficacy* and *response efficacy*. Explain what these concepts mean. Does the proposed protective action in this fear appeal argument display self-efficacy and response efficacy?

(2) The ingestion of mercury and related compounds through fish consumption is a significant public health problem in many parts of the world. There is evidence that pregnant women, nursing mothers, and young children are at particular risk from the adverse health effects of exposure to mercury. Zhang et al. (2018) reported that a mother's consumption of aquatic products (at 6 ounces a day) from offshore farms in China is associated with a loss of 0.38 IQ points in their newborns. These 'at risk' groups are at the forefront of public health efforts to raise awareness about safe fish consumption. The following poster, which is also available in Chinese and Spanish, is used by public health authorities in California to warn about elevated mercury levels in certain types of fish. Examine the poster in Fig. 4.14 carefully, and then answer the following questions:

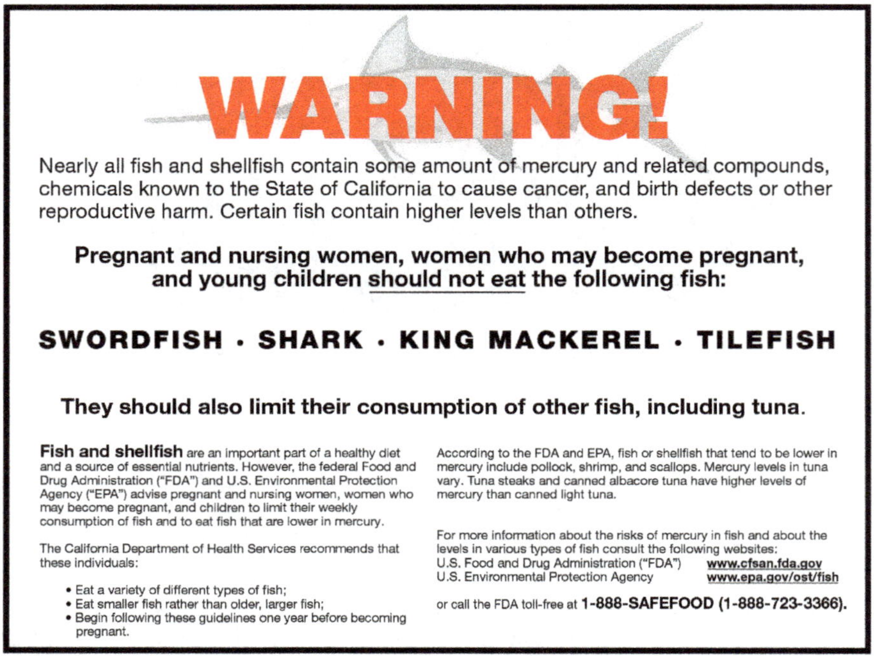
WARNING!
Nearly all fish and shellfish contain some amount of mercury and related compounds, chemicals known to the State of California to cause cancer, and birth defects or other reproductive harm. Certain fish contain higher levels than others.
Pregnant and nursing women, women who may become pregnant, and young children should not eat the following fish:
SWORDFISH · SHARK · KING MACKEREL · TILEFISH
They should also limit their consumption of other fish, including tuna.
Fish and shellfish are an important part of a healthy diet and a source of essential nutrients. However, the federal Food and Drug Administration ("FDA") and U.S. Environmental Protection Agency ("EPA") advise pregnant and nursing women, women who may become pregnant, and children to limit their weekly consumption of fish and to eat fish that are lower in mercury.
The California Department of Health Services recommends that these individuals:
• Eat a variety of different types of fish;
• Eat smaller fish rather than older, larger fish;
• Begin following these guidelines one year before becoming pregnant.
According to the FDA and EPA, fish or shellfish that tend to be lower in mercury include pollock, shrimp, and scallops. Mercury levels in tuna vary. Tuna steaks and canned albacore tuna have higher levels of mercury than canned light tuna.
For more information about the risks of mercury in fish and about the levels in various types of fish consult the following websites:
U.S. Food and Drug Administration ("FDA") www.cfsan.fda.gov
U.S. Environmental Protection Agency www.epa.gov/ost/fish
or call the FDA toll-free at 1-888-SAFEFOOD (1-888-723-3366).

Fig. 4.14 A Proposition 65 warning in California about mercury in fish (the official name of Proposition 65 is the Safe Drinking Water and Toxic Enforcement Act of 1986)

Questions

(a) All the essential elements of a fear appeal argument are present in this poster. These elements are the *initial action* that leads to an *adverse outcome*, the *fear arousal* that is associated with this outcome, and the recommended *protective action* that can avert the adverse outcome and its associated fear. Identify each of these elements in the above poster.

(b) It has been argued that much of the guidance on fish consumption in pregnancy fails to make women aware of the nutritional benefits of eating fish (Taylor et al. 2018). Is this an accurate characterization of the above poster?

(c) Explain how an assessment of the benefits of fish consumption might play a role in the evaluation of the fear appeal argument in this poster. In what other type of argument that we have encountered must the positive and negative consequences of an action be considered during argument evaluation?

(d) Expertise is used extensively in this warning about fish consumption. What form does this expertise take? Which of the elements in a fear appeal argument (see [a] above) does this expertise make the greatest contribution to?

(e) Which aspect of the advice recommended by the agencies that you identified in your response to (d) permits women to derive nutritional benefits from fish consumption while reducing their risk of mercury exposure?

(3) We saw in Exercise 4.3 that a public health campaign that arouses fear but that does not convey readily accessible protective actions is unlikely to be effective. In that case, the public health issue was antibiotic resistance, and the protective actions could only be accessed through a website—they were not stated in the poster that aroused fear. Like the posters in Exercise 4.3, the following poster is also produced by the Public Health Agency of Canada. Examine this poster and then answer the questions below it:

(a) In ▸ Sect. 4.4, one of the logical pitfalls in the use of fear appeal argument was described as the error of representing the negative consequence of an action in terms of deductive consequence, so that if action *A* occurs it is inevitably the case that consequence *C* will follow. What words in the poster in ◘ Fig. 4.15 indicate that the relation between an action and its consequence is *not* construed in this case in terms of deductive consequence?

(b) An argument may state the negative consequence of an action without thereby arousing fear. Is this an accurate description of the poster in ◘ Fig. 4.15? Provide a justification of your response.

(c) Four protective actions are described at the bottom of the poster in ◘ Fig. 4.15. What specific conditions must be in place in order for someone to comply with these actions?

(d) Does the person who can comply with the conditions stated in your response to (c) display high self-efficacy or high response efficacy?

(e) Two of the recommended protective actions concern the protection of people other than the person who is reading the poster. What are the actions in question? What other fear appeal argument that we have examined in this chapter recommends actions that protect people other than the recipient of the argument?

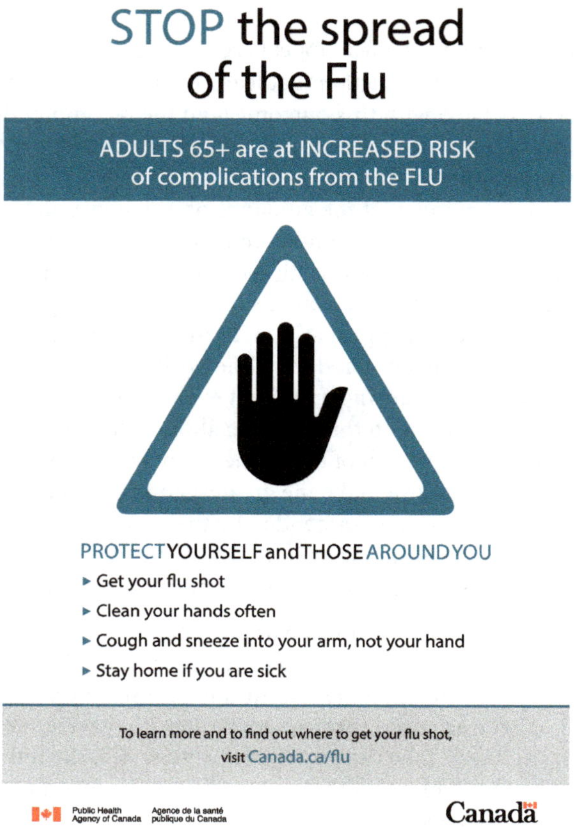

Fig. 4.15 A public health poster about influenza that targets people 65 years and older (© All rights reserved. *Stop the spread of the Flu*. Public Health Agency of Canada. Adapted and reproduced with permission from the Minister of Health, 2018)

Answers

Exercise 4.1

(1)

(a) The fearful consequence is accidental death, and (b) the action that causes it is the use of the opioid oxycodone. The consequence and action in this case are the same as in the CDC poster.

(2) The poster contains the words *college party* where it can be expected that alcohol will be consumed. The consumption of alcohol increases the likelihood that an opioid like oxycodone will cause respiratory depression and death.

(3) In the CDC poster, it was strongly implied that readers should avoid the use of opioid drugs altogether or at least restrict their use. In this case, however, it appears to be accepted that combined alcohol and opioid use *will* occur—the avoidance of

this behaviour is *not* the recommended protective action. Instead, the protective action that is recommended is the use of naloxone by a college friend.

(4) This poster differs from the CDC poster in that the agent of the initial action is the student who takes oxycodone while the agent of the protective action is a college friend who is able to administer naloxone. The agents of these two actions are different people, while in the CDC poster the same person is the agent of both initial and protective actions.

(5) This poster is *not* advancing a fear appeal argument. Although there is a fearful consequence (death) of an action (use of oxycodone), the fearful consequence is not used as a reason to avoid the action that caused it. Instead, the fearful consequence is used to prompt another agent to perform a quite separate action (the administration of naloxone).

Exercise 4.2

(1)

(a) The action that leads to a negative consequence or bad outcome is the use of lead-based paints in the decoration of homes.

(b) The individuals who are most likely to sustain damage related to the use of lead-based paints are children. This is implied by the word 'generations'. It is also explicitly stated at the bottom of the poster where a telephone number is given so that members of the public can find out how to protect their children from lead poisoning.

(c) The protective action that is implied by the poster is clearly the avoidance of lead-based paints in homes. For other protective actions, readers of the poster are advised to use the telephone number at the bottom of the poster.

(2) The intended recipients of this fear appeal argument are the parents of children. However, it is children who are most likely to sustain damage from lead-based paints. The logical feature of fear appeal argument that ensures that parents will be motivated to undertake protective actions is that it is in their *interests* to ensure that no harm comes to their children. The interests of the recipient are explicitly articulated in *P2* of the logical structure of a fear appeal argument.

(3) The poster poses the question 'What's on your walls?'. This question contributes to fear arousal by making readers aware that the threat to their children's health does not exist at a distance from them but lurks within the home.

(4) The significant difference between the poster in Fig. 4.7 and the posters in Fig. 4.6 is that the lead poisoning poster does not make use of visual imagery. Fear arousal in premise *P3* of a fear appeal argument is most likely to be affected (probably diminished) in the absence of visual imagery.

(5) The expression that creates an ambiguity is the noun phrase *lifetime guarantee*. Normally, we associate this phrase with the guarantee of the quality of a product (e.g. *John's new watch has a lifetime guarantee*). However, in this poster the typical or expected meaning of the phrase is reworked to mean a product that will cause health damage on an indefinite basis.

Exercise 4.3

(1) The *initial action* in this fear appeal argument is the misuse of antibiotics especially for the treatment of conditions like cold or flu (poster [c] in ▣ Fig. 4.12). The *negative consequence* of this action is the development of antibiotic resistance (posters [a] and [b] in ▣ Fig. 4.12). This consequence *arouses fear* in readers through the suggestion in posters (a) and (b) that someday their own children may develop a bacterial infection that cannot be effectively treated by the use of antibiotics. The recommended *protective action* is to take antibiotics only as directed by a doctor, and to keep hands clean and vaccinations updated in order to avoid contracting bacterial infections (and the need to take antibiotics) in the first place (poster [c] in ▣ Fig. 4.12).

(2) Posters (a) and (b) convey a negative consequence, namely, antibiotic resistance, and arouse fear in readers. Neither of these elements of a fear appeal argument is conveyed by poster (c).

(3) Poster (c) conveys an initial action, namely, the use (or misuse) of antibiotics to treat conditions such as cold and flu. Poster (c) also conveys protective actions such as using antibiotics only as directed by a doctor and not to treat ailments like cold and flu. Further protective actions include hand washing and vaccination. Neither of these elements is conveyed by posters (a) and (b).

(4) The fear aroused by posters (a) and (b) is unlikely to lead to the type of behaviour modification that is needed to address antibiotic resistance. This is because the protective actions that can reduce antibiotic resistance, such as not taking antibiotics for colds and flu, are not stated in the posters. Instead, readers are recommended to visit a website 'to learn more about what [they] can do'.

(5) The campaign adopted by the Public Health Agency of Canada appears somewhat disjointed and is not strongly rationally warranted. No single campaign poster captures all the elements that are required for members of the public to make a positive contribution to the reduction of antibiotic resistance. Posters (a) and (b) make it difficult for readers to undertake protective actions. Meanwhile, poster (c) fails to state the very serious negative consequence that results from incorrect use of antibiotics, namely, antibiotic resistance, and fails to arouse the legitimate sense of fear that should attend this consequence.

End-of-Chapter Questions

(1)

(a) The fear appeal argument in the poster can be reconstructed as follows:

Premise 1: If you (a person with asthma) contract flu, then there is an increased likelihood that serious complications will occur.
Premise 2: The development of serious complications is a very bad outcome for you.
Premise 3: The development of serious complications arouses considerable fear in you.
Conclusion: Therefore, you should avoid contracting flu by getting a flu vaccination.

(b) In this case, the initial action that leads to a fearful consequence is the development of flu. Contracting this infectious disease appears not to be under a person's volitional control, unless in the unusual case where someone has deliberately undertaken efforts to become infected. But even when the initial action is contracting flu, we must assume that the person with asthma is able to exercise some degree of volitional control over this action. If we could not make this assumption, then the protective action that is recommended in the conclusion of a fear appeal argument would not make sense, as it would encourage the recipient of the argument to take steps to control an action or process that cannot be controlled.

(c) The boxer and boxing are serving as a metaphor in this case. This permits a number of metaphorical comparisons to be drawn between the boxer and the person with asthma who develops flu. For example, the person with asthma may be *knocked out* or *floored* by the flu in the same way that the boxer can be knocked out or floored by a single punch. The person with asthma may *lose consciousness* and even *die* as a result of flu in the same way that a boxer may lose consciousness and die as a result of a severe blow to the head. However, in the same way that the boxer may be able to pick himself up and *fight back*, so too may the person with asthma be able to fight back against the flu.

(d) The 'boxer' metaphor has a logical function in that it allows us to conceive of the consequence and protective action in the fear appeal argument in concrete terms. The flu in a person with asthma can have particularly adverse consequences in the form of serious complications. These complications are equivalent to the boxer who has been knocked out. The protective action to be taken by the person with asthma is to have a flu vaccination. The vaccination is equivalent to the fight back of the boxer.

(e) Self-efficacy is a person's belief that they can undertake the recommended action. Response efficacy is a person's belief that the recommended action will successfully avert the undesirable consequence. The recommended protective action in this case is getting a flu vaccination. The intended readers of this poster—people with asthma—know that flu vaccinations are readily available and that they can easily access them, in most cases for no cost. So self-efficacy is satisfied in this particular fear appeal argument. People with asthma generally trust their healthcare providers to give them expert advice. When doctors and others in the medical community recommend the flu vaccination as the most effective way of averting serious complications of flu, they believe that this is indeed the case. So this fear appeal argument also displays response efficacy.

(2)

(a) The *initial action* is the consumption of fish and particularly certain types of fish (e.g. swordfish). The *adverse outcome* is the development of cancer, birth defects in babies, and other reproductive harm. The process of thinking about the development of serious disease (e.g. cancer) in oneself and birth defects in one's children leads to *fear arousal*. There are several *protective actions* recommended for pregnant and nursing women, women who may become pregnant, and children. These groups should avoid eating certain fish altogether. They should also eat a variety of different types of fish, and eat smaller fish rather than larger, older fish. Women are advised to start taking these protective actions a year before getting pregnant.

(b) This is not an accurate characterization of the poster. This is because the poster explicitly states that there are nutritional benefits from the consumption of fish: "Fish and shellfish are an important part of a healthy diet and a source of essential nutrients."

(c) This fear appeal argument about fish consumption is only rationally warranted to the extent that the fear aroused by the negative outcome of consumption (e.g. birth defects) exceeds any nutritional and other benefits that derive from consumption. The same weighing up of positive and negative consequences of actions is central to an evaluation of slippery slope argument (see Sect. 3.3 in ▶ Chapter 3).

(d) The expertise in this warning about fish consumption takes the form of recommendations from three expert agencies, namely, the Food and Drug Administration, the Environmental Protection Agency, and the California Department of Health Services. The expertise of these bodies makes the most significant contribution to the *protective actions* that pregnant women and nursing mothers are urged to take.

(e) The Food and Drug Administration and the Environmental Protection Agency are not advising women to avoid eating fish altogether, only to 'limit their weekly consumption'. These agencies also recommend types of fish and shellfish that have lower mercury, including pollock, shrimp, scallops, and some types of tuna.

(3)

(a) The words 'increased risk' in the poster in ◘ Fig. 4.15 indicate that the relation between the action in this case (namely, contracting flu) and the consequence (developing complications) is a probabilistic relation and is not one of deductive consequence.

(b) The poster in ◘ Fig. 4.15 states a negative consequence of contracting flu, namely, the development of complications. But, in addition, it also attempts to arouse fear. This is achieved through the use of a warning symbol. This symbol is similar to those found on construction sites and on roadsides where their function is to warn pedestrians and others of danger.

(c) In order to comply with the recommended protective actions in this poster, readers must be able to bear the costs of vaccination (if such costs exist), and be able to sustain the loss of pay if they stay at home (many people aged 65 years and older are still in paid employment). They must also be able to travel to health facilities that offer vaccinations, and have access to hand cleansing facilities and products. These financial and practical conditions must be satisfied if these protective actions are to be carried out by members of the general public.

(d) The person who can comply with the financial and practical conditions described in the response to (c) will believe that they can undertake the recommended protective actions. That is, this person will have high self-efficacy.

(e) The two recommended actions that protect people other than the reader of the poster are the recommendation to cough and sneeze into your arm and not your hand, and to stay at home if you are unwell. These actions are intended to reduce the transmission of influenza to others. The 'second hand smoke' example is the other fear appeal argument examined in this chapter that recommends actions that are protective of someone other than the recipient of the argument.

References

Bastien, S. (2011). Fear appeals in HIV-prevention messages: Young people's perceptions in northern Tanzania. *African Journal of AIDS Research, 10*(4), 435–449.

Carcioppolo, N., Jensen, J. D., Wilson, S. R., Collins, W. B., Carrion, M., & Linnemeier, G. (2013). Examining HPV threat-to-efficacy ratios in the Extended Parallel Process Model. *Health Communication, 28*(1), 20–28.

Carcioppolo, N., John, K. K., Jensen, J. D., & King, A. J. (2018). Joking about cancer as an avoidance strategy among US adults. *Health Promotion International, 34*(3), 420–428.

Centers for Disease Control and Prevention. (2016). *Wide-ranging online data for epidemiologic research (WONDER)*. Atlanta, GA: National Center for Health Statistics. ► http://wonder.cdc.gov. Accessed December 2016.

Centers for Disease Control and Prevention. (2017). *Prevent childhood lead poisoning*. Available online: ► www.cdc.gov/nceh/lead/infographic.htm. Accessed 15 May 2018.

Choi, H. J., Krieger, J. L., & Hecht, M. L. (2013). Reconceptualizing efficacy in substance use prevention research: Refusal response efficacy and drug resistance self-efficacy in adolescent substance use. *Health Communication, 28*(1), 40–52.

Cummings, L. (2012). Scaring the public: Fear appeal arguments in public health reasoning. *Informal Logic, 32*(1), 25–50.

Davis, K. C., Patel, D., Shafer, P., Duke, J., Glover-Kudon, R., Ridgeway, W., et al. (2018). Association between media doses of the *Tips From Former Smokers* campaign and cessation behaviors and intentions to quit among cigarette smokers, 2012–2015. *Health Education & Behavior, 45*(1), 52–60.

Drope, J., Liber, A. C., Cahn, Z., Stoklosa, M., Kennedy, R., Douglas, C. E., et al. (2018). Who's still smoking? Disparities in adult cigarette smoking prevalence in the United States. *CA: A Cancer Journal for Clinicians, 68*(2), 106–115.

Fernández, M. E., Diamond, P. M., Rakowski, W., Gonzales, A., Tortolero-Luna, G., Williams, J., et al. (2009). Development and validation of a cervical cancer screening self-efficacy scale for low-income Mexican American women. *Cancer Epidemiology, Biomarkers & Prevention, 18*(3), 866–875.

Flammer, A. (2001). Self-efficacy. In N. J. Smelser & P. B. Baltes (Eds.), *International encyclopedia of the social & behavioral sciences* (pp. 13812–13815). Amsterdam and New York: Elsevier.

Guignard, R., Gallopel-Morvan, K., Mons, U., Hummel, K., & Nguyen-Thanh, V. (2018). Impact of a negative emotional antitobacco mass media campaign on French smokers: A longitudinal study. *Tobacco Control, 27*(6), 670–676.

Handley, M. A., Nelson, K., Sanford, E., Clarity, C., Emmons-Bell, S., Gorukanti, A., et al. (2017). Examining lead exposures in California through state-issued health alerts for food contamination and an exposure-based candy testing program. *Environmental Health Perspectives, 125*(10), 104503.

Haroutounian, S., Ratz, Y., Ginosar, Y., Furmanov, K., Saifi, F., Meidan, R., et al. (2016). The effect of medicinal cannabis on pain and quality-of-life outcomes in chronic pain: A prospective open-label study. *Clinical Journal of Pain, 32*(12), 1036–1043.

Huang, Y. M., Shiyanbola, O. O., & Smith, P. D. (2018). Association of health literacy and medication self-efficacy with medication adherence and diabetes control. *Patient Preference and Adherence, 12*, 793–802.

Lee, M. J. (2018). College students' responses to emotional anti-alcohol abuse media messages: Should we scare or amuse them? *Health Promotion Practice, 19*(3), 465–474.

Melvin, C. L., Jefferson, M. S., Rice, L. J., Cartmell, K. B., & Halbert, C. H. (2016). Predictors of participation in mammography screening among non-Hispanic Black, non-Hispanic White, and Hispanic women. *Frontiers in Public Health, 4*, 188.

Murray-Johnson, L., Witte, K., Liu, W.-Y., Hubbell, A. P., Sampson, J., & Morrison, K. (2001). Addressing cultural orientations in fear appeals: Promoting AIDS-protective behaviors among Mexican immigrant and African American adolescents and American and Taiwanese college students. *Journal of Health Communication, 6*(4), 335–358.

Orbell, S., Szczepura, A., Weller, D., Gumber, A., & Hagger, M. S. (2017). South Asian ethnicity, socioeconomic status, and psychological mediators of faecal occult blood colorectal screening participation: A prospective test of a process model. *Health Psychology, 36*(12), 1161–1172.

Pechmann, C., & Reibling, E. T. (2000). Anti-smoking advertising campaigns targeting youth: Case studies from USA and Canada. *Tobacco Control, 9*(Suppl. II), ii18–ii31.

Rhodes, F., & Wolitski, R. J. (1990). Perceived effectiveness of fear appeals in AIDS education: Relationship to ethnicity, gender, age, and group membership. *AIDS Education and Prevention, 2*(1), 1–11.

Roskos-Ewoldsen, D. R., Yu, J. H., & Rhodes, N. (2004). Fear appeal messages affect accessibility of attitudes toward the threat and adaptive behaviors. *Communication Monographs, 71*(1), 49–69.

Ruiter, R. A. C., Kessels, L. T. E., Peters, G.-J. Y., & Kok, G. (2014). Sixty years of fear appeal research: Current state of the evidence. *International Journal of Psychology, 49*(2), 63–70.

Shi, J. J., & Smith, S. W. (2016). The effects of fear appeal message repetition on perceived threat, perceived efficacy, and behavioral intention in the extended parallel process model. *Health Communication, 31*(3), 275–286.

Taylor, C. M., Emmett, P. M., Emond, A. M., & Golding, J. (2018). A review of guidance on fish consumption in pregnancy: Is it fit for purpose? *Public Health Nutrition, 21*(11), 2149–2159.

Tversky, A., & Kahneman, D. (2004). Belief in the law of small numbers. In E. Shafir (Ed.), *Preference, belief and similarity: Selected writings by Amos Tversky* (pp. 193–202). Cambridge: MIT Press.

Wakefield, A. J., Murch, S. H., Anthony, A., Linnell, J., Casson, D. M., Malik, M., et al. (1998). Ileal-lymphoid-nodular hyperplasia, non-specific colitis, and pervasive developmental disorder in children. *The Lancet, 351*(9103), 637–641.

Walton, D. N. (2000). *Scare tactics: Arguments that appeal to fear and threats*. Dordrecht: Kluwer Academic.

Weinstein, N. D. (1980). Unrealistic optimism about future life events. *Journal of Personality and Social Psychology, 39*(5), 806–820.

Weinstein, N. D. (1984). Why it won't happen to me: Perceptions of risk factors and susceptibility. *Health Psychology, 3*(5), 431–457.

Witte, K., & Allen, M. (2000). A meta-analysis of fear appeals: Implications for effective public health campaigns. *Health Education & Behavior, 27*(5), 591–615.

Witte, K., Meyer, G., & Martell, D. (2001). *Effective health risk messages: A step-by-step guide*. Thousand Oaks, London, and New Delhi: Sage.

Xi, B., Veeranki, S. P., Zhao, M., Ma, C., Yan, Y., & Mi, J. (2017). Relationship of alcohol consumption to all-cause, cardiovascular, and cancer-related mortality in U.S. adults. *Journal of the American College of Cardiology, 70*(8), 913–922.

Zhang, W., Zhang, X., Tian, Y., Zhu, Y., Tong, Y., Li, Y., et al. (2018). Risk assessment of total mercury and methylmercury in aquatic products from offshore farms in China. *Journal of Hazardous Materials, 354*, 198–205.

Appeals to Expertise

L. Cummings, *Fallacies in Medicine and Health*,
https://doi.org/10.1007/978-3-030-28513-5_5

LEARNING OBJECTIVES: Readers of this chapter will

- be able to distinguish appeals to expertise in argument from other non-logical uses of expertise in discourse.
- be able to identify various linguistic markers of expertise, and recognise when these markers reflect actual expertise in argument.
- be able to characterise the logical structure of the argument from expertise, and understand the individual contribution of each of the three premises of this argument to the support of the conclusion.
- be able to recognise and describe the many different ways in which arguers may use expert appeals erroneously in argument, or use these appeals to deceive an opponent into accepting a conclusion in argument.
- be able to give an account of some of the main findings of social scientific research on expertise, and understand the complex array of factors that influence our trust in experts.
- be able to explain how expertise can be used as a shortcut or mental heuristic through complex deliberations that are costly for reasoning agents in terms of time and cognitive effort.

5.1 Introduction

Knowledge generation and assimilation are shared social enterprises. Each of us has knowledge of certain people, events, and things in the world around us. But each of us must also defer to others when our knowledge is incomplete or is not sufficiently specialized to address a question or issue. The reliance on others for knowledge is an important division of cognitive labour that has been necessitated by the rapid expansion of all forms of knowledge in modern societies. Each of us is charged with knowing *certain things*, but none of us is responsible for knowing *everything*. In this chapter, we will examine how the knowledge of others is used in argumentation. In the context of medicine and health, appeals to the knowledge, or expertise of others is a very common practice. This is because most issues in medicine and health involve specialized or high-level knowledge that is acquired over many years of formal education and training that only some of us can undertake. So we must appeal to the knowledge and expertise of others in order to make decisions and arrive at judgements, or be left in a state of ignorance and inaction. But even as we rely on others for knowledge that guides our decision-making, we can interrogate that reliance, and make judgements about when it is more or less rationally warranted. In other words, not every appeal to the knowledge or expertise of others in argument is rationally warranted. We will have occasion in this chapter to examine a number of appeals to expertise in medicine and health where it would be best to disregard the knowledge or expertise of others. But before addressing the rational evaluation of these appeals, a number of other introductory remarks are in order.

Knowledge and expertise are highly prized attributes of those who are judged to possess them. In all societies, these attributes are valued and revered. A tribal elder may receive the respect of others because he has wisdom and knowledge that have been acquired over many years of experience and learning. A lawyer, medical specialist, or academic may acquire wealth and achieve high social status on account of his or her knowledge and expertise. In each of these cases, individuals with knowledge and expertise are regarded by others as having *authority* to make pronouncements on certain issues. These pronouncements carry weight or have significance for others exactly because they originate in someone who has cognitive authority to make them based on their knowledge and expertise. When other people use these pronouncements in argument, they are making an appeal to expertise. The appeal to expertise in argument has a long history in logic and philosophy where it is called *argumentum ad verecundiam*. The literal translation of this term is 'argument from modesty'. In *An Essay Concerning Human Understanding*, John Locke describes how it is judged to be a 'breach of modesty' to challenge the authority of someone 'whose parts, learning, eminency, power, or some other cause has gained a name, and settled their reputation in the common esteem with some kind of authority' (Book IV, Chapter XVII: Of Reason). While Locke was not prepared to subscribe to the view that a man's opinion is right 'because I, out of respect, or any other consideration but that of conviction, will not contradict him', it nevertheless remains the case that the opinions of people with knowledge and expertise can carry substantial weight in argument and elsewhere. This assumption is a starting point of the current chapter.

In the discussion that follows, the various ways in which appeals to expertise are used in argument are examined at length. This includes an analysis of the logical form of these appeals and how they may be used to achieve persuasion in argument. A person's cognitive authority to make pronouncements on an issue can be established incrementally through markers of expertise. Authority may be established by means of competence markers like formal qualifications, and personal attributes such as integrity and trustworthiness. Researchers in social science have had much to say about people's perceptions of the competence and integrity of authorities and the relative importance that they attach to these factors. For example, there is evidence that personal integrity and trustworthiness are afforded greater significance than competence in an assessment of an individual's credibility and authority, at least in certain study populations. The widespread use of appeals to expertise in medicine and health is a reflection of the distribution of epistemic resources among different actors in the medical and health domains. The epistemic resources of doctors and patients cannot be characterized in terms of the presence and absence of expertise, respectively. Such a distinction overlooks the fact that even within the medical profession there are widely differing levels of knowledge and expertise between general medical practitioners, and those who have specialized in sub-disciplines of medicine such as cardiology and neurology. Meanwhile, there can be considerable expertise among members of the public who have no medical training or qualification whatsoever. We begin by examining logical and non-logical uses of expertise before focusing our discussion on the logical use of expertise in argument.

5.2 Logical and Non-logical Uses of Expertise

Expertise is part of our daily lives. I get up in the morning and switch on the television. I learn that a report has just been published by a group of international climate scientists. These scientists have concluded that many coastal regions and island nations around the world will be totally submerged by water within the next 20 years if immediate action is not taken to curb CO_2 emissions. As I travel to work on the bus, I read a warning on a billboard about smoking by the Chief Medical Officer for England. It states that every 50 cigarettes smoked causes one DNA mutation per lung cell. A colleague with asthma at work tells me that his doctor has advised him to get vaccinated against pneumococcal infection, and that he will be leaving the office early to attend an appointment at his local health clinic. As I wait at the bus stop to make my journey home after work, I read a poster in the bus shelter that says a government scientific advisory committee recommends a reduction in the number of units of alcohol that men and women can safely drink each week. I finally get home and settle down to read the newspaper. The headline story that day has been the publication of the findings of an independent review panel tasked with investigating the safety of the MMR vaccine. These scenarios are so commonplace in our lives that we are seldom aware of them, or the extent to which they embody medical and scientific expertise. But only some scenarios in which expertise is employed involve its use in the context of an argument. In this section, we examine how expertise may be used in a logical way as a premise in an argument. We also distinguish this use of expertise from the many non-logical ways in which language users may employ expertise.

In the above scenarios, expertise is represented through different individuals and bodies. Expertise may come in the form of one's doctor or physician who recommends a particular vaccination. Alternatively, expertise may be embodied by a government-appointed Chief Medical Officer or scientific advisory committee. Expertise may involve geographically dispersed individuals such as a group of international climate scientists, or it may involve an independent review panel that stands apart from any government influence or interference. Different types of expertise, and the markers that signify them, will be examined in ▶ Sect. 5.3. For our present purposes, we want to explore if the use of medical and health expertise as in the above scenarios is always with a view to supporting a conclusion in argument, or if appeals to expertise can serve other functions as well. To this end, consider the following article that appeared online in the *Belfast Telegraph* on 8 May 2018. The article describes failings in Ireland's cervical screening programme.

UK health expert to investigate cancer testing in Ireland

Dr Gabriel Scally will bring real experience to the probe into the handling of cervical smear screening, Irish health minister Simon Harris said.

A UK health expert who investigated abuse at the Winterbourne care home for the disabled will lead an inquiry into the misinterpretation of cancer tests in Ireland.

Dr Gabriel Scally is an eminent individual who will bring real experience to the preliminary probe into the handling of cervical smear screening, Irish health minister Simon Harris said.

He contributed to a serious case review of Winterbourne View Hospital where staff were shown to be mistreating and assaulting adults with learning disabilities and autism.

Mr Harris said: "We need to establish the facts and we need to get answers quickly for Irish women."

He has asked Dr Scally to give early feedback by the start of next month and a full report by the end of June.

An audit by CervicalCheck – Ireland's national screening programme – of 1,482 women diagnosed with cervical cancer since 2008 had found potential errors in 208 cases, as tests showed no abnormality when they should have been given a cancer warning.

The majority of the 208 women – 162 – were not initially told of the outcome of the audit. Of the 208, 17 have since died.

It then emerged that a further 1,518 women with the cancer in the same period have not been audited, though health chiefs stress the number affected by potential errors in this group is likely to be lower.

The head of Ireland's health service has faced calls to go.

Vicky Phelan, a 43-year-old mother of two from Co Limerick, took legal proceedings after a 2011 smear test which returned no abnormalities was found three years later to be incorrect. She was diagnosed with cervical cancer in 2014.

Mr Harris said it was a "horrific and worrying" time for women and ministers had agreed to order the scoping inquiry.

The minister said Dr Scally had experience in reviews of this type as a senior public health doctor and adviser to the UK Department of Health and the NHS.

The inquiry will independently examine details of the non-disclosure to patients relating to CervicalCheck clinical audits and the management and level of knowledge of various parties including the Health Service Executive and the Department of Health.

It will also examine the tendering, contracting, operation of the labs contracted by CervicalCheck.

An international expert panel review led by the Royal College of Obstetricians and Gynaecologists, and the British Society for Colposcopy and Cervical Pathology will review the results of screening tests of all women who have developed cervical cancer who participated in the screening programme since it was established.

This will provide independent clinical assurance to women about the timing of their diagnosis and any issues relating to their treatment and outcome, Mr Harris said.

Dr Scally said he believed he did not know anyone involved in the screening services but could not rule out the possibility.

He drew comparisons with the Northern Ireland inquiry into hyponatraemia-related deaths, in which he assisted.

Dr Scally said: "That was difficult for me to do because I knew a lot of the people involved in that.

"But I don't think anyone would question my expert advice to that, at all.

"It will play no part in my considerations.

"My primary responsibility is to the women involved and to the population as a whole."
(Reproduced courtesy of the Press Association)

Expertise is developed on two fronts in this article. The expertise of Dr Gabriel Scally, the medical specialist charged with leading the inquiry into the cancer screening programme, is established from the outset of the article. Dr Scally is described as an 'eminent individual' who has 'experience in reviews of this type'. His experience is based on the fact that he conducted an inquiry into the abuse by staff of adults with learning disabilities and autism at Winterbourne View Hospital. Dr Scally's expertise is further established by his description as a 'senior public health doctor' and an 'adviser to the UK Department of Health and the NHS'. We might wish to query how experience in conducting an inquiry into the social care of adults qualifies someone to lead an inquiry into cancer screening. Indeed, we will see in ▶ Sect. 5.4 that a lack of *relevant* expertise is a common criticism of appeals to expertise in argument. This issue aside, it is clear that the article is attempting to set out the nature and extent of Dr Scally's expertise. But this expertise is not being used to support a claim in argument. Towards the end of the article, another issue is raised that might affect the objectivity of Dr Scally's expertise. That issue concerns personal relationships to people who are involved in the cancer screening service that he has been tasked with investigating. But here again, the potential conflict of interest that such relationships may pose to the independence of Dr Scally's expertise is concerned only with establishing the legitimacy of his claim to expertise. The fact remains that Dr Scally's expertise is doing no argumentative work whatsoever within this article.

Expertise is developed on a second front in this newspaper article. Alongside Dr Scally's inquiry into the cancer screening service, there will also be an international expert panel review of the screening tests of all women who developed cervical cancer and participated in the screening programme since it was first established. This review will be led by two expert bodies, namely, the Royal College of Obstetricians and Gynaecologists, and the British Society for Colposcopy and Cervical Pathology. The experts who constitute these bodies will undoubtedly have the medical knowledge and training that are required to review the cases of all screened women who have developed cervical cancer. The decision by the Irish health minister to place these bodies in charge of the international review panel is clearly intended to provide reassurance to women about the accuracy of their test results. But establishing the credibility of this review panel through the use of expertise is *not* the same as using expertise to support a claim in argument. When the inquiry and review have been conducted by Dr Scally and his team, certain conclusions and findings will undoubtedly be reported. The logical standing of these conclusions will be based on the expertise of those who draw them. But this article is not reporting the findings of the inquiry into cervical screening. Instead, it is exploring for readers how the Irish health minister intends to address the crisis of confidence in the cervical screening programme through the use of the best available medical expertise. This does not constitute an appeal to expertise *in argument*, even though it is expertise that is in the thematic foreground of the entire article.

This article illustrates that it is possible to discuss expertise and to reflect on its nature and extent without using expertise as a ground or reason to support a claim in argument. Expertise may be the dominant theme of discourse which has no argumentative purpose whatsoever. As a discourse theme, expertise can be explored and interrogated with no implications for the rational standing of, or our epistemic commitment to, a thesis or claim. When we turn to the use of expertise in argumentative discourse, however, quite different considerations come into play. Appeals to expertise in argumentative discourse involve logical relations that are lacking in other types of discourse. The logical inference that takes us from an 'expertise' premise to the conclusion that a particular thesis or claim is true is the most significant of these relations. To illustrate the characteristics of discourse in which an argumentative appeal to expertise is made, consider the following extracts from a newspaper article that appeared in *The Guardian* on 8 August 2017. The article is entitled 'A danger to public health? Uproar as scientist urges us to eat more salt'. *The Guardian*'s health editor, Sarah Boseley, is describing the reaction of public health experts in the UK to the publication of a book by New York scientist James DiNicolantonio in which he claims that people need to consume more, not less, salt. These extracts are part of a wider dialectical exchange in which DiNicolantonio is arguing that salt is good for one's health, while public health experts are claiming that salt is bad for one's health. Five appeals to expertise appear in the article. They are reported here in the order in which they occurred:

» (1) "**Prof Louis Levy, head of nutrition science at Public Health England**, said: "Diet is now the leading cause of ill health. By advocating a high-salt diet this book is putting the health of many at risk and it undermines internationally recognised evidence that shows a diet high in salt is linked to high blood pressure, a known risk for heart disease.""

(2) "But the evidence on salt is incontrovertible, according to Graham MacGregor, **a professor of cardiovascular medicine**, who led the campaign for action on salt and health."

(3) "But DiNicolantonio, who is an **associate editor of the journal BMJ Open Heart and a cardiovascular research scientist at Saint Luke's Mid America Heart Institute**, says the evidence does not stack up, whatever bodies such as Public Health England and the American Heart Association say."

(4) "**The government's scientific advisory committee on nutrition (SACN)**, which backed a reduction to 6g of salt a day in the UK diet from around 9g, lists a number of trials in animals and humans that suggest high salt levels do lead to higher blood pressure in its 2003 report."

(5) "But the **National Institute for Health and Care Excellence**, which looked at the impact of salt reduction for the population in 2013, said the government's strategy could lead to 20,000 fewer heart deaths each year."

By arguing that people should increase their dietary intake of salt, DiNicolantonio is challenging a long-standing medical view that salt is bad for health. This unorthodox stance is reflected in the fact that most appeals to expertise in this article support the dominant medical view that salt is damaging to health. Expertise is marked in these appeals in various ways. The expertise of individuals is indicated through the use of academic titles (*professor*), medical disciplines (*cardiovascular medicine*), and affiliations with health agencies (*Public Health England*). As well as these markers of expertise, DiNicolantonio accrues expertise through his role as an associate editor of the academic journal *BMJ Open Heart*. Expertise is also represented by government-appointed bodies such as the scientific advisory committee on nutrition, and agencies that are operationally independent of government such as the National Institute for Health and Care Excellence. Markers of expertise will be examined further in ▶ Sect. 5.3. In the meantime, it is the use of expertise in these extracts to provide claims with rational warrant which sets the appeals to expertise in this article apart from the appeals to expertise in the article on cervical screening. In appeal (1), for example, Professor Levy asserts a number of propositions, including *Diet is the leading cause of ill health* and *This book is putting the health of many at risk*. Professor Levy's authority to make these **assertions** is based entirely on his expertise as the head of nutrition science at Public Health England. It is this expertise that confers rational warrant on these claims—we can be certain that they are *true* claims exactly because Professor Levy is an expert and he is asserting them to be true (◘ Fig. 5.1).

In each of the appeals to expertise displayed above, the veracity of one or more propositions is based on the assertion of an individual expert or a body of experts. In (2), we can be confident that the evidence on salt truly is incontrovertible because a professor of cardiovascular medicine has asserted this to be the case. In (4), we can be certain that high salt levels cause high blood pressure because an expert scientific advisory committee has examined the relevant evidence and has concluded that this is the case. Even a dissenting scientific viewpoint, if it is uttered by a reputable expert, has a claim on truth. So when DiNicolantonio states in (3) that the evidence that salt is bad for our health 'does not stack up', the truth of this claim is based on his perceived expertise. (Truth is an absolute concept while perceived expertise is a relative concept. We will see in ▶ Sect. 5.4 that somehow we manage to bridge the two when we make assessments of expertise in argument.) Finally, we can be reasonably certain in (5) that 20,000 fewer heart deaths each year will be the impact of the UK government's

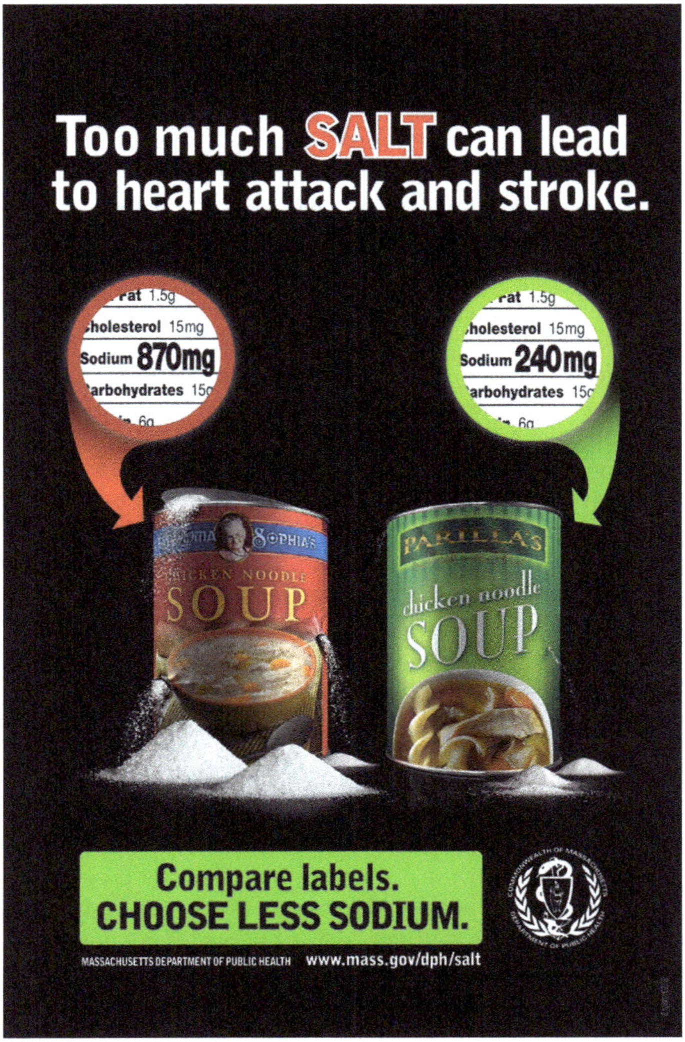

Fig. 5.1 The dominant medical view is that high salt intake increases the risk of heart attack and stroke (Reproduced courtesy of the Massachusetts Department of Public Health)

salt reduction strategy because an expert agency, the National Institute for Health and Care Excellence, has considered the matter and has arrived at this conclusion. In each of these appeals to expertise, the truth of a proposition is based on the expertise of the individual who asserts the proposition. The logical relation can be expressed as follows: proposition *P* is true *because* it is asserted by expert *E*. In non-logical uses of expertise, this logical relation does not exist. In the cancer screening article, it was not possible to identify a proposition that owed its truth to the assertion of an expert.

It is now time for you to get practice in identifying logical and non-logical uses of expertise in discourse by attempting Exercise 5.1.

EXERCISE 5.1: Logical and non-logical uses of expertise

We described above how the use of expertise in argument involves a logical relation between the truth of a proposition and the expertise of an individual or group of individuals who assert the proposition. Where this logical relation cannot be identified, expertise is performing some other, non-logical function in discourse. The following extracts are taken from articles that appear in national newspapers. Use your knowledge of expertise to identify which of these extracts is making logical use of expertise and which is making non-logical use of expertise:

(a) "The academics, led by Theresa Marteau, director of the Behaviour and Health Research Unit at Cambridge University, believe there is little evidence that nudging alone will help people shun unhealthy choices in favour of more healthy ones." ('It'll take more than a nudge, say public health experts', *The Telegraph*, Stephen Adams, 26 January 2011)

(b) "The lead investigator, Dr. Kenneth J. Mukamal, an associate professor of medicine at Harvard Medical School, discussed the methods with alcohol groups by email in August 2014, responding to questions raised by Diageo, Anheuser Busch InBev, and trade groups like the Distilled Spirits Council." ('Major study of drinking will be shut down', *The New York Times*, Roni Caryn Rabin, 15 June 2018)

(c) "'There is really not strong evidence that coffee does cause cancer', says Dr Kathryn Wilson, Harvard Medical School epidemiologist, who served on the committee of the World Health Organization that decided to downgrade coffee to an unlikely carcinogen." ('Should you be worried about cancer in your coffee? Expert breaks down the science behind California's new law which says a cup of Joe could kill you', *Daily Mail Online*, Natalie Rahhal, 30 March 2018)

(d) "The Hong Kong government has commissioned the first local study on breast cancer risks to determine if women in the city should receive universal screening. The University of Hong Kong will helm the project, with a report expected in March next year. Led by Professor Gabriel Leung from HKU's school of public health, the study will develop a risk prediction model specifically for Hong Kong and identify risk factors for a disease that claimed the lives of 702 local women in 2016." ('HKU assigned to launch study on breast cancer risk and pave way for local universal screening', *South China Morning Post*, Emily Tsang, 10 March 2018)

(e) "Doctors must stop telling patients to finish an entire course of antibiotics because it is driving antimicrobial resistance, a group of eminent specialists has warned [...] Prof Mark Woolhouse, Professor of Infectious Disease Epidemiology, University of Edinburgh, said: 'It is very clear that prescribing practices do need to change; there is every indication that current volumes of antibiotic usage are too high to be sustainable'." ('"Don't finish the course of antibiotics"—experts turn medical advice on its head', *The Telegraph*, Sarah Knapton, 27 July 2017)

5.3 Logical Structure of Expert Appeals

In the last section, it appeared that appeals to expertise in argumentation are a type of one-premise argument. A proposition *P* is presumed to be *true* because it is asserted or uttered by an expert *E*. The fact of the expert assertion seemed to be the only ground on which the logic of the argument rests. But what appears to be a one-premise argument is, in fact, a three-premise argument in which certain premises are left implicit. Walton (1997: 258) characterizes the logical structure of the argument from authority or expertise as follows. In this schema, *A* is a proposition, *E* is an expert, and *D* is a domain of knowledge:

E is an expert in domain *D*.
E asserts that *A* is known to be true.
A is within *D*.
Therefore, *A* may (plausibly) be taken to be true.

In the logical appeals to expertise that we examined in the last section, only the second premise in this schema was explicit. The various contributors to the debate on the health implications of dietary salt intake were represented as asserting that certain propositions or claims are true. The first and third premises in the above **argument schema** were suggested by the article that described the public health reaction in the UK to the publication of James DiNicolantonio's book. But a suggestion does not amount to an assertion on the part of the article's author. At no point, for example, did the author directly assert that any of the individuals named in the article is an expert on health and salt consumption. It was left to the reader of the article to infer both these premises based on other information that was supplied in the article. By providing various linguistic markers of expertise, the author was able to lead readers to conclude that each protagonist in the debate has *some* claim on expertise, however dubious that claim may be found to be upon further examination. These markers trigger the inference that each named contributor to the debate has some degree of expertise on the question of the health effects of salt consumption. The article also leads readers to draw the inference that makes explicit the third premise in the above argument schema. The various propositions and claims advanced by the experts in the article must relate to the issue of the health effects of salt consumption. Otherwise, readers might reasonably query why the author is presenting these claims at all in the article. So the author of the article is effectively setting up inferences that allow readers to make the first and third premises in Walton's argument scheme fully explicit.

So a logical appeal to expertise is a three-premise argument in which on most occasions only the second premise is explicitly stated. The supply of missing or implicit premises in this argument is not as straightforward as it might at first seem. Let us consider the first premise of this argument, namely, that *E* is an expert in domain *D*. We saw in ► Sect. 5.2 how expertise is assessed in a particular case on the basis of linguistic markers. These markers include academic and medical titles, professional affiliations, and areas of specialization. These markers can be used as quick 'rules of thumb' that allow people who lack specialist knowledge to make assessments of expertise. But even an assessment of the significance of these markers can be very complex in individual cases. Imagine a scenario in which we are trying to assess an argument from authority or expertise relating to the safety of the MMR vaccine. We read a newspaper article that reports the views of three medical experts. Two of these experts claim the vaccine is safe, while the third expert raises concerns about its safety. The experts are a professor of virology, a professor of immunology, and a professor of pharmacology. Each expert is affiliated with one or more academic and/or medical institutions.

The question naturally arises: which, if any, of these experts is qualified to make assertions about the safety of the MMR vaccine? The fact that they are all professors certainly confers some expertise on each of them. But is it the right type of expertise to address the issue of MMR safety? For this we must know something about the areas of specialization of each professor. At this point, judgements of expertise become particularly challenging. For while an individual with medical knowledge may be able to decide if an expert in virology can competently make pronouncements about MMR safety, the same cannot be said of many lay people. For such individuals, they must fall back on other markers of expertise to aid their judgement making. So an individual's area of specialization may be assessed alongside professional experience, academic and medical qualifications, and the type of affiliation that an 'expert' may have. Considered in combination, these different markers may settle the issue of whether a professor of virology is expertly placed to make pronouncements about the safety of the MMR vaccine. Otherwise, this professor's expertise, as valid as it may be on its own terms, may remain something of an open issue in relation to MMR safety, at least as far as the lay person is concerned.

It can be seen that supplying a missing first premise in an argument from expertise is quite a difficult task. In the absence of specialist knowledge, it can also be difficult to supply the third premise in an argument from expertise. That premise states that the proposition asserted by an expert falls within a particular domain of knowledge. Once again, this judgement can be more easily made by some individuals than by others. Imagine a scenario in which two oncologists are taking part in a television program in which they are discussing the risk factors that predispose women to develop breast cancer. Among the factors they address are alcohol consumption, smoking, obesity, and the hormone oestrogen. A medical student who is in the audience and is listening to the discussion may understand the relationship between endocrine (specifically, ovarian) function and breast cancer development. As a result, he or she may have little difficulty in establishing the relevance of claims about ovarian oestrogen to the domain of knowledge that is addressed by the discussion, namely, risk factors for breast cancer development. This student will be well positioned to supply the missing third premise in the appeals to expertise that occur during the discussion. However, the same cannot be said of other individuals in the audience who have little or no medical knowledge. For these individuals, it will be difficult or impossible to establish the relevance of claims about oestrogen to breast cancer development. In the absence of background knowledge, these members of the audience will be unable to supply a missing third premise. Once again, the supply of missing premises in appeals to expertise is shown to involve complex judgements that often lie beyond the competence of those to whom these appeals are directed.

So the first and third premises that are often implicit in expert appeals are not always readily supplied by those who are the intended recipients of these appeals. Some remarks are also in order about the second premise in the argument from expertise. This premise states that an expert *E asserts* that *A* is known to be true. Assertion is a special type of speech act that entails the truth of the asserted proposition. If someone asserts that it is raining outside, then we can reasonably expect to open the door and see that it is actually raining outside. Assertion is the speech act that we use to describe states of affairs and report events in the world. The truth orientation of this speech act has made it a favourite for analysis by generations of philosophers and logicians. Certainly, no appeal to expertise would be possible if we could not assume the truth of the propositions that an expert asserts. But here we must be careful. This is because experts can also advance propositions in a range of other speech acts where the assumption of truth does not hold. An expert may *propose* that *P* or may *suggest* that *P*. In neither of these cases can the truth of *P* be assumed. An expert may also *presume* that *P* in which there is only a tentative commitment to the truth of a proposition. These additional speech acts allow experts (and other language users) to express quite different epistemic commitments to propositions. This is important because even experts need to be able to make uncertain or tentative statements on occasion. But it is only the speech act of assertion that involves an absolute commitment to the *truth* of a proposition. And it is, after all, to establish the truth of propositions that we defer to the pronouncements and opinions of experts.

We have described logical features of each of the three premises that constitute an argument from expertise. Some remarks should also be made about the conclusion of this argument. According to Walton's scheme, the conclusion states that a proposition *A* may (plausibly) be taken to be true. The word 'plausibly' in parenthesis is important. It reflects the fact that the conclusion of an argument from expertise can be accepted as true until such times as the rejection of a proposition becomes necessary. In medicine and health, we have become familiar with (or maybe overwhelmed by) how quickly the opinions of experts can be overturned by the emergence of new evidence. Until recently, medical experts in general expressed the view that a course of antibiotics should be taken in its entirety in order to ensure that a bacterial infection was completely eliminated. This expert opinion was printed on each antibiotic information leaflet. It was also verbally reinforced by doctors who prescribed antibiotics for patients and by pharmacists who dispensed these medications. With growing antimicrobial resistance, the overuse of antibiotics has become an issue of considerable concern to the medical community. As a result, the expert advice to complete a course of antibiotics is now beginning to be questioned and challenged. In a recent article in the *British Medical Journal*, Llewelyn et al. (2017) stated that:

> » The idea that stopping antibiotic treatment early encourages antibiotic resistance is not supported by evidence, while taking antibiotics for longer than necessary increases the risk of resistance. Without explicitly contradicting previous advice, current public information materials from the US Centers for Disease Control and Prevention (CDC) and Public Health England have replaced "complete the course" with messages advocating taking antibiotics "exactly as prescribed."

The marked change in expert opinion illustrated by this case is not at all uncommon in medicine and health. It is possible because appeals to expertise are a type of defeasible argument that may be overturned by the emergence of contrary evidence. A plausible or presumptively true expert opinion is exactly that—it stands until new evidence defeats or overturns it. It is not held aloft and protected in the face of countervailing considerations. We will examine this point further in the next section when we consider the type of criteria that are used in a rational evaluation of expert appeal.

It is now time for you to get practice in identifying the logical components of expert appeals by attempting Exercise 5.2.

EXERCISE 5.2: E-cigarettes, vaping and human health

The use of e-cigarettes and vaping as an alternative to the smoking of tobacco has raised new human health concerns. In an article published in *The Guardian* on 29 January 2018, science editor Ian Semple discussed the findings of a study that purported to find evidence that vaping may raise the risk of certain cancers and heart disease. The study by a team of scientists examined the effects of e-cigarette smoke on healthy mice and human cells. In the extract from the article that follows, the views of two 'experts' on this issue are represented. One expert is the professor who led the study into the health effects of e-cigarette smoke. The other expert is another academic who believes the study's findings have few, if any, implications for human health. Examine the extract in detail and then answer the questions that follow:

» Vaping may raise the risk of certain cancers and heart disease, according to a team of scientists who studied the effects of e-cigarette smoke on healthy mice and human cells.

Moon-shong Tang, professor of environmental medicine at New York University, said the DNA changes [related to e-cigarette smoke] were similar to those linked to secondhand smoke, but added that more work was needed to see whether vaping really did increase cancer rates.

The researchers have now launched long-term experiments to look at the development of tumours in mice exposed to vapour from e-cigarettes, but Tang does not expect to have answers any time soon. "The results may take years to come in because cancer is such a slow process," he said.

While some researchers said the work was important, others all but dismissed it as irrelevant to humans. The mice were exposed to high levels of e-cigarette smoke and the effects may be very different in people who inhale nicotine from vaping, critics caution.

"This study shows nothing at all about the dangers of vaping," said Peter Hajek, director of the Tobacco Dependence Research Unit at Queen Mary University of London. "It doesn't show that vaping causes cancer."

"This is one in a long line of false alarms which may be putting people off the switch from smoking to vaping which would undoubtedly be of great benefit to them," he added. "The best current estimate is that vaping poses, at worst, some 5% of risks of smoking."

('Vaping may raise cancer and heart disease risk, study suggests', *The Guardian*, Ian Semple, 29 January 2018)

Questions

(a) What *three* linguistic markers of expertise are used in relation to the lead investigator of the e-cigarette study, Moon-shong Tang?

(b) Linguistic markers of expertise are also used in relation to the other expert in this article, Peter Hajek. How do these markers differ from those used in relation to Tang?

(c) For each of the experts in this article, identify *one* proposition or claim that is asserted to be true.

(d) The conclusions of the study led by Tang relate to the harmful effects of e-cigarette smoke on mice. Some researchers challenged the relevance of these findings to human health. Which of the three premises in an argument from expertise is this challenge intended to weaken?

(e) The argument from expertise has been characterized as a plausible or presumptive argument in which conclusions are held on a tentative basis until such times as contrary evidence emerges. What evidence is there in this extract that Tang regards the current evidence base on the health effects of e-cigarette smoke as provisional in nature and subject to change?

5.4 Logical Pitfalls in Arguing from Expertise

An appeal to expertise can prove to be very powerful in terms of encouraging an opponent in argument to accept a proponent's claim. It should come as no surprise, therefore, that expert appeals can often be exploited by a proponent who may use them to gain ground illegitimately in argument by hoodwinking an opponent into accepting a claim. There are almost limitless ways in which arguers can abuse or misuse expertise. The proponent of a claim may exaggerate the extent of someone's expertise in an area. A lay person's knowledge of astronomy, genetics, and reproductive medicine does not amount to the knowledge of an expert, no matter how much a proponent in argument claims otherwise. A proponent may claim that expert *E* has expertise in area *A* when *E*'s only expertise is in area *B*. Expertise in electrical engineering is not the same as expertise in aeronautical engineering or mechanical engineering, even if a proponent forcefully argues that expertise in one of these engineering disciplines amounts to expertise in all three disciplines. A proponent may appeal to an expert in argument who has the requisite specialization in a particular field or discipline, while all the time knowing that this person accepts bribes and other incentives to express certain opinions and views. A proponent may misrepresent certain claims as assertions of an expert when the expert in question only tentatively offered his or her opinions as **presumptions** or suppositions. Finally, a proponent may advance an expert's opinion without using any of the qualifications that the expert used when he or she advanced the opinion. These errors and deceptions in the use of appeals to expertise in argument will be examined further in this section.

One of the most common abuses of expertise in argument occurs when a proponent of a claim exaggerates an individual's expertise. Exaggeration of expertise can take several forms. An individual may have certain qualifications, but they are not as numerous or as specialized as the proponent of an expert appeal claims. An 'expert' may have five years of experience in a particular field or discipline. However, when their opinion is reported in argument, five years' experience may be increased to 20 years or may be described using words like 'extensive'. A proponent who states that an 'expert' has spent his 'entire career' investigating the carcinogenic effects of a food additive may not utter a falsehood. But if we were to discover that this career amounted to only three years of study into the additive, we may rightfully feel duped and misled. Arguers who exaggerate an individual's expertise often do so in the belief that their exaggeration will pass undetected. More often than not, this belief is warranted. On hearing an appeal to expertise in argument, most of us cannot undertake the verification that is required to check if a person's expertise is as extensive as it is claimed to be. And so we must operate on **trust** that the expert is qualified and experienced to exactly the extent that the proponent claims is the case. Of course, our trust may be misplaced, and we may discover that the 'expert' we are urged to defer to has minimal expertise. At that point, the expertise that previously appeared to support a claim in argument no longer does so, and the proponent's appeal to expertise lacks rational warrant. The exaggerated use of expertise to achieve some gain in argument has been effectively exposed.

Exaggeration is only one of the ways in which the extent of an individual's expertise may be misrepresented. A proponent may also seek to undermine a claim of his opponent in argument by minimizing the expertise of the authority who asserts it. The expert, to whom the opponent appeals in argument, may have the necessary qualifications and experience to warrant the title of expert. And yet the proponent may set out to diminish this individual's qualifications and experience as a means of undermining his or her claim to expertise. A proponent may claim, for example, that expert *E* did not attend a prestigious medical school in a high-ranking university. For this reason, the proponent argues, we must doubt the quality of any medical training received and the standing of any qualifications obtained. An expert's experience may also be misrepresented. A proponent may claim that an expert has limited clinical experience and that this compromises his ability to assert particular opinions. It may be argued, for example, that an expert only has clinical experience of patients with child-onset epilepsy and so he or she cannot competently assert opinions about the treatment of adult-onset epilepsy. In each of these scenarios, the extent of an individual's expertise is purposefully minimized with a view to invalidating the claims or opinions that an expert can competently assert. The minimization and exaggeration of an individual's true expertise are two of the most common deceptive strategies in the use of expert appeals. The misrepresentation of the extent of an individual's expertise is the first logical pitfall in the use of the argument from expertise:

Logical pitfall 1: The extent of expertise is misrepresented

The proponent and opponent in argument may selectively exaggerate and minimize the expertise of authorities with a view to securing acceptance of a proposition or claim.

By way of illustration of this logical pitfall, let us consider an article about talc-related cancers that appeared in the *Mail Online* on 22 June 2018. In this article, reporter Simon Lennon describes how Phillip Gower, a British solicitor, has teamed up with an attorney in the US who has mounted numerous successful legal challenges against the manufacturers of talcum powder. The basis of these challenges is that the powder is responsible for the development of mesothelioma and ovarian cancer in a significant number of people, particularly middle-aged women, who used the product as a toiletry during their teenage years. Mesothelioma is an aggressive cancer that is associated with exposure to asbestos, most often in the construction industry. It develops in the lining of the heart, lungs, and abdomen. Talcum powder is made from talc which is often located near asbestos deposits. It is believed that talc became contaminated with asbestos during earlier mining techniques which have since been modified.

Talcum powder cancer 'ticking timebomb': Solicitor warns middle-aged women at risk of disease due to use of toiletry in their teens

» A solicitor has warned of a 'ticking timebomb' of cancer among middle-aged women due to them using talcum powder as teenagers.

Phillip Gower fears thousands of British women could have deadly cancer linked to extensive use of talc sold by popular high street brands [...]

Mr Gower, of Simpson Millar solicitors, has teamed up with a US attorney, who has a string of court victories for women with talc-related cancer under his belt.

The news comes after a New Jersey investment banker was awarded $117 million (£88m) in damages in April after developing mesothelioma through asbestos dust in Johnson and Johnson talcum powders.

Mr Gower, who estimates thousands of British men and women have been affected, told Mail Online: 'It's a massive scandal and is only going to get bigger.'

'There is a big problem out there. So far we are just scratching the surface. This is a ticking timebomb.'

'We believe many women were unaware that using talcum powder could have been bad for them and some of them are now seriously ill.'

'Others have unfortunately died and their families only found out about the potential link afterwards.'

Mr Gower, an expert on asbestos-related mesothelioma, heavily linked to the use of talc, added: 'People are rightly worried and concerned.'

'It was an incredibly popular product among women just a few decades ago and now unfortunately they and their children are paying the price.'

'They should have been told about the risks but they were kept in the dark.'
(Simon Lennon, *Mail Online*, 22 June 2018)

Mr Gower is reported to be an 'expert on asbestos-related mesothelioma, heavily linked to the use of talc'. It is undoubtedly the case that Mr Gower has *some* expertise. He is, after all, a solicitor who will have the requisite academic and professional qualifications that are needed to practice law. Mr Gower probably also has *some* training and qualification in medicine. This is because many lawyers who specialize in complex medical cases have dual training and professional qualifications in medicine and law. But to describe Mr Gower as an 'expert' on asbestos-related mesothelioma linked to the use of talc would appear to be an exaggeration by any reasonable standard. If Mr Gower does have formal medical training—and we may even be charitable in attributing this much to him—it is by no means certain that this would amount to the level of medical specialization that would be needed in order to be described as an 'expert' in talc-related mesothelioma. By way of comparison, it is worth noting how the article reports the views of various *actual* experts who have investigated the purported link between use of talcum powder and cancers such as mesothelioma. One such expert is Professor Paul Pharoah, an epidemiologist at Cambridge University, who is reported not to have found a strong link between talc and ovarian cancer. Meanwhile, Dr Daniel Cramer, an epidemiologist at Harvard University and a consultant for one of the legal trials against Johnson & Johnson, is reported to have found that some talcum powders increase the risk of developing ovarian cancer by 30%. These are the true experts on talc-related cancers, not Mr Gower, regardless of how well versed he is in the scientific literature on the issue.

As well as misrepresenting the extent of an individual's expertise, a proponent in argument may also misrepresent the field or discipline in which an individual's expertise has been gained. Expertise in geriatric medicine does not qualify someone to make pronouncements about the containment of Ebola virus disease or about the treatment of anorexia nervosa in adolescents. Even within medical disciplines, an expert in one aspect of a field is not necessarily qualified to advance an opinion about an issue in another aspect of a field. For example, a neonatal cardiologist who asserts opinions about the heart problems of elderly people may stray beyond the limits of his or her expertise. It is not difficult to see how this particular error or deception in the use of expert opinion may pass undetected in argument. Many lay people do not understand that cardiology is the branch of medicine that diagnoses and treats diseases and abnormalities of the heart. Even among those who do recognize the term, they may struggle to identify *neonatal* cardiology as the sub-discipline in cardiology that specializes in the diagnosis and treatment of heart defects in neonates or newborns. Against this lack of knowledge, a logical sleight of hand is particularly easy to perpetrate against an opponent in argument. Such an opponent may simply hear the word 'cardiologist' and assume that this individual is qualified to make expert statements about any type of heart condition whatsoever, including conditions that are never encountered in neonates. Worse still is a situation in which an opponent simply assumes that the title of cardiologist qualifies an individual to make expert statements on *any* medical as well as non-medical issue in a type of **halo effect** (see Walton [1997] for discussion). An error of this type is the basis of our second logical pitfall in the use of argument from expertise:

Logical pitfall 2: Expertise is specific to a field or domain

It may be wrongly assumed (or actively promoted) by proponents and opponents in argument that expertise in one field or discipline entails expertise in another field or discipline. Expertise is discipline-specific, and should be evaluated as such in argument.

The understanding of many complex medical and health conditions requires the involvement of experts from a range of different fields. Autism is a case in point.

Because of the wide array of symptoms in this neurodevelopmental disorder, autism is investigated by geneticists, epidemiologists, cognitive scientists and neuroscientists, psychologists, linguists, and many other experts. This combined expertise is not just important in terms of studying autism, it is vital to our understanding of the condition. This is because no single individual can embody the vast knowledge that is required to understand this complex neurodevelopmental disorder. Collaboration between different experts who converge on a disorder or problem often makes possible new and productive lines of inquiry. But difficulties can arise in a large, interdisciplinary area of research such as that into autism when one group of experts make claims or pronouncements about an aspect of autism that lies beyond their area of expertise. We would be rightly concerned, for example, if epidemiologists who study the incidence and prevalence of autism began to assert statements about the language and communication skills of people with this condition. However, we might view it as appropriate that a geneticist should attempt to explain aspects of the behavioural phenotype of autism typically studied by psychologists in terms of certain defective genes. In short, experts in one discipline that investigates autism can appropriately assert views on issues that lie within another discipline on only some occasions. On other occasions, an expert who asserts such views is overstepping the boundaries of his or her legitimate expertise.

DISCUSSION POINT: Gene editing and autism

Does expertise in gene-editing technology qualify someone to express views about the behavioural symptoms of autism? At least one team of researchers at the University of Texas thinks so. As reported in the *Mail Online* on 26 June 2018, this team believes that it is able to manipulate behavioural symptoms of autism. This belief is based on a study of behavioural changes in mice that were brought about by the use of CRISPR gene editing (see Sect. 3.3 in Chapter 3 for discussion of CRISPR gene editing). By editing genes in mice, these scientists were able to reduce the mice's digging behaviour by around 30% and their jumping by around 70%. Study leader Hye Young Lee from the University of Texas said:

> There are no treatments or cures for autism yet, and many of the clinical trials of small-molecule treatments targeting proteins that cause autism have failed. This is the first case where we were able to edit a causal gene for autism in the brain and show rescue of the behavioral symptoms.
> ('Autism traits may be edited out in the future using new genetic techniques: Scientists complete successful trial to change the way the brain works', Sam Blanchard, *Mail Online*, 26 June 2018)

You should discuss this study and its findings in a small group. In your discussion, you might want to consider if this is appropriate transference of expertise from one discipline (genetic engineering) with a scientific interest in autism to another discipline (psychology), also with a scientific interest in autism. (It is typically psychologists who study the behavioural traits of autism.) Alternatively, you might want to debate with your group members whether experts in the CRISPR gene-editing technology are overstepping the limits of their own expertise when they make statements about the recovery of the behavioural symptoms of autism.

It is a sign of the value and prestige that are attached to expertise that there are many individuals, companies, and organizations that seek to influence it. This influence may be achieved in more or less subtle and significant ways. It may involve pharmaceutical companies providing financial rewards and gifts to doctors who recommend certain drugs to their patients. Alternatively, influence of expertise may be achieved by the financial support of scientific research. This type of influence is particularly pernicious if a potential conflict of interest is not declared by researchers, or if commercial and other sponsors attempt to modify findings or prevent the publication of unfavourable results. Less subtle exploitation of expertise is used in the advertising and marketing of products of various kinds to consumers. We might be persuaded to buy a certain vitamin supplement because it has been recommended by a nutritionist, or to use a particular brand of toothpaste because a dental expert in a television commercial gives his approval to the product. In each of these scenarios, expertise sits alongside a number of commercial and financial interests. The issue, then, for anyone assessing an appeal to expertise in argument is the extent to which these interests influence the opinions and views that are asserted by experts. In an ideal world, experts would only be motivated to produce certain opinions because they believe those opinions to express objective and true 'facts'. But this is not an ideal world, at least as far as the use of expertise in argument is concerned. Expertise can be very malleable depending on who is sponsoring the expert to produce certain claims. The intrusion of external interests on expertise is the basis of the third logical pitfall in the use of expert argument:

Logical pitfall 3: Expert opinion is influenced by external interests

An expert may assert certain opinions because of commercial or other interests, not because he believes these opinions to be true. Where external interests can be shown to influence the views of an expert, the claims of that expert must be rejected.

When the expertise of scientists is compromised by external interests, the penalties are often appropriately severe. On 15 June 2018, *The New York Times* reported that the National Institutes of Health (NIH) had closed down a major global study of the health effects of alcohol that had received $100 million in funding when it was discovered that the National Institute on Alcohol Abuse and Alcoholism, which is part of the NIH, had solicited funding from alcohol manufacturers. An investigation revealed that various interactions had taken place between the study researchers and industry representatives. For example, alcohol industry officials were found to have offered input into the design of the trial. An advisory panel to Dr Francis Collins, director of the NIH, concluded that:

> The early and frequent engagement with industry representatives calls into question the impartiality of the process and thus casts doubt that the scientific knowledge gained from the study would be actionable or believable.

It is with a view to protecting the integrity of researchers and the objectivity of their findings that actions such as those of the NIH are taken. The very credibility of the institution of science requires that we are able to trust experts and the claims that they make. This credibility is threatened when there is inappropriate industry or commercial involvement in scientific research. In this case, an assertion from a scientific expert has no more logical force or weight than an assertion from someone who has no scientific training or knowledge. The fundamental commitment of an expert to the truth of his or her claims is effectively eroded.

It is not always immediately apparent to participants in an argument if an appeal to expertise is compromised as a result of external interests. In the above case, it was an investigation by *The New York Times* that revealed a serious conflict of interest on the part of the researchers in the alcohol study. But the investigative resources of a large national newspaper far exceed the resources that are available to participants in an argument. For these arguers, they must establish if an expert is biased by posing a number of critical questions à la Walton (1997). They should interrogate if an individual or organization stands to benefit from the results of an investigation. If so, it is reasonable to ask if the individual or organization in question is funding the expert's research. This is because we should be sceptical about a study, for example, that reports no adverse health effects of vaping if the study has been funded by manufacturers of e-cigarettes. In the absence of financial gain, arguers should also interrogate if an expert is motivated to produce opinions or arrive at conclusions for other reasons. For example, an expert with conservative religious views may exaggerate his or her findings about the capacity of a foetus to experience pain in utero with a view to resisting the relaxation of the anti-abortion law in a country or state. Similarly, a medical expert with strong political views may argue that population-level health interventions such as vaccination programmes and water fluoridation schemes should not be implemented. This is not because of a lack of proven health benefits, but because the expert views these interventions as a violation of an individual's liberty. In all these cases, targeted critical questions that interrogate the basis of an expert's views and opinions have the potential to uncover bias, should it exist.

SPECIAL TOPIC: Human papilloma virus (HPV) vaccine safety

There are undeniable benefits of vaccinations for human health. However, trust in the safety and effectiveness of vaccines is damaged when public health experts find their integrity challenged by accusations of commercial interests and other conflicts of interest. Many of these accusations are false or exaggerated. They are often advanced by so-called anti-vaxxers, a group of people who are trenchant in their opposition to vaccination, particularly of their own children. One vaccine in particular has been damaged by the claims of anti-vaxxers. This is the vaccine that provides protection against HPV, a virus that is linked to cervical cancer in women and other cancers (e.g. oral and throat cancers) in men. On 3 December 2017, *The Guardian* in the UK reported that Japan, Ireland, and Denmark had all seen significant reductions in the uptake of HPV vaccine as a result of anti-vaccine campaigns. These campaigns, which allege adverse health effects of the vaccine, are often waged on social media:

> Japan, Ireland and Denmark have already witnessed sustained campaigns that have seen take-up rates plummet. (UK take-up rates are high.) In each case, the vaccine – which scientists insist is safe – has been linked to alleged cases of seizures, walking problems, and neurological issues. Photographs have been exchanged and video clips uploaded to YouTube.
> ('Fears for women's health as parents reject HPV vaccine', *The Guardian*, Robin McKie, 3 December 2017)

Often what lies behind these allegations is fervent opposition to the pharmaceutical industry that manufactures and markets Gardasil and Cervarix, the two trade names of the HPV vaccine. A frequent accusation against so-called Big Pharma is that it exercises inappropriate influence over the public health experts who advise parents to have their children vaccinated against HPV. This view is evident in the following comment that was posted in response to an earlier article on the HPV vaccine that also appeared in *The Guardian*:

> Countries which have banned Gardasil include India, France and Japan. The numbers of young girls showing serious side effects from this vaccine should raise alarm bells in all parents. Big pharma cannot be trusted, neither can those in the pockets of big pharma.
> (Comment on: 'We know it's effective. So why is there opposition to the HPV vaccine?', *The Guardian*, David Robert Grimes, 11 January 2016)

Views like that above arise when a challenge to the objectivity and integrity of experts is not based on evidence. An expert and his claims are discredited by an opponent who has adopted an entrenched position in argument. From this position, every opinion that is asserted by experts is biased and is not to be trusted. This entrenched stance about health experts is common among anti-vaxxers, and not just in relation to HPV vaccine. When it is not challenged and overturned by sound scientific argument, it can cause considerable damage to safe, effective immunization programs.

There is a final logical pitfall in the use of expert appeal in argument. When an expert advances a view or opinion, there is normally some qualification on how it is expressed and on how it may be interpreted or understood. If a public health expert claims that all cases of dengue fever in Hong Kong between 1 April 2018 and 31 March 2019 are linked to dengue virus serotype 4, then we would not expect this claim to be reported without any temporal qualification: *All cases of dengue fever in Hong Kong are linked to dengue virus serotype 4.* By the same token, we would not expect to hear this expert's claim reported without any geographical qualification: *All cases of dengue fever between 1 April 2018 and 31 March 2019 are linked to dengue virus serotype 4.* The removal of temporal and geographical qualification from this expert's statement has the effect of changing the proposition that the expert asserts. The expert's expressed view or opinion has been misrepresented in the act of reporting it. We would also not expect a view or opinion that is expressed tentatively by an expert to be reported with all the certainty that the expert's original formulation was intended to avoid.

The expert who asserts that an avian virus *may* mutate and *may* transmit to humans is definitely not asserting that an avian virus *will* mutate and *will* transmit to humans. Even experts are entitled to express their views with greater or lesser certainty, and to have these different levels of epistemic commitment to a proposition reflected accurately when their views are reported in argument. The misrepresentation of an expert's views illustrated by these examples is the basis of the fourth logical pitfall in the use of argument from expertise:

Logical pitfall 4: Expert opinion is inaccurately reported

The qualification and certainty with which an expert expresses an opinion is misrepresented at the point at which the opinion is reported in argument. Misrepresentation of this type substantially alters the proposition that the expert asserts.

Experts' views are frequently misrepresented when they are reported by others. This occurs most commonly in the print media. It is not difficult to see why this is the case. Newspaper editors want to publish sensationalist claims that arouse the interest of readers. The tentative claims of an expert may be an accurate representation of the current state of scientific knowledge. But cautious, measured statements do not sell newspapers. A headline that states EXPERTS WARN THAT AN AVIAN VIRUS WILL TRANSMIT TO HUMANS is certain to engage the attention of readers. If the same headline were expressed tentatively using the auxiliary verbs *may* and *might*, readers could query its newsworthiness. Caveats, qualifications, and uncertainty are an integral part of many expert opinions. However, their significance is diminished in newspaper editorial processes that subordinate scientific accuracy to hard-hitting headlines and attention-grabbing statements. In an article in the *British Medical Journal*, Margaret McCartney, a general practitioner from Glasgow in the UK, identifies press releases as a source of much of the misrepresentation of the views and findings of scientists. She argues that although they provide journalists with easy articles, they do so at the expense of distorting the claims of scientists. As a way forward, she asks: 'Should we formalise press release writing to highlight uncertainties and caveats?' Awareness that uncertainty and caveats are *part of* the message that experts wish to convey, and not aspects of meaning and language that can simply be jettisoned in the reporting of experts' views, would go some way to addressing this particular logical error in the use of the argument from expertise.

You can now get practice at identifying logical pitfalls in the use of the argument from expertise by attempting Exercise 5.3.

EXERCISE 5.3: Scientists develop a new insulin pill

On 29 June 2018, an article about an insulin pill appeared in the *Mail Online*. The article reported how scientists had developed an insulin pill that could signal the end of injections for diabetics. All previous attempts to develop oral diabetes medications had failed. The newly developed pill, however, survived the acidic environment of the stomach to release insulin into the bloodstream. The views of two experts are reported in the article. One expert is described as having no involvement in the study. The other expert is the author of the study. Examine the following extracts from the article, and then answer the questions below:

» Dr Mark Prausnitz, from the Georgia Institute of Technology, who was not involved in the study, said: 'This study shows remarkable results where insulin given by mouth works about as well as a conventional injection'. […]

Study author Professor Samir Mitragotri, from Harvard, said: 'Once ingested, insulin must navigate a challenging obstacle course before it can be effectively absorbed into the bloodstream'.

'Our approach is like a Swiss Army knife, where one pill has tools for addressing each of the obstacles that are encountered.' […]

Speaking of the benefits of such a drug, Professor Mitragotri said: 'Many people fail to adhere to [the injection] regimen due to pain, phobia of needles, and the interference with normal activities'.

'The consequences of the resulting poor glycemic control can lead to serious health complications.'

Dr Prausnitz added: 'It has been the holy grail of drug delivery to develop ways to give protein and peptide drugs like insulin by mouth, instead of injection'.

'The implications of this work to medicine could be huge if the findings can be translated into pills that safely and effectively administer insulin to humans'. ('Could this be the end of painful injections for diabetics? Scientists create an insulin pill with "remarkable results"', *Mail Online*, Alexandra Thompson, 29 June 2018)

Questions

(a) The academic titles and university affiliations of both experts in this article are indicated. What other linguistic marker might also help readers to establish the expertise of these scientists?

(b) The article states that Dr Mark Prausnitz is 'not involved in the study'. However, a background examination reveals that Dr Prausnitz has previously co-authored scientific articles with the lead investigator of the study, Professor Mitragotri. Does the joint publication of scientific articles with the lead investigator of the study pose a conflict of interest for Dr Prausnitz? Provide a justification of your response.

(c) When they report expert views, newspapers often omit caveats or qualifications that are integral to the opinions expressed by experts. Does this happen when Dr Prausnitz's claims are reported?

(d) A frequent criticism of experts is that they are unable to express their views in a manner that can be readily understood by lay people. What linguistic device does Professor Mitragotri use to convey clearly to readers how this new drug works?

(e) Identify *one* proposition about insulin that is asserted by each of the experts in this article.

5.5 Expert Appeal in the Social Sciences

We have argued that the relation between an expert and his or her assertions is a rather special one. Any assertion involves the truth of the claim or proposition that is asserted. But when an assertion is produced by an expert, it comes with an additional guarantee of veracity and scientific accuracy. Put simply, when an expert asserts that *p*, we can be certain that *p* really is the case. Or at least this is what we have believed, or have been led to believe, to date. More recently, expertise has lost some of its special status. It no longer comes with a cast-iron guarantee of scientific objectivity and truth. In fact, in some quarters, the term 'expert' has become a derogatory designation. This was particularly evident in the period leading up to the UK's referendum on 23 June 2016 on the future place of the United Kingdom in the European Union. Campaigners who wanted the UK to leave the EU (so-called Brexit campaigners) were keen to dismiss the views of experts, many of whom warned of serious economic consequences if the UK voted to leave. In a Sky News question-and-answer session on 3 June 2016, the UK's justice secretary, Michael Gove (a prominent Brexit campaigner), even went as far as to declare that "people in this country have had enough of experts" ('Britain has had enough of experts, says Gove', *Financial Times*, 3 June 2016). Aside from political manoeuvring, expertise has been damaged by continually changing scientific advice and by notable public health failures (e.g. the failure to predict the transmission of BSE to humans). Scientific and medical experts have also been tarnished by accusations (many of them validated) that they are unduly influenced by industry. Expertise, it seems, has never before experienced such a crisis of public confidence.

SPECIAL TOPIC: Scientific experts under the spotlight

There is intense scrutiny of scientific experts, and with some justification. In the domain of public opinion, experts still exercise considerable influence on the decisions we make and courses of action that we take. In order to warrant this position of influence, experts must have their beliefs, motivations, and claims interrogated. Where expert claims are found to be problematic, the individuals who promote them should be exposed in order that bogus experts and fraudulent claims can be completely rejected. Only then can it be said that scientific experts are 'under the spotlight' from the public that they serve.

It was described in ▶ Sect. 5.4 how the investigators of a major global study of the health effects of moderate alcohol consumption were exposed by *The New York Times* for their receipt of funding from the alcohol industry. In return for this funding, alcohol industry representatives were given significant involvement in the design of the study, including the selection of participants. This egregious violation of scientific procedure and professional conduct is, unfortunately, not uncommon. On 2 August 2011, an article that appeared in *The Guardian* revealed the extent of a practice in which 'independent, influential academics' would appear as guest authors of papers that had been written by pharmaceutical companies. One pharmaceutical company called Wyeth had used so-called ghostwriters to prepare

26 medical articles that had emphasized the benefits and downplayed the risks of taking HRT for conditions such as heart disease and dementia. The article reported calls for scientists who engaged in the practice of ghostwriting to be charged with fraud. Trudo Lemmens, a law professor at the University of Toronto, remarked of the practice:

» It's a prostitution of their [scientists'] academic standing. And it undermines the integrity of the entire academic publication system. ('Scientists credited on ghostwritten articles "should be charged with fraud"' *The Guardian*, Ian Semple, 2 August 2011)

Fraudulent authorship of academic work is not the only abuse of scientific expertise that would appear to be widespread. On 7 April 2009, the *Independent* reported that the Law Commission for England and Wales was publishing preliminary proposals that would aim to prevent scientists, doctors, and other experts from giving misleading evidence in court. Such evidence, it was argued, was responsible for a series of miscarriages of justice. The most prominent miscarriage happened to Sally Clark, a solicitor who was wrongfully convicted of murdering her two infant sons after the jury heard the chances of the babies dying of natural causes was just one in 73 million. Clark's conviction was quashed in 2003 by the Court of Appeal after it was heard that this statistic grossly misrepresented the chance of two sudden deaths within the same family from unexplained but natural causes.

The article in the *Independent* went on to report the cases of several fraudulent 'expert' witnesses who had previously been convicted, including Godwin Onubogu, a bogus medical doctor convicted in 1998, Barian Baluchi, a bogus psychiatrist convicted in 2005, and Gene Morrison, a bogus psychologist convicted in 2007. Professor Jeremy Horder, the commissioner leading the work of the Law Commission on expert testimony, explained the rationale behind the proposals in the following terms:

» The parties in criminal trials are relying increasingly on the evidence of expert witnesses. Expert evidence, particularly scientific evidence, can have a very persuasive effect on juries. It is vital that such evidence should be used only if it provides a sound basis for determining a defendant's guilt or innocence. There have been miscarriages of justice in recent years where prosecution expert evidence of doubtful reliability has been placed before Crown Court juries. There may also have been unwarranted acquittals attributable to such evidence. We want to ensure the criminal courts have the means to authenticate expert evidence and be satisfied the information before them is sound. ('Crackdown on expert witnesses', *Independent*, Robert Verkaik, 7 April 2009)

Fraudulent expert testimony in court is a further way in which scientific expertise can fall short of high standards of objectivity and truthfulness. It reminds us once again that the credentials of experts may not be what they seem, and that the only expertise that we should trust is the expertise that can withstand scrutiny.

One of the ways in which we may begin to restore public confidence in experts is by examining the factors that influence our *trust* in them (Cummings 2014). It goes without saying that experts who conduct themselves in an unethical manner by accepting financial incentives to assert certain claims will nearly always experience reduced public trust when their lack of integrity is exposed. But there are many other, more subtle issues involving trust in experts that are not so easily established. For example, the emphasis placed on academic attainment and learning in many societies has encouraged us to defer to people like doctors, lawyers, and university professors on issues that require certain types of expertise. The perceived competence of these individuals may be a key motivation for our trust in them. But academic attainment and high-level learning may not be particularly influential considerations in an assessment of trust for those who lack extensive formal education, for those who have strong kinship relations, or for those who belong to certain age groups. For these individuals, the perceived integrity of an expert may be more influential than competence in an assessment of trust. Also, a lack of personal integrity may have different consequences for our trust in experts depending on their area of expertise. Medical and health experts may be held to higher standards of personal integrity than experts in finance and business, for example. A doctor may suffer irreparable damage in public trust over a financial conflict of interest that has little impact on trust in a finance or business expert. It is on these questions of what *actually* influences how we assess trust in experts that social scientists stand to make their most significant contribution. This section examines some of these scientists' findings.

At the heart of trust in scientists and other experts is the public's credibility in their communication. However, as Fiske and Dupree (2014) have stated '[s]cientists as communicators have earned audiences' respect, but not necessarily their trust' (p. 13593). The public respects the competence and expertise of scientists but may doubt their integrity and trustworthiness. This combination of high competence and low trust has serious consequences for scientific communicators, whose credibility rests not just on their perceived competence but also on their perceived integrity and trustworthiness (warmth[1]). Fiske and Dupree asked adults to rate 42 jobs, including scientists, researchers, professors, and teachers, on warmth and competence dimensions, as well as relevant emotions. Lawyers, chief executive officers, engineers, accountants, scientists, and researchers were ambivalently perceived as having high competence and low warmth. They were also perceived as 'envied' professions. The ability of these professionals to be viewed as credible communicators is compromised by their lack of warmth (and possibly envy). When we appeal to the expertise of scientists and researchers in argument, we may also expect this perceived lack of warmth to have a negative effect on their credibility as communicators of truthful claims. However, for other experts whose views we appeal to in arguments on medicine and health, the situation is quite different. Fiske and Dupree found that doctors are perceived as warm and trustworthy *as well as* capable and competent. Doctors also elicit emotions of admiration and pride. These empirical findings suggest that when we appeal to the expertise of doctors in argument, this professional group's opinions are most likely to be accepted and believed by the public.

So competence or expertise and warmth both contribute to the credibility of scientific communicators. But it is pertinent to ask if there are circumstances in which one of these dimensions outweighs the other in an assessment of credibility. The results of some investigations indicate that there are occasions when study participants subordinate competence or expertise to factors associated with integrity and trustworthiness (warmth). Eiser et al. (2009) found that openness and shared interests were more important predictors of trust in individual sources than perceived expertise. Two sources in their study—resident groups and friends/family—were trusted by participants despite being perceived as relatively inexpert. Allum (2007) found that shared values are more important for citizens' judgements of trust in scientists involved in the development of genetically modified food than beliefs about competence and expertise. The weighting of these dimensions also varies with the issue under consideration. Nakayachi and Cvetkovich (2010) examined determinants of public trust in the government's control of tobacco in Japan. These investigators surveyed 1394 Japanese adults over 20 years old. Determinants of trust were found to vary in accordance with the issue that the participants were asked to assess. On the affirmatively supported issue of prohibiting smoking among minors, competency was a stronger predictor of trust than fairness. By contrast, fairness was a stronger predictor of trust than competency when the contentious issue of increasing tobacco tax was considered. These issue-dependent variations in our trust of experts can also be expected to influence when the opinions of experts are accepted in argument.

Finally, trust in experts also varies significantly with the socio-demographic characteristics of audiences. In a study of survey data from 4845 respondents, Bleich et al. (2007) found that women and more educated individuals had significantly higher odds of trusting scientific experts on obesity. Distrust in scientific experts was associated with Hispanic race and older age (over 50 years). Armstrong et al. (2007) examined the relationship between physician distrust and race/ethnicity, gender, and socioeconomic status in the United States. Socioeconomic status was based on income, education level, and health insurance. Blacks and Hispanics reported higher levels of physician distrust than did Whites. Lower socioeconomic status was in general associated with higher levels of distrust, with men generally reporting more distrust than women. Wada and Smith (2015) examined associations between mistrust for governmental vaccine recommendations and socio-demographic characteristics of 3140 Japanese people aged 20–69 years. A total of 893 (28.4%) individuals reported general mistrust towards the Japanese government's recommendations for vaccination. Relatively poor health in men was associated with general mistrust of vaccination recommendations. Worsening self-rated health conditions for women were significantly associated with mistrust for governmental recommendations on vaccination. Age and differences in education levels were not significantly associated with vaccination mistrust. Similar socio-demographic variables are likely to play a significant role in audience acceptance of a conclusion in an argument from expertise. Empirical studies of this type thus serve to complement a logical analysis of expert appeals in argumentation.

DISCUSSION POINT: The public's trust in non-experts

A significant minority of people place their trust in individuals with no medical expertise when they make decisions relating to their health. Freed et al. (2011) examined parental trust in various sources of information about vaccine safety in 1552 parents of children aged ≤17 years. There were high levels of trust in traditional sources of information about vaccine safety such as family physicians (76% endorsed a lot of trust), other health care providers (26%), and government vaccine experts and officials (23%). However, individuals with no evident medical expertise were also trusted by the participants in this study. Family and friends were trusted by 15% of respondents. Even celebrities were trusted a lot by 2% of respondents. In Wada and Smith's (2015) study of 3140 Japanese adults, the single most trusted information source on vaccination was health care workers (44.1%). Family members were also a significant trusted source for 8.5% of participants, a percentage that was nearly as large as that for government as a trusted source of information (9.1%). Brown-Johnson et al. (2018) conducted phone surveys of a cross-sectional sample of 1001 Oklahoma adults aged 18–65 years to assess their trust in seven media sources. The highest trust was recorded for interpersonal sources: health providers; health insurers; and family/friends. Health providers and health insurers were reported to be trustworthy by 81% and 48% of respondents, respectively. Family and friends received a higher trust rating than health insurers, with 55% of respondents reporting them to be trustworthy.

These figures demonstrate that a significant proportion of people look to sources other than conventional experts in matters relating to health. In a small group, discuss the various factors which might explain why this is occurring. What factors may be pushing people away from conventional experts as a trusted source on health issues? Also, what factors may be pulling people towards trust in individuals and groups with little or no medical expertise on questions of health?

5.6 Expertise as a Cognitive Heuristic

We conclude this chapter by continuing to develop the view that informal fallacies can function as cognitive heuristics during medical and health reasoning. When we have discussed the argument from expertise in this chapter, we have argued that expertise is a powerful tool of rational persuasion in argument, notwithstanding historical accounts of *ad verecundiam* as a weak or fallacious form of reasoning. By advancing the opinion of an expert, a proponent or opponent can effectively gain the upper hand in argument. But there are even stronger grounds why it is a good idea to appeal to expertise in argument. Those grounds relate to the fact that most of us lack the expert knowledge that is required to make pronouncements about a range of issues in medicine and health. I may have very limited knowledge of measles. I may know that it is an infectious disease that can be prevented by vaccination. However, I may know nothing about its incidence and prevalence, its route(s) of transmission, the serious complications that it may cause, and the people who are most at risk of developing these complications. But in reality I need to know none of these things if I can appeal to an expert on measles. I am able to compensate for my knowledge deficit about measles by drawing on the expertise of someone whose knowledge of this infectious disease is particularly well developed. If I can bridge one or more gaps in my knowledge by drawing on a trusted expert, I can make decisions and take courses of action that would otherwise not be possible in the absence of knowledge. Moreover, I can achieve all this while avoiding the need to embark on my own investigation into measles. Appealing to expertise liberates me from this onerous inquiry.

Like ignorance and fear, expertise can achieve certain cognitive efficiencies for those who know how to employ it effectively. It is a one-stop shop for a number of epistemic virtues that we hold dear. When a claim is asserted by a genuine expert, it comes with a guarantee that it is based on the best available evidence. Its truth is assured and we can confidently base our decisions and actions on its propositional content. The expert can stand over the truth of the claims that he asserts because he or she has undertaken the exhaustive inquiries that we cannot pursue for cognitive or practical reasons. The expert's heavy lifting allows the individual who appeals to expertise in argument to have immediate access to a body of knowledge without expending significant cognitive effort. But this individual is not relieved of all epistemic responsibility when he or she makes an expert appeal. An appeal to expertise in argument still carries the significant responsibility of ensuring that the expert that we have chosen to hold aloft merits the title of an expert. This is where the individual who appeals to expertise is required to expend some cognitive effort. But the effort that is required to verify markers of expertise such as academic titles and professional qualifications is altogether less than that required to study vast literatures and to undertake experiments. Academic titles and qualifications are proxies for expertise, the verification of which lies within most individuals' competence and practical resources. An appeal to expertise is an effective shortcut or heuristic through resource-intensive inquiries into an issue or question. A rational agent that must attend to the allocation of its cognitive resources takes this shortcut whenever possible.

Yet again, we see a form of argument that was once condemned as a fallacy resurrected as a cognitive heuristic that facilitates our reasoning about complex issues in health. There is no greater need for this heuristic than in the health domain. As a parent of a child, I cannot engage in extensive deliberation about the safety of a vaccine like the HPV vaccine. I must act within the relatively short period of time that I have been given to sign the consent form for my child to be vaccinated by the school nurse. I also have no special knowledge, experience, or training with which to assess the safety of the HPV vaccine. I have no option but to listen to different experts who make claims about this vaccine's safety. So this is exactly what I do. My expertise heuristic allows me to reject quite quickly the views of two of these experts. They are not credible experts because they also act as consultants for the pharmaceutical company that manufactures the HPV vaccine. A further 'expert' is a family doctor who opposes the use of the vaccine on religious grounds. This doctor believes the vaccine encourages early sexual activity in young girls and that this behaviour must be avoided at all costs. My expertise heuristic guides me away from the views of this individual also. Meanwhile, my expertise heuristic is positively inclining me towards the views of two other experts who support the use of the HPV vaccine. Both experts are senior public health physicians at a highly respected government health agency in the UK. I decide to accept their reassurances about the safety of the HPV vaccine, and proceed to sign my child's vaccination consent form. The entire deliberative process guided by an expertise heuristic reaches a conclusion within a reasonable timeframe.

This scenario is typical of many everyday situations where we are compelled to make judgements about complex medical and health issues in the absence of expert knowledge. And yet we make these judgements and, for the most part, do so quite competently. This is only possible because we are able to press an expertise heuristic into action. This heuristic is a vital adaptation of our rational procedures to the problem of reasoning in the practical sphere, where knowledge can be scarce and time is often limited. In this sphere, quick rules of thumb or mental shortcuts are needed in order to bypass the vast bodies of knowledge that are possessed by experts. The systematic reasoning of experts, in which evidence is carefully scrutinised and weighed up, is a cognitive luxury that the practically situated agent cannot afford. But we can still glean some of the benefits of expertise, particularly the above average propensity to be accurate, by being guided by an expertise heuristic. This heuristic is attuned to certain markers of expertise which have **cognitive salience** for us as a result. So we attend to features of experts like academic titles, qualifications, and areas of specialization, and leave aside the bodies of knowledge that they have accrued over many years of formal education and professional experience. Because the heuristic is an adaptation (evolutionary or otherwise) of more systematic processes of reasoning, we can be sure that its dictates—*Attend to this! Ignore that!*—will lead us on most occasions to an accurate (truthful) conclusion. Error is still a *possible* outcome of the use of an expertise heuristic in exactly the same way that systematic reasoning can result in an erroneous conclusion. But error is not a *more likely* outcome as the result of the use of an expertise heuristic.[2]

The rationale for an expertise heuristic is certainly clear enough. However, specific proposals about the form that this heuristic should take have largely not been forthcoming. One exception is Walton (2010) who proposes the concept of a parascheme. A parascheme is part of an older cognitive system which is fast and automatic and uses heuristics to jump to conclusions. Each parascheme is associated with an argumentation scheme. This is part of a newer (in evolutionary terms) cognitive system that is slow, controlled, and conscious. The person who reasons according to an argumentation scheme addresses critical questions that are aimed at exposing logical weaknesses in an argument, if such weaknesses exist. Applied to the argument from expertise, a heuristic in an expertise parascheme permits us to leap directly from the premises *E is an expert* and *E asserts that A* to the conclusion that *A is true* (see ◘ Fig. 5.2). An expertise heuristic bypasses assumptions such as *E is sufficiently knowledgeable as an expert source* and *E is an expert in the field that A is in*. The processing of such assumptions requires considerable cognitive effort on our part, and is a feature of the slower, deliberative processes that are associated with an argumentation scheme. Walton's proposal that expertise can be effectively interrogated by the posing of critical questions certainly seems intuitively correct. When we evaluated the nature and extent of an individual's expertise in the cases examined in earlier sections of this chapter, we were essentially posing and responding to critical questions. But whether critical questions can be integrated into a framework that befits the cognitive orientation of an expertise heuristic awaits further development of the program of fallacies-as-heuristics.

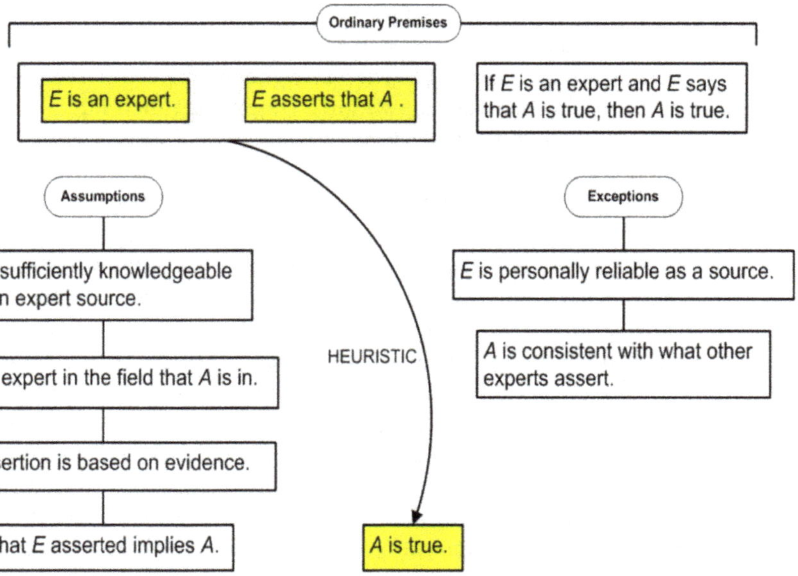

Fig. 5.2 Heuristic of argument from expert opinion according to Walton (2010) (Reproduced courtesy of Douglas Walton and *Informal Logic*)

NOTES

1. Fiske and Dupree (2014) define warmth as follows: "The warmth/trustworthiness judgment assesses the other's perceived intent for good or ill (friend or foe)" (p. 13596).
2. Heuristics are no more prone to error than more complex reasoning strategies, as Todd and Gigerenzer (2000) remark: "[S]imple heuristics perform comparably to more complex algorithms, particularly when generalizing to new data" (p. 727).

Chapter Summary

Key points

- The opinion of an expert can carry substantial weight in argument. This was not always considered to be the case, however. The idea that we should accept as true the opinion of a man because he has 'learning, eminency, and power' seemed to Locke and many earlier (and later) generations of philosophers the weakest of all reasons to accept a claim as true. The *argumentum ad verecundiam* was thus set on its course as a logical fallacy.
- Expertise is not only used in argumentative discourse. There are many non-logical uses of expertise. It is possible to describe, interrogate, and even evaluate an individual's expertise without thereby using that expertise to support a claim in argument. These non-logical uses of expertise may occur as part of argumentative discourse or as separate forms of discourse.

- The logical structure of the argument from expertise can be variously characterized. At a minimum, the argument contains a single premise that states that an expert *E* asserts that a proposition *A* is known to be true. Additional premises, which often remain implicit, state that *E* is an expert in domain *D*, and that *A* is within domain *D*. Reflecting the presumptive character of the argument, the conclusion states that *A* may plausibly be taken to be true.
- There are various ways in which the argument from expertise may be abused and misused. These logical errors and pitfalls include misrepresenting (usually exaggerating) the extent of an individual's expertise. They can also include misrepresenting the field or domain in which an individual's expertise lies. Expertise in one medical domain (e.g. cardiology) does not necessarily qualify someone to make pronouncements in another medical domain (e.g. neurology).
- Expertise can also be compromised by external interests. We are rightly inclined not to trust statements about vaccine safety from a scientific expert who is funded by vaccine manufacturers. The opinions of experts may also be distorted or misrepresented in the process of reporting them. Vital caveats and qualifications may be omitted.
- Social scientists have produced an extensive body of empirical findings on what influences our trust in experts. Competence and expertise can be subordinated to judgements of personal integrity and trustworthiness, with some study participants prioritising the honesty of friends and family over the competence of experts. Socio-demographic features of audiences such as age, gender, and ethnicity also influence trust in experts.
- Expertise is an effective heuristic during reasoning about complex health issues. It allows us to bypass vast literatures and experimentation which are costly for agents in terms of time and cognitive effort. By attending to salient markers of expertise, we can rapidly form judgements about the statements that we can accept as true.

Suggestions for Further Reading

(1) Kutrovátz, G. (2012). Expert authority and ad verecundiam arguments. In F. H. van Eemeren & B. Garssen (Eds.), *Exploring argumentative contexts* (pp. 195–212). Amsterdam: John Benjamins Publishing Company.

This chapter contrasts a number of approaches to the study of *ad verecundiam* arguments. These approaches include the work of pragma-dialecticians, who treat fallacious uses of the argument as a violation of rules of rational discussion, and Douglas Walton who characterizes expert appeals in terms of argument schemes. Empirical considerations relating to appeals to authority are also addressed through an examination of Internet blog discussions of the case of H1N1 (swine flu).

(2) Cummings, L. (2015). Argument from authority. In *Reasoning and public health: New ways of coping with uncertainty* (pp. 67–92). Cham: Springer.

This chapter examines the argument from expertise or authority in the context of public health. The discussion includes the logical structure of the argument, historical views of logicians, and dialectical and epistemic analyses of expert appeals. The chapter also addresses the role of expert argument in systematic and heuristic reasoning, and considers the findings of an empirical study of arguments from expertise in 879 members of the public.

(3) Walton, D. (1997). *Appeal to expert opinion: Arguments from authority*. University Park: Pennsylvania State University Press.

5

This is the only book-length treatment of arguments from authority from the perspective of informal logic. Walton undertakes a wide-ranging discussion that includes the historical background of these arguments, the different forms of the argument, and dialectical aspects of expert appeals. Scientific expertise as expert testimony in legal settings is examined in ▸ Chapter 6. Other contexts for the examination of this argument are advertising, political debate, and health.

Questions

(1) We have seen in this chapter how logical and non-logical uses may be made of expertise. Only in the former use is it possible to identify a proposition that is *true* on account of the fact that it is uttered by an expert. The following extract is taken from an article that appeared in *The Sydney Morning Herald*. The article is discussing a once-a-month injection that helps stop the onset of migraines. The injection is already approved in the United States and there are plans to make the treatment available in Australia. The views of two neurologists about the new migraine treatment are reported. Your task is to identify *three* propositions or claims that are *true* because they are asserted by these neurologists.

New drug offers relief for millions of migraine sufferers

The current preventive treatments for migraines involve combinations of drugs and other therapies not designed for headache disorders, including antidepressants, anti-epileptic drugs and botox.

"Patients using [botox] were telling their doctors their headaches were getting better", Professor Tissa Wijeratne, a leading neurologist, said. "Initially the doctors were laughing at them, then trials were done and sure enough it was found to be beneficial." [...]

Professor Wijeratne said many of these medications had unpleasant side effects preventing them from being taken long term, while there were some patients who did not respond to them at all. [...]

Melbourne neurologist David Williams said he was anxiously awaiting the drug for his patients who had not responded to other treatments.

"People with chronic migraine can be in a state where they are working less than 50 per cent of their brain capacity all the time", he said.
(*The Sydney Morning Herald*, Aisha Dow, 16 June 2018)

(2) The relationship between coffee consumption and heart health is quite often discussed in newspaper articles. While some scientific studies demonstrate a protective effect of coffee and caffeine on heart function, other studies suggest that caffeine may cause heart damage. The following extract is taken from an article that appeared in *Mail Online* on 21 June 2018. In this article, health reporter Sam Blanchard is describing the findings of a study by a group of German researchers based at the Heinrich Heine University and IUF-Leibniz Research Institute for Environmental Medicine in Dusseldorf. The extract reports the views of two 'experts', one of whom is the study author. Examine the extract in detail, and then answer the questions below:

Drinking four cups of coffee a day could help the heart grow stronger and repair itself from damage, study suggests
Pensioners should drink four cups of coffee a day to protect and repair their heart muscle, research suggests. [...]

Study author Professor Judith Haendeler of the IUF-Leibniz Research Institute for Environmental Medicine in Dusseldorf said: 'Our results indicate a new mode of action for caffeine, one that promotes protection and repair of heart muscle'.

'These results should lead to better strategies for protecting heart muscle from damage, including consideration of coffee consumption or caffeine as an additional dietary factor in the elderly population.' [...]

'With respect to ageing and thus to the elderly population, our data demonstrate that the mitochondrial capacity of the old heart is improved by caffeine to that of the adult heart.' [...]

Professor Tim Chico from the University of Sheffield said: 'These researchers have discovered that a protein called p27 is important for recovery after heart attack in mice, and that p27 function is boosted by caffeine'.

'These are very interesting findings but need to be confirmed in clinical trials before we can tell whether caffeine is truly helpful after a heart attack in humans.'

'There is already some evidence suggesting coffee might protect against some diseases, which if true could be due to the effect of caffeine on p27.'

'I do not think people need to drink more coffee in response to this study, but that people who already drink coffee can be reassured that it might have health benefits (as long as they don't use it to wash down an enormous muffin, cake, or doughnut).'
(*Mail Online*, Sam Blanchard, 21 June 2018)

Questions

(a) What *two* linguistic markers are used to confer cognitive authority on the two experts in this article?

(b) To what extent is your view of the expertise of these authorities influenced by the geographical location of their academic institutions? Provide a justification of your response.

(c) The utterances of experts (and other language users) can contain more than one proposition. For each of the experts in this article, identify an utterance that contains more than one proposition. For each utterance, state what these propositions are.

(d) Professor Tim Chico states that the findings of the German study need to be confirmed in clinical trials before it is possible to say if caffeine is helpful after a heart attack in humans. Which premise in an argument from expertise is this comment particularly relevant to?

(e) Often, practical advice and recommendations are based on appeals to expertise. Identify *one* recommendation offered by each of the experts in this article as a result of this study's findings.

(3) We rely on experts to tell us facts. Facts are taken to represent how things *actually* are in the world. They are *the truth* unmediated by any particular viewpoint, bias, or other influence. Many public health messages place an emphasis on presenting facts about disease and illness. The source of these facts is expert individuals and institutions. Examine the following messages and the facts that they convey. Then answer the questions below (Fig. 5.3).

Questions

(a) The source of these facts about Hepatitis C and Ebola virus are two public health agencies. Both agencies are widely regarded as expert bodies. Describe the factors that contribute to their expertise.

(b) The argument from expertise was described as a three-premise argument in ▶ Sect. 5.3. To which of these premises do the facts in the above posters relate?

(c) The third premise in an argument from expertise states that a proposition *A* is within domain *D*. What is the domain to which these posters relate? Is it true to say that each of the propositions conveyed by the facts in these posters relate to this domain?

(d) An epistemic distinction is often made between *propositional* knowledge (knowledge *that* something is the case) and *procedural* knowledge (knowledge *how* to do something). To which of these types of knowledge do the facts in these posters contribute?

(e) Hepatitis C infection is a treatable condition. Currently, Ebola virus disease cannot be directly treated, although symptoms can be more or less successfully managed. How does this difference between these infectious diseases alter the expert advice that is offered by these public health agencies?

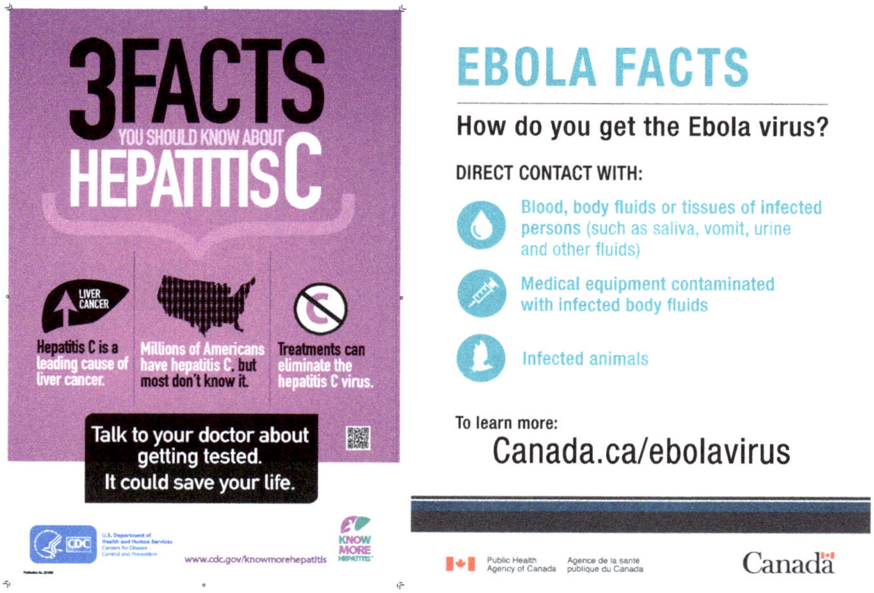

Fig. 5.3 The facts about Hepatitis C infection and Ebola virus disease (© All rights reserved. *Ebola Facts: How do you get the Ebola virus?* Public Health Agency of Canada, 2016. Adapted and reproduced with permission from the Minister of Health, 2018)

Answers

Exercise 5.1

(a) Logical use of expertise – it is *true* that there is little evidence that nudging people alone will help them shun unhealthy choices because academics, led by Theresa Marteau of Cambridge University, believe that this is the case.

(b) Non-logical use of expertise.

(c) Logical use of expertise – it is *true* that there is not strong evidence that coffee does cause cancer because Dr Kathryn Wilson of the Harvard Medical School says that this is the case.

(d) Non-logical use of expertise.

(e) Logical use of expertise – it is *true* that current volumes of antibiotic usage are too high to be sustainable because Professor Mark Woolhouse of the University of Edinburgh says that this is the case.

Exercise 5.2

(a) Three linguistic markers of expertise: (i) academic title (*professor*); (ii) area of specialization (*environmental medicine*); and (iii) academic affiliation (*New York University*).

(b) Like Tang, Hajek's academic affiliation (*Queen Mary University of London*) is given. However, in place of an academic title and area of specialization, Hajek's directorship of a research unit (the *Tobacco Dependence Research Unit*) is presented.

(c) Tang asserts the proposition *the DNA changes related to e-cigarette smoke are similar to those linked to secondhand smoke*. Hajek asserts the proposition *this study does not show that vaping causes cancer*. Other propositions include *cancer is a slow process* (Tang) and *vaping poses some 5% of risks of smoking* (Hajek).

(d) This challenge is intended to weaken the third premise in an argument from expertise: *A* is within *D*. These researchers are arguing that propositions (*A*) about the effects of e-cigarette smoke on mice are not within the domain (*D*) of knowledge about the effects of e-cigarette smoke on human health.

(e) Tang states that more work is needed to establish if vaping really does increase cancer rates. He also states that the results of experiments may take 'years to come in'. Both statements indicate that Tang is aware that the evidence base in this area is incomplete and will change, albeit slowly, as further experimental results become available.

Exercise 5.3

(a) The area of specialization would also help readers establish the expertise of Dr Prausnitz and Professor Mitragotri.

(b) Dr Prausnitz does have a conflict of interest in this case. Given that he has jointly published scientific articles with the lead investigator of the study, Dr Prausnitz cannot offer an impartial view on the significance of the study's findings.

(c) A caveat expressed by Dr Prausnitz is *not* omitted by the newspaper. The caveat occurs when Dr Prausnitz states that the implications of the study could be huge 'if the findings can be translated into pills that safely and effectively administer insulin to humans.'

(d) Professor Mitragotri uses a simile to convey to readers how the new drug works: 'Our approach is *like a Swiss Army knife*'. The professor is saying that the drug contains a number of tools, each of which is designed to address a specific problem en route to insulin absorption by the bloodstream.

(e) Two propositions asserted by the experts in the article:
Dr Prausnitz: Insulin given by mouth works about as well as conventional injection.
Professor Mitragotri: Insulin must navigate a challenging obstacle course before it can be effectively absorbed into the bloodstream.

End-of-chapter questions

(1) Three propositions or claims that are true by virtue of their assertion by an expert:

(i) Many migraine medications have unpleasant side effects that prevent their long-term use (uttered by neurologist Professor Tissa Wijeratne).

(ii) Some patients do not respond to migraine medications at all (uttered by neurologist Professor Tissa Wijeratne).

(iii) People with chronic migraine can be in a state where they are working less than 50% of their brain capacity all the time (uttered by neurologist David Williams).

(2)

(a) Two linguistic markers of expertise: (i) academic title (*professor*); and (ii) academic affiliation (*IUF-Leibniz Research Institute for Environmental Medicine in Dusseldorf; University of Sheffield*).

(b) The geographical locations of the academic institutions with which these authorities are affiliated have a significant influence on judgements of their expertise. Professors Haendeler and Chico are based at universities in Germany and the UK, respectively. Both countries are recognized for having well developed academic and scientific communities. This confers greater cognitive authority on both individuals than would be the case if they worked in countries with poorly developed academic and scientific communities.

(c) Professor Haendeler produces the utterance: "With respect to ageing and thus to the elderly population, our data demonstrate that the mitochondrial capacity of the old heart is improved by caffeine to that of the adult heart." This utterance contains the propositions: (i) our data demonstrate that the mitochondrial capacity of the old heart is improved by caffeine to that of the adult heart; and (ii) the mitochondrial capacity of the old heart is improved by caffeine to that of the adult heart. Professor Chico produces the utterance: "These researchers have discovered that a protein called p27 is important for recovery after heart attack in mice, and that p27 function is boosted by caffeine." This utterance contains the propositions: (i) a protein called p27 is important for recovery after heart attack in mice, and (ii) p27 function is boosted by caffeine.

(d) Professor Chico is stating that a proposition or claim about the effects of caffeine on recovery following heart attack in mice may not be relevant to recovery following heart attack in humans. This note of caution relates to premise 3 in an argument from expertise. This premise states that a proposition *A* is within domain *D*. Professor Chico is claiming that a proposition about the recovery effects of caffeine following heart attack in mice (proposition *A*) need not relate to recovery following heart attack in humans (domain *D*).

(e) Professor Haendeler's recommendation is that coffee, or at least caffeine, might be included in the diets of elderly people. Professor Chico's recommendation is that people do not need to drink more coffee as a result of this study, but that those who already drink coffee should be reassured that it might have health benefits.

(3)

(a) The expertise of these public health agencies is related to (i) the knowledge and competence of the individuals who work for these agencies, and (ii) their integrity and trustworthiness. Each of these two main components of expertise contains further sub-components. Knowledge and competence are based on high standards of formal education, academic and professional qualifications, and clinical experience. Integrity and trustworthiness are based on high standards of professional behaviour and ethical conduct which are enshrined in the working practices and goals and missions of these agencies.

(b) The second premise in an argument from expertise states that an expert *E* asserts that a proposition *A* is known to be true. Each of the facts in the posters serves as proposition *A* in this premise. For example, expert *E* (the CDC) asserts that a proposition *A* (hepatitis C is a leading cause of liver cancer) is known to be true.

(c) The domain to which these posters relate is infectious diseases. Each of the propositions conveyed by the facts in these posters relates to infectious diseases.

(d) The facts in these posters contribute to propositional knowledge. For example, it is known *that* Ebola can be contracted by direct contact with blood, body fluids or tissues of infected persons. It is also known *that* millions of Americans have hepatitis C.

(e) Because Ebola virus disease (EVD) is not currently a treatable condition, the expert advice offered by the Public Health Agency of Canada focuses on prevention (e.g. EVD can be prevented by avoiding infected animals and contaminated medical equipment). Hepatitis C is a treatable condition, and so the CDC's expert advice focuses on treatment. Readers are advised, for example, to talk to their doctor about getting tested for hepatitis C with a view to beginning treatment.

References

Allum, N. (2007). An empirical test of competing theories of hazard-related trust: The case of GM food. *Risk Analysis, 27*(4), 935–946.

Armstrong, K., Ravenell, K. L., McMurphy, S., & Putt, M. (2007). Racial/ethnic differences in physician distrust in the United States. *American Journal of Public Health, 97*(7), 1283–1289.

Bleich, S., Blendon, R., & Adams, A. (2007). Trust in scientific experts on obesity: Implications for awareness and behavior change. *Obesity, 15*(8), 2145–2156.

Brown-Johnson, C. G., Boeckman, L. M., White, A. H., Burbank, A. D., Paulson, S., & Beebe, L. A. (2018). Trust in health information sources: Survey analysis of variation by sociodemographic and tobacco use status in Oklahoma. *JMIR Public Health Surveillance, 4*(1), e8.

Cummings, L. (2014). The 'trust' heuristic: Arguments from authority in public health. *Health Communication, 29*(10), 1043–1056.

Eiser, R. J., Stafford, T., Henneberry, J., & Catney, P. (2009). "Trust me, I'm a scientist (not a developer)": Perceived expertise and motives as predictors of trust in assessment of risk from contaminated land. *Risk Analysis, 29*(2), 288–297.

Fiske, S. T., & Dupree, C. (2014). Gaining trust as well as respect in communicating to motivated audiences about science topics. *Proceedings of the National Academy of Sciences of the United States of America, 111*(suppl. 4), 13593–13597.

Freed, G. L., Clark, S. J., Butchart, A. T., Singer, D. C., & Davis, M. M. (2011). Sources and perceived credibility of vaccine-safety information for parents. *Pediatrics, 127*(Suppl. 1), S107–S112.

Llewelyn, M. J., Fitzpatrick, J. M., Darwin, E., Tonkin-Crine, S., Gorton, C., Paul, J., et al. (2017). The antibiotic course has had its day. *BMJ, 358,* j3418.

Nakayachi, K., & Cvetkovich, G. (2010). Public trust in government concerning tobacco control in Japan. *Risk Analysis, 30*(1), 143–152.

Todd, P. M., & Gigerenzer, G. (2000). Simple heuristics that make us smart. *Behavioral and Brain Sciences, 23*(5), 727–741.

Wada, K., & Smith, D. R. (2015). Mistrust surrounding vaccination recommendations by the Japanese government: Results from a national survey of working-age individuals. *BMC Public Health, 15,* 426.

Walton, D. N. (1997). *Appeal to expert opinion: Arguments from authority.* University Park: Pennsylvania State University Press.

Walton, D. N. (2010). Why fallacies appear to be better arguments than they are. *Informal Logic, 30*(2), 159–184.

Arguments from Analogy

L. Cummings, *Fallacies in Medicine and Health*,
https://doi.org/10.1007/978-3-030-28513-5_6

6

LEARNING OBJECTIVES: Readers of this chapter will

- be able to distinguish when an analogy is used to argue in support of a claim (logical use of analogy) and when an analogy is used to explain an issue or illuminate a problem (non-logical use).
- be able to identify the logical form of an analogical argument, and recognize the different ways in which this form may be represented in logic textbooks.
- be able to identify significant similarities and dissimilarities between two analogues, and understand the relevance of these features to a target property in argument.
- be able to identify the conditions under which use of an analogical argument can provide rational warrant for a proponent's claim in argument.
- be able to recognize different ways in which a proponent may use analogical argument fallaciously, either as a deceptive tactic in argument with an opponent or as a logical error.
- be able to explain how analogical argument can function as a cognitive heuristic during reasoning, and report some findings from experimental studies of analogical reasoning.

6.1 Introduction

Humans are very skilled at detecting similarities in the world around them. We observe likenesses between people and places on a daily basis. Just think about the occasions when you have confused a complete stranger for a friend based on similarities of facial appearance, hair color, and body type. In fact, you may be so convinced based on physical similarities that a person on the street is your friend that you proceed to greet them, only to realize that you have been mistaken. Humans have such a strong propensity to establish similarities between features of their environment that they see a child's face in the pattern on a curtain, they think a cloud in the sky looks like a poodle, and they believe that the shadow of a tree on the ground has the appearance of a monster. Our tendency to observe similarities with objects and people in some of our most basic perceptual experiences reflects the extent to which thinking has evolved to establish analogies between features of our environment. The ability to detect similarities has considerable survival value for humans. It allows us to avoid situations, people and objects that pose a risk to our safety. If an approaching object has the same or similar form to one that previously caused us injury, we would do well to avoid it. Rapid detection of similarities also allows humans to take advantage of opportunities that might otherwise not be exploited. I might pursue a financial course of action because it is similar in important respects to one that I previously pursued and that secured some monetary gain for me. If I cannot even see how my current situation is similar to my former one, I am unlikely to do anything at all.

Throughout this book, we have taken the view that at least certain informal fallacies function as cognitive heuristics. As heuristics, these arguments confer a range of benefits on the cognitive processes in which they participate. They may increase the speed of cognitive processing so that decisions can be taken and courses of action can be pursued more quickly than would otherwise be the case. They may allow us to conserve valuable cognitive resources by deferring to the opinion of an expert rather than storing large bodies of knowledge in memory. The **argument from analogy** can also be characterized as a cognitive heuristic. By relating a current situation or object to one that is similar to it in essential respects, I can achieve a number of cognitive gains. I can use similarities between the two situations or objects to guide decision-making, without undertaking the more extensive deliberations that would be needed if the situation or object were genuinely novel. By mapping a new scenario onto one that is similar to it, the costs of cognitive processing can be reduced. The template onto which we map a new scenario or object is already familiar to a cognitive agent. This familiarity allows for the rapid identification of features of the novel situation that require our attention or to which we should be alert. We can conserve our cognitive resources by using a previously familiar situation or object to increase the salience of features of a new situation or object. We will return later in the chapter to the cognitive efficiencies that can be achieved through use of **analogical argument** as a heuristic during reasoning. In the meantime, suffice it to say that analogical argument is a type of cognitive heuristic *par excellence*.

This chapter will examine the use of analogies in reasoning and argumentation. We will see that we can reflect on all sorts of similarities that we perceive in the world around us without employing those similarities during reasoning. So **analogical reasoning** is only one type of thinking that is based on similarities. Like other arguments that we have examined in this book, argument from analogy has been viewed by some logicians as a rather weak form of reasoning. One of the chief criticisms of the argument is that similarity between two objects, people, or situations (so-called **analogues**) is a weak basis upon which to base any conclusion in argument. Just because two objects, *A* and *B*, are similar in certain respects does not mean that they will also be similar in relation to another feature that is of interest to us. Indeed, this feature may be the crucial attribute that distinguishes *A* from *B* and is the reason why we say that *A* and *B* are *similar* rather than the *same*. The chapter will examine the logical structure of analogical argument. This structure is variously characterized but in general contains two premises. One premise establishes several features in respect of which *A* and *B* are similar. The other premise introduces a further attribute of *A* which we may go on to conclude is also an attribute of *B*. The rational standing of analogical argument rests ultimately on how well each of these premises is supported by evidence. We will examine instances of the rationally warranted use of analogical argument in medical and health contexts. Medicine and health remain almost completely unexplored in an otherwise large literature on **analogy** (Guarini et al. 2009). We will also consider various logical pitfalls into which analogical argument may lead. Analogical reasoning has been the focus of many experimental studies in both children and adults, and we briefly consider some of the findings of this research. But we begin by examining some views that exist about analogies. We will see that for many commentators, analogy is anything but a beneficial concept.

6.2 Preliminary Remarks

Before we embark on a logical analysis of analogical argument, it will be useful to make a few preliminary remarks about the use of analogies. It is fair to say that not everyone is positively inclined towards analogies. For some commentators, analogies are used fraudulently, sometimes egregiously so. Writing in *The New York Times*, Adam Cohen stated that "[w]e are living in the age of the false, and often shameless, analogy". Cohen continued:

> Intentionally misleading comparisons are becoming the dominant mode of public discourse. The ability to tell true analogies from false ones has never been more important. ('An SAT without analogies is like: (A) A confused citizenry…', *The New York Times*, 13 March 2005)

For other commentators, analogies achieve little in the way of illumination of a problem or concept. Instead, they serve only to entertain an audience, and 'enliven' or 'adorn' an issue. Writing in *The Chronicle of Higher Education*, Alexander Stern discusses an analogy between Donald Trump and the blond alien in the movie *Species*, and between Australia and the basketball player Robert Horry and actor Philip Baker Hall:

> Our understanding of Trump is unlikely to benefit from an attentive viewing of *Species*. The careers of the basketball player Robert Horry and the actor Philip Baker Hall, admirable though they may be, leave Australia similarly unilluminated. This kind of analogy – which often consists of an ostensibly funny pop-culture reference or of objects between which certain equivalences can be drawn (x is the y of z's) – has become increasingly common.
> You can also find it in academic writing. For example, from the journal *Cultural Critique*: "Attempting to define multiculturalism is like trying to pick up a jellyfish – you can do it, but the translucent, free-floating entity turns almost instantly into an unwieldy blob of amorphous abstraction." The analogy aims not to enlighten, but to enliven, adorn, divert. ('When Analogies Fail', *The Chronicle of Higher Education*, 11 September 2016)

Other, more positive attitudes towards analogies do exist. In a blog by *The Guardian* to accompany the 2013 Wellcome Trust Science Writing Prize, Jacob Aron, a physical sciences reporter on *New Scientist*, recognizes the value of analogies, while also being cognizant of the damage they can cause:

> Analogies in science writing are like forklift trucks – when used correctly they do a lot of heavy lifting, but if you don't know what you're doing you'll quickly drive them into a wall of laboured metaphors and cause some major damage.

Aron highlights the value of analogies in explaining complex concepts in the physical sciences. But analogies also have an important role to play in medicine and health, where they can help patients understand medical conditions and their treatment. Pat Harrold, a general practitioner in County Galway in Ireland, makes this very point along the following lines:

» When you are confronted by the task of condensing a medical condition and treatment options into a memorable and effective statement, you just can't beat the analogy. It takes the threat out of the message and gives the patient something to think over before the message is dismissed. ('Does your GP overdose on analogies too?', *The Irish Times*, 6 April 2010)

It will not surprise readers that similarly positive and negative views exist about the use of analogy in reasoning. We will see in subsequent sections that for some logicians, similarities are a weak basis on which to base any conclusion in argument. In using such similarities to support a conclusion, analogical argument is a weak or fallacious form of reasoning. However, within the pragmatic approach to fallacies that is developed in this book, it will be argued that there are contexts in medicine and health (and elsewhere) where a strongly warranted similarity between two entities can (and should) be used to support a conclusion in argument. In the meantime, it is worth remarking on another issue that is raised by the use of the term 'analogy' by various commentators. As the above statement by Jacob Aron indicates, the term 'analogy' is often used interchangeably with 'metaphor'. On other occasions, 'analogy' is treated as a synonym of 'simile'. In an article in *The Guardian* entitled 'Terrible Analogies', Oliver Burkeman uses all three terms—'analogy', 'metaphor' and 'simile'—as synonymous expressions:

» According to an investigation I've been conducting – based on visiting a couple of those gift shops that sell fridge magnets, key rings and wooden plaques with hand-painted slogans – life is like a river, but also like a pizza, a butterfly, a box of chocolates, a patchwork quilt and good wine ("best enjoyed with friends") [...] Even those of us who rightly shun the world of cheesy fridge magnets rely on certain governing similes or metaphors to conceive our lives. ('Terrible Analogies', *The Guardian*, 21 November 2009)

This is not the place to undertake an analysis of the conceptual distinctions between these terms. Literary scholars and linguists have done exactly that (Steen and Gibbs 2004; Dancygier and Sweetser 2014). Suffice it to say that similes (e.g. *He was as brave as a lion*) and metaphors (e.g. *The children were angels*) involve figurative comparisons that are not a feature of the type of logical analogies that will be studied in this chapter. The conflation of these terms by Burkeman and other authors is best avoided.

DISCUSSION POINT: Analogies in the public sphere

In an article in *The New York Times*, Owen Harries provides the following cautionary remark about the role of analogies in our lives:

» Analogies are probably indispensable but are also hazardous to intellectual health and tend to take on a life of their own. They need to be carefully scrutinized, especially when advanced by influential opinion-makers. ('As ideology dies, analogies rise', *The New York Times*, 29 October 1989)

In a small group, you should think of analogies that have been used by 'influential opinion-makers' in at least *four* of the following domains: politics; law; medicine; science; sport; literature; popular culture; and economics. Which aspects of

these analogies do you find persuasive? Are there any aspects that you do not find logically compelling? Discuss with your group members why some of the analogies you have identified encourage you to think in a different way about a problem while others do little to illuminate an issue.

6.3 Logical and Non-logical Uses of Analogy

In previous chapters, we have seen how ignorance, fear, and expertise may have logical and non-logical uses in discourse. Determining which of these uses applies in a particular case is often complex and requires considerable judgement. Analogy operates in a similar fashion. Analogies can be used in discourse in a myriad of ways. They may have an explanatory or descriptive function in the discourses in which they appear. They might help us to grasp a dimension of a problem or issue that is difficult to understand or that might be overlooked and not properly examined. But in none of these scenarios is an analogy advanced with a view to supporting a claim in argument. Indeed, there may be no argument at play whatsoever. In this section, we examine two examples of the use of analogy in discourse. It will be seen that in only one of these cases is analogy undertaking logical work in the form of supporting a claim in argument.

Consider the following extract from an article that appeared in the *Evening Standard* on 10 January 2014. The article describes the response of the then UK health secretary, Mr Andrew Lansley, to an analogy between sugar and smoking tobacco used by doctors in a health campaign. The campaign is designed to achieve a reduction in the amount of sugar in the diet of consumers (◘ Fig. 6.1).

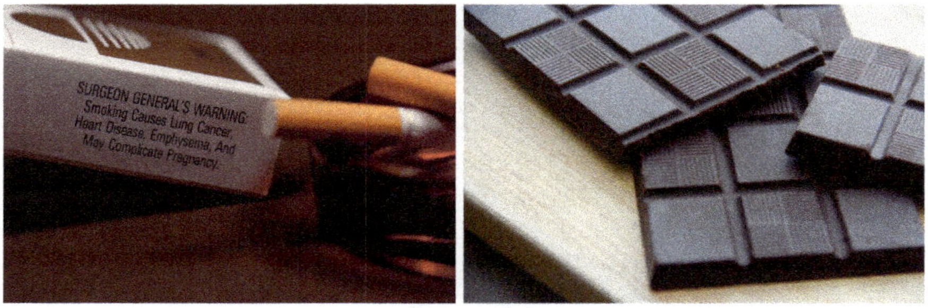

◘ **Fig. 6.1** Is smoking really a good analogy for the health consequences of consuming sugary foods like chocolate? (Photo by Debora Cartagena is reproduced courtesy of CDC, 2012)

Lansley backs food sector on sugar

» It is inaccurate to claim a sugary diet is as dangerous as smoking, former health secretary Andrew Lansley has said.

Mr Lansley said that instead of slashing the amount of sugar in consumers' diets, the food industry should be allowed to reduce the level incrementally, otherwise people would not accept it.

> The Commons Leader […] said the analogy between sugar and tobacco was not appropriate, telling MPs the food industry had already reduced the amount of salt in food.
>
> His comments came as a group of doctors likened the danger posed by sweet foods to smoking tobacco as they launched a campaign to cut the amount of sugar in consumers' diet.
>
> Speaking during his weekly question and answer session in the Commons, Mr Lansley said: "We have had significant success in the reduction of salt in food but it has to be understood that this can only be achieved working with the industry on a voluntary basis … and it can only be done on an incremental basis."
>
> "You can't simply slash the sugar in food otherwise people simply won't accept it. That is what they are looking for. I don't think it is helped by what I think are inaccurate analogies. I just don't think the analogy between sugar and tobacco is an appropriate one.
>
> "I think we have to understand that sugar is an essential component of food, it's just that sugar in excess is an inappropriate and unhelpful diet."
> (*Evening Standard*, 10 January 2014)

The analogical argument that is central to the doctors' stance in this article remains implicit for the most part. However, it can be reconstructed as follows:

P1: Sugary food and tobacco can seriously damage health.
P2: Manufacturers of tobacco have faced strict government restrictions.
C: Manufacturers of sugary food should face strict government restrictions.

Mr Lansley is clearly contesting the soundness of this particular argument. The first premise is the target of his challenge. He describes the analogy that doctors are drawing between sugar and tobacco as 'inaccurate' and not 'appropriate'. The thrust of his objection appears to be that while no amount of tobacco use is considered to be safe, a certain amount of dietary sugar is essential to maintain good health. Health problems only arise when sugar is consumed to excess. Mr Lansley proposes a different analogy as a way forward in tackling the public health implications of excessive sugar consumption. This analogy is based on the Government's prior experience of working with the food industry to reduce the amount of salt in consumers' diets. Mr Lansley's alternative analogical argument can be reconstructed as follows:

P1: Salty food and sugary food when consumed to excess can seriously damage health.
P2: Manufacturers of salty food have reduced incrementally its salt content.
C: Manufacturers of sugary food should reduce incrementally its sugar content.

Analogical arguments clearly pervade this article. One analogical argument is central to the position taken by doctors who wish to see immediate regulation of the food industry in order to achieve a reduction of the consumption of sugar. This argument is challenged by Mr Lansley who wants to see a different regulatory approach taken to the food industry in relation to sugar. That approach should replicate earlier actions taken by the Government and the food industry to achieve a reduction of the salt content of food. Both in his challenge to the doctors and in his support of a different regulatory approach to sugar, Mr Lansley is guided by logical considerations. The first logical consideration is that the analogy doctors are drawing between sugar and tobacco is unwarranted, according to the health secretary. Sugar and tobacco are dissimilar in an essential respect, in that there is a safe level of sugar consumption but no safe level of tobacco use. The second logical consideration is that Mr Lansley believes there is a much stronger analogy to be found between sugar and salt consumption than between sugar consumption and tobacco use. The much stronger rational warrant of the former analogy is what motivates Mr Lansley to pursue a different regulatory approach in relation to sugar from the one proposed by doctors. In his rejection of the doctors' analogy, and in his proposal of an alternative analogy, Mr Lansley is guided by what he believes is the most rationally warranted position to hold. We may contest the rational warrant of his stance. But that it is guided by logical considerations is beyond doubt.

The above extract exemplifies the logical use of analogy to support two different claims about the regulation of the food industry in relation to sugar consumption. Analogy may also be used in discourse for a non-logical purpose such as explanation or illustration. Consider the following extract that appeared in *The Guardian* on 19 February 2002. The author of the article is Dr Ron Roberts of the Institute of Psychiatry at King's College London. Dr Roberts is attempting to explain the poor mental health of the student population. Also, he is expressing his opinion about the use of support services to address the deteriorating mental health of students.

Prevention is better than the cure

» A major cause of the poor mental health of the student population has come from the removal of the safety net of the maintenance grant, and the introduction of tuition fees. Looking to support services as a cure-all is a retrogressive step—it is applying a sticking plaster after the damage has been done—it is hardly preventative in nature. As an analogy, it would be akin to relying on antibiotics in a situation where the government was actively engaged in germ warfare on its own population.
(*The Guardian*, 19 February 2002)

Dr Roberts attributes the cause of poor mental health of students to financial pressures that have been brought about by the removal of the maintenance grant and the introduction of tuition fees. He is unconvinced that the Government's proposal to use support services to reduce the mental health difficulties of students will be effective. In fact, he believes this is a 'retrogressive step' that is disproportionate to the scale of the challenge. The use of support services also does not prevent these difficulties which, he argues, should be the aim of the Government. In order to illustrate just how retrogressive the use of support services would be, Dr Roberts adopts the analogy of the Government using antibiotics to treat the adverse health effects of germ warfare on its own population. Support services, Dr Roberts is claiming, would be as ineffective a response to students' mental health difficulties as the use of antibiotics to treat the adverse health consequences of germ warfare. This analogy vividly illustrates the point that Dr Roberts is attempting to make. To this extent, it is an effective discourse strategy. But what this analogy does not achieve is the logical work of supporting a claim in argument. The analogy does not provide *evidence* that support services are unlikely to be effective—there is no argument that could be made about the effectiveness of these services that might draw on germ warfare and antibiotics. Instead, the analogy merely *illustrates* the scale of the challenge that is faced by these services. In summary, this illustration is an important non-logical use of analogy in a discourse that aims to *explain* (rather than *argue* about) the cause of students' poor mental health.

6.4 Logical Structure of Argument from Analogy

Most logic textbooks represent the logical structure of the argument from analogy in one of two ways. Some authors use the first premise of the argument to present the analogy between two objects, people, or situations, represented here by *A* and *B*. The second premise states a further attribute or feature *N* of *A*. These combined premises are the logical grounds for the conclusion that *B* also exhibits *N*. This logical structure is used by Munson and Black (2017: 111), among other authors:

A is similar to *B* in possessing features 1, 2, 3, …
A also possesses feature *N*.

B possesses feature *N*.

In other logic textbooks, the analogy that is expressed in the first premise in the above argument is not directly stated but remains implicit. The shared attributes or features of *A* and *B* are presented in separate premises. It is then implicit propositions that take us from these premises to the conclusion of the argument. One of these propositions is the analogy <*A* is similar to *B* in respect of features *a*, *b* and *c*>. This logical structure is adopted by Hurley (2015: 525):

Entity *A* has attributes *a*, *b*, *c*, and *z*.
Entity *B* has attributes *a*, *b*, *c*.
Therefore, entity *B* probably has attribute *z* also.

Hurley's logical structure illustrates another important characteristic of the argument from analogy. The conclusion of this argument is not a deductive consequence of the premises. It is possible for *A* and *B* to be similar in respect of attributes *a*, *b*, and *c* and yet for *B* not to have attribute *z*. In any argument from analogy, the conclusion can only be expressed in terms of probability—*B probably* has attribute *z*. The probabilistic nature of analogical argument is one of the main reasons why the argument has been negatively characterized by many logicians. Baronett (2008: 321) writes that "[i]t is important to acknowledge at the outset that analogical inferences contain a specific weakness. Generally speaking, the conclusions of analogical inferences do not follow with logical necessity from the premises." In ▶ Sect. 6.5, we will see that there are many ways in which arguments from analogy can commit logical errors. However, simply being a type of probabilistic argument is not one of them. The tendency to treat as defective any argument that falls short of deductive standards of **soundness** and **validity**, as Baronett is doing, is the hallmark of deductivism in logic (see ▶ Sect. 1.4). The logical features of analogical argument will be examined further in the remainder of this section. But first, you should attempt the task in Exercise 6.1.

EXERCISE 6.1: The logical structure of analogical argument

Authors of logic textbooks can present the logical structure of analogical argument in different ways. The two most common ways are shown below. Examine these different structures and then answer the questions that follow:

Argument 1
Object *A* has features *v*, *w*, *x*, *y*, and *z*.
Object *B* has features *v*, *w*, *x*, and *y*.
Therefore, object *B* probably also has feature *z*.
(Watson and Arp 2015: 259)

Argument 2
A is similar to *B*.
B has property *P*.
So, *A* has property *P*.
(Howard-Snyder et al. 2009: 534)

Questions

(a) Which of these arguments contains an explicit analogy premise? Is the argument that you have identified similar to the argument used by Hurley or by Munson and Black?
(b) In which of the above arguments is the conclusion treated as a probabilistic consequence of the premises?
(c) Identify the implicit analogical premise or proposition in argument 1 that is essential to the inference generated by the argument?
(d) In what way does the first premise of argument 2 differ from the first premise of the argument used by Munson and Black? How does the difference that you have identified affect the evaluation of argument 2?
(e) In which of these arguments does the conclusion have the certainty of a deductive consequence of the premises?

To facilitate our discussion of the logical features of argument from analogy, consider the following extract that appeared in an editorial in *EBioMedicine* in 2015. The editorial is describing the approach to the regulation of new psychoactive substances that is taken by New Zealand:

> In July 2013, instead of a blanket ban on new psychoactive substances, New Zealand enacted a different approach: testing. Any new molecule that is chemically related to or intended to have similar physiological effects as another psychoactive compound is subject to the same rigorous testing as other pharmaceuticals before being publically available, with manufacturers and experimenters being strictly regulated.

The analogical argument that underpins New Zealand's strategy to new psychoactive substances can be represented as follows:

Psychoactive compound *A* and new molecule *B* have similar chemical nature and physiological effects.
Psychoactive compound *A* had to undergo rigorous testing.
Therefore, new molecule *B* has to undergo rigorous testing.

This argument has the two-premise structure of an analogical argument. The first premise expresses the analogy between *A* and *B*—they both have similar chemical natures and produce similar physiological effects. The second premise expresses a further feature or attribute of *A*—it is subject to rigorous testing—that we are led to conclude should also apply to *B*. The argument has the same logical structure as the argument represented in schematic form by Munson and Black. But unlike the abstract form used by Munson and Black, the content of the current argument allows us to make a number of other logical observations. The strength of the analogy expressed in the first premise rests on the number and type of attributes which *A* and *B* are taken to share. In general, strong analogies can demonstrate several attributes or features that *A* and *B* have in common. Where there is only one feature in common between *A* and *B*, the analogy is weaker. However, even this general statement must be immediately qualified. We might be prepared to describe an analogy as strong on the basis of a single attribute that carries considerable weight. For example, if two organisms *A* and *B* have the same genetic makeup, and *A* belongs to a particular animal species, then we would be very inclined to conclude that *B* belongs to the same species. The single attribute of genetic makeup is enough to convince that there is a strong analogy between *A* and *B*. By the same token, *A* and *B* can share several attributes, and yet these attributes may give rise to a weak analogy. For example, I may purchase two drugs *A* and *B* from the same pharmacist who dispenses the drugs in the same type of bottle and issues the same advice not to exceed the stated dose. The two drugs may be manufactured by the same pharmaceutical company and have the same trading license from regulatory authorities. Notwithstanding all these shared attributes, we would not be inclined to conclude that drug *B* treats hypertension just because drug *A* treats hypertension. The similarities, numerous though they may be, are not the right type of similarities to convince us that we have a strong analogy. These observations about the number of attributes that support an analogy can be summarized as follows:

> ***Logical feature 1***
>
> The number of attributes has *some* bearing on the strength of an analogy. *In general, the more attributes that A and B have in common, the stronger the analogy.*

Returning to our example of psychoactive substances, there are two attributes or features that the psychoactive compound *A* and new molecule *B* have in common. These attributes are chemical nature and physiological effects. Although there are only two attributes, they provide very convincing grounds for claiming that there is a strong analogy between *A* and *B*. This is because both attributes—and chemical nature in particular—carry considerable weight in an assessment of the similarity of two psychoactive substances. In this case, the *type* of attribute carries more logical weight in deciding the strength of the analogy than the *number* of attributes present. This gives rise to the second logical feature of analogical argument:

> ***Logical feature 2***
>
> The *type* of attribute(s) that *A* and *B* have in common may be more important than the *number* of attributes in deciding the strength of an analogy. Even a single shared attribute can be the basis of a strong analogy between *A* and *B* if that attribute has particular significance to the similarity of these entities.

There really is no better attribute than chemical nature that we can use when we are considering the potential similarity of a new molecule to a pre-existing psychoactive substance. If two substances share chemical constituents then their similarity is effectively guaranteed. The result is a particularly strong analogy that can be used as a basis for further comparisons. But even a strong analogy will fail to support additional comparisons if the attributes that are the basis of the analogy are not relevant in a significant way to a new property. Imagine that we are using an analogy between *A* and *B* based on chemical structure and physiological effects to support the claim that *B* has property *P* because *A* has property *P*. Property *P* may be <*is trading illegally in Brazil*>. But there is no connection between attributes such as chemical structure and physiological effects and the property <*is trading illegally in Brazil*>. So even though there is a strong analogy between *A* and *B*, this analogy does not support a new comparison based on property *P* because there is no evident connection between <*is trading illegally in Brazil*> on the one hand and chemical structure and physiological effects on the other hand. However, there *is* a connection between chemical structure and physiological effects and the property <*undergoes rigorous testing*>. Substances that have certain chemical structures and physiological effects may have damaging consequences for human health. It is the aim of rigorous testing to establish if such health consequences exist so that actions may be taken to avoid them. These considerations are the basis of the third logical feature of argument from analogy:

Logical feature 3

The shared attributes between *A* and *B* that are the basis of the analogy must exhibit a high degree of relevance to a new property *P*. Even a strong analogy cannot support further comparisons between *A* and *B* if the attributes that are the basis of the analogy are not relevant to a new property *P*.

To illustrate further this particular logical feature, consider the following argument from analogy that was prominent during the emergence of BSE in British cattle in the late 1980s. The argument was used extensively by government ministers and health officials to reassure members of the public that this new disease in cattle had no implications for human health:

BSE in cattle and scrapie in sheep have similar pathological and epidemiological features.
Scrapie has not transmitted to humans.
Therefore, BSE will not transmit to humans.

As we now know, BSE did transmit to humans to cause variant Creutzfeldt-Jakob disease (vCJD). So the conclusion of this argument is false. But the argument was nevertheless rationally warranted when it was used to allay public anxiety about the potential risks of BSE to human health. Early scientific investigations revealed pathological and epidemiological similarities between BSE and scrapie. These similarities led investigators to conclude that BSE was a transmissible spongiform encephalopathy (TSE) like scrapie in sheep. This was a strong analogy that drew support from several pathological and epidemiological similarities between these diseases. Moreover, these similarities were highly relevant to a further property of these diseases, namely, their transmissibility to other species such as humans. To appreciate this relevance, we need only consider how the transmissibility of a disease to other species is established. It is established by means of pathological studies that attempt to demonstrate that a previously unrecognized disease in a species has all the hallmarks of a disease that is already known to investigators and that is associated with one or more other species. Epidemiological studies also play a key role in determining if a disease has transmitted to other species. The distribution of cases of a new disease can reveal important information about its source or origin of transmission. It is this high degree of relevance between pathological and epidemiological features on the one hand and the property of transmission to species on the other hand that permitted scientists and others to draw the conclusion based on an analogy with scrapie that BSE was unlikely to transmit to humans (Fig. 6.2).

(a) (b)

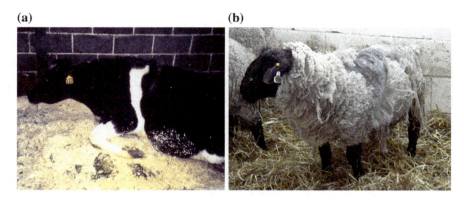

6

Fig. 6.2 **a** Cattle affected by BSE experience progressive degeneration of the nervous system. Infected animals display behavioural changes in temperament (e.g. nervousness or aggression), abnormal posture, incoordination and difficulty in rising, decreased milk production, and/or loss of weight despite continued appetite (Photo by Dr Art Davis is reproduced courtesy of the U.S. Department of Agriculture—Animal and Plant Health Inspection Service, APHIS, 2003); **b** A sheep with scrapie. An intense itching sensation (pruritus) is one of the symptoms of the disease. This causes the animal to engage in rubbing, scraping or chewing behaviour with resulting deterioration of the fleece (Photo © Moredun Photo Library)

The analogy between BSE and scrapie illustrates another important logical feature of argument from analogy. It is possible for the premises of this argument to be strongly warranted and for the conclusion to be false. Even a strongly warranted analogical argument is not a deductive argument. The conclusion of an analogical argument expresses a probabilistic consequence of the premises which may, in the end, prove to be false. It was eventually established that BSE did transmit to humans, and was the cause of a new spongiform encephalopathy called vCJD. What appeared to be a strong analogy between BSE and scrapie when it was first used by government ministers and health officials to allay public anxiety was later shown by strain-typing studies to be weak and unwarranted (Cummings 2010). So no conclusion about BSE's transmissibility to humans could be drawn based on the fact that scrapie had not transmitted to humans. Even a strong analogy is still in the end an analogy that is based on similarities. Similarities that might at first appear to provide convincing grounds for an analogy can weaken over time as new evidence emerges. When this happens, the conclusion must be overturned or rejected. This is exactly the situation that arose during the BSE epidemic in the UK. Pathological and epidemiological similarities that initially grounded the analogy between BSE and scrapie were shown ultimately to be false and to give rise to an erroneous conclusion about the transmissibility of BSE to humans. These considerations give rise to the final logical feature of analogical argument which can be summarized as follows:

Logical feature 4

In an argument from analogy the premises may be strongly warranted and yet the conclusion may be false. Argument from analogy is not a deductive argument. Its conclusion expresses a probabilistic consequence of the premises that may ultimately have to be overturned.

SPECIAL TOPIC: Analogies during the BSE epidemic

It is important to be aware that one and the same analogy can support a range of conclusions in analogical arguments. These conclusions sometimes express not just different, but contrary, claims. For example, opponents of the UK Government strategy of using scrapie as an analogue of how BSE would behave turned this analogy on its head by showing that it could support a quite different conclusion about the transmissibility of BSE. Their argument can be represented as follows:

BSE is similar to scrapie in sheep.
Scrapie has transmitted to other species.
Therefore, BSE will transmit to other species.

It was argued by detractors of the Government's approach to BSE that as long as there was the possibility of BSE transmission to other species—as indeed there was, based on this analogy with scrapie—the risk that humans would be one of the species to which the disease might transmit could not be excluded. The Government's repeated reassurances that BSE would not transmit to humans and posed no risk to human health were consequently misguided. The same analogy was central to other analogical arguments that emerged during the BSE crisis. In July 1990, the Spongiform Encephalopathy Advisory Committee (SEAC) sent a letter to the Chief Medical Officer that contained advice about the safety of beef. SEAC's advice was arrived at by analogical reasoning, which can be reconstructed as follows:

BSE is similar to scrapie in sheep.
Low doses of scrapie agent are insufficient to transmit disease.
Therefore, low doses of BSE agent will be insufficient to transmit disease.

BSE is similar to scrapie in sheep.
The oral route of transmission is inefficient in scrapie.
Therefore, the oral route of transmission will be inefficient in BSE.

These analogical arguments concern the dose of infectious agent that would be required to achieve transmission, and the efficiency of the oral route of transmission. In a later meeting of SEAC held on 27 February 1992, the analogy was used yet again to consider if there were any human health implications of the finding that BSE had been experimentally transmitted by inoculation to marmosets. SEAC advised that this finding was expected given what was already known about the transmissibility of scrapie to marmosets, and that no new guidance in relation to BSE was required. The argument at the centre of SEAC's deliberations can be represented as follows:

BSE is similar to scrapie in sheep.
Scrapie is transmissible to marmosets by inoculation.
Therefore, BSE will be transmissible to marmosets by inoculation.

These arguments demonstrate the many different ways in which the analogy between BSE and scrapie was pressed into action during the BSE epidemic. The analogy was repeatedly used during risk assessments about all aspects of BSE, including routes of transmission, the host range of the disease, and the dose of infectious agent that would be required to achieve transmission. With such heavy reliance on this analogy, it is hardly surprising that there was widespread consternation among health officials and government ministers when they began to realise that BSE and scrapie were dissimilar in significant respects. The once unshakeable analogy that had been integral to the Government's response to BSE could no longer support claims of safety about British beef.

6.5 Logical Pitfalls in Analogical Argument

Historically, logicians and philosophers have taken a rather dim view of arguments that are based on analogies. In 1883, Alfred Sidgwick remarked as follows of analogical argument:

> The argument from analogy is, properly speaking, not so much a mode of attempting proof, as a mode of attempting to dispense with the serious labour of proving. It lies at the end of the scale of cogency which is furthest from Demonstration. (Chap. VI, Part II, p. 232)

For Sidgwick, argument from analogy is nothing more than the attempt to avoid the serious work of proving or demonstrating a thesis. Many pejorative characterizations of this argument are related to deductivism in logic, the idea that in order for an argument to be a good argument, it must be deductively valid and have true premises (the so-called soundness doctrine). But even for those who do not subscribe to deductivism, we still want to be able to describe the various ways in which this argument can go awry and lead us into error. These pitfalls in the use of analogical argument stem not from any deductive disappointment on our part, but from the recognition that despite their best intentions, proponents of these arguments may commit certain logical flaws.

One such flaw is to attribute too much weight to similarities in an analogy, and insufficient weight to dissimilar features that suggest the analogy may not be warranted. This situation arose during the BSE epidemic in the UK. Similarities based on the findings of early pathological and epidemiological studies were afforded too much significance in the analogy between BSE and scrapie. Meanwhile, findings that suggested BSE and scrapie may be dissimilar in significant respects were largely overlooked. In May 1990, scientists discovered a spongiform encephalopathy in a domestic cat for the first time. Domestic cats were not susceptible to scrapie. Around the same time, cases of spongiform encephalopathy began to appear in exotic ungulates. Exotic ungulates like the eland, Arabian oryx and the greater kudu were also not susceptible to scrapie. These reports suggested that BSE may have a different host range from scrapie. If that were the case, then an analogy with scrapie would not be warranted and could not be used to support the claim that BSE would not transmit to humans. A further dissimilarity between BSE and scrapie that was not afforded due significance emerged in November 1990. The Neuropathogenesis Unit in Edinburgh confirmed that it had succeeded in orally transmitting BSE to 'negative' line sheep that were not susceptible to scrapie. Here again was further evidence that the analogy between BSE and scrapie may not be warranted. However, none of these dissimilarities between BSE and scrapie prompted health officials to revise the scrapie analogy that was integral to the British Government's approach to BSE. The logical flaw in the use of analogical argument can be summarized as follows:

Logical pitfall 1

In establishing an analogy, too much logical weight may be attached to similarities between *A* and *B* and insufficient weight may be attached to dissimilarities. The proponent of an analogy misrepresents its strength by selecting only similarities and downplaying the significance of dissimilarities.

When dissimilarities are overlooked, it is not always intentionally so. Sometimes an analogy can appear so strong that those who subscribe to it may be blinkered to the possibility that dissimilarities even exist. Alternatively, the analogy may be a long-standing one that has been used so extensively that it can appear to be incontestable. When SEAC scientists failed to abandon the analogy between BSE and scrapie as findings emerged that these diseases had different host ranges, these scientists were in the grip of an analogy. The analogy between BSE and scrapie appeared so firmly established that they could not challenge or contest it. On other occasions, the neglect of dissimilarities is anything but inadvertent. It may be in the commercial interests of a pharmaceutical manufacturer to suppress certain dissimilarities between two drugs *A* and *B*. Imagine that both these drugs may be used to treat hypertension and have similar active ingredients. The manufacturer uses these similarities between the drugs to argue that drug *B* will be safe based on the long safety record of drug *A*. However, a significant dissimilarity between the drugs is suppressed. The newly developed drug *B* has a chemical compound that is not found in drug *A* and that is known to increase the risk of deep vein thrombosis. This dissimilarity is sufficiently important that it invalidates the use of the analogy to make any safety claim about drug *B*. Drug *B* may well be safe, but we cannot make this claim on the basis of an analogy where a key difference of chemical structure is actively suppressed. The logical flaw in this case is not inadvertent. It is a deliberate attempt to suppress a significant dissimilarity between the drugs that are the basis of the analogy.

Another logical pitfall in the use of argument from analogy arises when the proponent uses similarities of *A* and *B* that have low relevance to a further property *P*. For example, a proponent may state that drugs *A* and *B* have the following similarities. They are both produced by the same French pharmaceutical manufacturer, the formula for their production was developed by British and American chemists, and they can both be shipped for delivery to destinations in North American and Europe in 6 weeks. However, these similarities between *A* and *B* have little bearing on the feature of *B* that is of concern to us, its safety for human use. To the extent that we are basing the safety of *B* on the long track record of safety of *A*, the similarities that we will want to see between *A* and *B* must have some relevance to safety. For example, instead of knowing how long it takes to ship the drugs, we would be better to know that the drugs contain similar chemical compounds, that they were subject to the same clinical trials, and that the results of these trials were reviewed by the same panel of independent experts. If these were the similarities at play, we might consider the following analogical argument to be very strongly warranted indeed:

> Drugs *A* and *B* have similar chemical compounds and underwent the same clinical trials.
> Drug *A* is safe for human use.
> Therefore, drug *B* will be safe for human use.

It is easy during argument to be misled into accepting similarities that have low relevance to a target property *P* if several of these similarities are used at the same time. On its own, the fact that both drugs can be shipped to their destinations in 6 weeks is unlikely to be accepted by anyone as a sufficiently strong basis for establishing an analogy between *A* and *B* that can then be used to ground claims about drug safety. However, if we add further superficial similarities such as the fact that they are produced by the same French pharmaceutical manufacturer and that the drugs were developed according to a formula produced by British and American chemists, then we may be led into thinking that the drugs are part of a stronger analogy than is actually the case and go on to draw unwarranted claims about their safety. These considerations are the basis of a second logical pitfall in the use of argument from analogy:

Logical pitfall 2

An analogy between *A* and *B* may be based on similarities that have low relevance to a target property *P*. This error is more likely to pass undetected in argument if several of these similarities are used at the same time. No conclusion about property *P* can be drawn based on similarities that have little or no relevance to *P*.

The relevance of similarities to a new property *P* is a highly context dependent matter. In the above example, the production of the two drugs by a French pharmaceutical manufacturer had little or no relevance to the property of drug safety. However, in a different context, the company that manufactures a drug or medical device may be a similarity that is highly relevant to the safety of the product concerned. In ▶ Sect. 2.4, it was described how the French medical device regulatory authority—Agence Française de Sécurité Sanitaire des Produits de Santé (AFSSAPS)—suspended the marketing, distribution, export, and use of PIP implants when an inspection of the company revealed that it was using silicone gel with a composition that was different from that which had been approved. It is not difficult to see how the identity of this particular company would be highly relevant to the property of product (implant) safety if this company were one of the similarities used to ground an analogy in an analogical argument. Even a similarity like the length of time that is needed to ship a drug to its destination may prove to be relevant to drug safety if it known that the drug cannot be safely stored for the 6-week period that it will be in transit. What these different scenarios demonstrate is that the relevance of any similarity to a new property *P* must be assessed on a case-by-case basis. One and the same similarity can be highly relevant to a target property *P* in one analogical argument, and have little or no relevance to property *P* (even the same property *P*) in a different analogical argument.

A further logical flaw of analogical argument arises when the proponent of this argument fails to refute counter-analogies or suppresses their existence. We saw in ► Sect. 6.4 that the analogy between BSE and scrapie could result in opposing conclusions when used in argument. When used by a government minister, the analogy resulted in the conclusion that BSE would not transmit to humans. However, a detractor of the government's approach to BSE drew a quite different conclusion from the same analogy, namely, that BSE could transmit to other species just as scrapie had done. Humans might very well be one of those species. Counter-analogies are often raised in challenge to an analogy in argument. Difficulties arise when they are suppressed by the proponent of an analogical argument because they undermine a particular thesis or claim. In February 1992, when SEAC members met to discuss the implications of the finding that BSE had been experimentally transmitted to marmosets, a **counter-analogy** was apparent to observers. That counter-analogy can be represented as follows:

Marmosets and humans are genetically close organisms.
BSE can be transmitted to marmosets.
Therefore, BSE can be transmitted to humans.

The fact that the transmission in question occurred under experimental conditions—a scenario that for ethical reasons could not be replicated in humans—did nothing to lessen the significance of this counter-analogy. For here was an indication that humans might, after all, be susceptible to BSE. If a genetically related organism had succumbed to the BSE agent, even if experimentally transmitted, then there was good reason to believe that humans might display the same susceptibility to BSE. However, such was the power of the dominant analogy between BSE and scrapie that the minutes of the meeting indicated that this counter-analogy did not occur to any of SEAC's members. The role of scrapie analogy in determining risk assessments of BSE was allowed to continue unabated. The failure of SEAC scientists to consider the implications of this important counter-analogy represented another lost opportunity to challenge the false analogy between BSE and scrapie. This third logical pitfall in the use of analogical argument can be summarized as follows:

Logical pitfall 3

The conclusion of an analogical argument can be overturned by a counter-analogy. A logical error occurs when a counter-analogy is suppressed because it supports an opposing claim or thesis in argument.

Counter-analogies are a particularly effective way of refuting a proponent's claim in argument. If a proponent is claiming that an emerging infectious disease will not transmit to certain species based on an analogy, and an opponent can show that it might very well transmit to these species based on an alternative analogy, then the opponent has achieved a very strong refutation of the proponent's claim. The burden of proof is then on the proponent to indicate why the opponent's counter-analogy does not hold, or to respond with a counter-analogy of his or her own that supports the original claim. When this burden of proof is not effectively discharged, and the proponent simply overlooks or deliberately suppresses a counter-analogy, then a logical flaw or error has been committed. The error is all the more conspicuous in this case because the proponent is refusing to yield to the very same logic in argument that he has used against his opponent.

A final logical error arises when the conclusion of an analogical argument is advanced with greater certainty than befits an argument based on analogy. The conclusion of an analogical argument is a probabilistic consequence of the premises. In some contexts, an analogical conclusion can be advanced with a high degree of probability. When the Centers for Disease Control and Prevention (CDC) concluded that a blood-borne virus was the likely causal agent of AIDS, this conclusion was highly probable based on epidemiological similarities between AIDS and another blood-borne disease, hepatitis B. But even this highly probable analogical conclusion only expressed a probability. It was still possible that evidence might emerge that would show that some other type of pathogen was the causal agent of AIDS. Alternatively, epidemiological similarities that suggested a strong analogy between AIDS and hepatitis B initially might appear less plausible over time as more knowledge about the cause of AIDS was acquired. In both scenarios, scientists may have had to revise or reject a once highly probable analogical conclusion. When a proponent continues to support an analogical conclusion in the face of contrary evidence, a logical error arises. The analogical conclusion is no longer treated as a probabilistic consequence of the argument's premises that is subject to revision, but as a certain claim that is essentially indefeasible. This fourth logical pitfall in the use of analogical argument can be summarized as follows:

Logical pitfall 4

A proponent may treat the conclusion of an analogical argument as a certain claim rather than a probabilistic consequence of the premises. This error may result in a proponent not rejecting a conclusion in the face of contrary evidence. The defeasibility that is a feature of a conclusion based on analogy is subverted by the proponent of an analogical argument.

This logical error replicates a now familiar pattern in the use of the arguments that we have examined in this book. A proponent tries to gain acceptance of his or her claim in argument by overstating the strength of the inference from the premises to the conclusion. An argument in which the premises and conclusion express claims that are presumptively true or probably true is made to shoulder the probative weight of a **deduction**. Because these arguments cannot shoulder this weight—they are not that *type* of argument—they are judged to be weak and fallacious. The only corrective to this pernicious tendency of evaluating all arguments against deductive standards is to assess arguments on their own logical terms. If we take this approach to argument from analogy, we will accept Hurley's assessment of the logical nature of this argument without acquiescing in his sense of disappointment: "The certitude attending such an inference is probabilistic *at best*" (2015: 37, italics added).

SPECIAL TOPIC: The AIDS-hepatitis B analogy

From today's perspective, it may seem that we have always known that HIV/AIDS was a blood-borne infectious disease. But this is not the case. On 4 March 1983, the CDC published an article in its *Morbidity and Mortality Weekly Report* in which it addressed the issue of the transmission of AIDS. Based on the available evidence, the view of the CDC was that AIDS was transmitted sexually and parenterally by means of blood and blood products. That the CDC was using the hepatitis B virus as a model for the transmission of AIDS was clearly evident in the article. The analogy between AIDS and hepatitis B is explicitly articulated in this extract from the article:

> » The distribution of AIDS cases parallels that of hepatitis B virus infection, which is transmitted sexually and parenterally. Blood products or blood appear responsible for AIDS among hemophilia patients who require clotting factor replacement. The likelihood of blood transmission is supported by the occurrence of AIDS among IV drug abusers. Many drug abusers share contaminated needles, exposing themselves to blood-borne agents, such as hepatitis B virus. Recently, an infant developed severe immune deficiency and an opportunistic infection several months after receiving a transfusion of platelets derived from the blood of a man subsequently found to have AIDS. The possibility of acquiring AIDS through blood components or blood is further suggested by several cases in persons with no known risk factors who have received blood products or blood within 3 years of AIDS diagnosis. These cases are currently under investigation.
> ('Current trends prevention of Acquired Immune Deficiency Syndrome (AIDS): Report of inter-agency recommendations', *Morbidity and Mortality Weekly Report, 32*(8), 101–103)

While acknowledging that "the cause of AIDS remains unknown", the article went on to say that the Public Health Service recommends that five actions be taken. These recommendations were based on pre-existing knowledge of the transmission properties of hepatitis B virus. For example, one recommendation advised members of groups at increased risk of AIDS to refrain from donating plasma and/or blood. Another recommendation stated that sexual contact should be avoided with persons who are known or are suspected to have AIDS. These recommendations were made in the knowledge that as long as the cause of AIDS remained unknown, "the ability to understand the natural history of AIDS and to undertake preventive measures [would be] somewhat compromised."

It is now time for you to get practice at identifying some logical errors in the use of argument from analogy by attempting Exercise 6.2.

EXERCISE 6.2: Liquor sales, breakfast cereal and toilet paper

The following extract is taken from an article that appeared in *The Sydney Morning Herald* on 17 July 2013. Journalist Gareth Hutchens is reporting government efforts in New South Wales, Australia to introduce a ban on supermarkets from using docket deals that offer 50% or more off the price of liquor. Hutchens argues that the supermarket and liquor industries are treating the people of New South Wales with contempt when they use fallacious arguments to defend the practice of selling heavily discounted alcohol (Fig. 6.3). His argument against three liquor industry representatives—Coles, Woolworths, and the Liquor Stores Association—unfolds as follows:

» Consider the fallacious arguments they use to try to convince government bureaucrats that coupon discounts offering 50 per cent or more off liquor will have no adverse social consequences.

From Coles: "We engaged [consultants] to review the available evidence on alcohol availability and pricing and, based on that review, are not aware of any conclusive evidence linking pricing/promotions, availability, and alcohol-related harm."

From Woolworths: "There is no evidence to support the contention that this promotion would somehow make customers purchase a product that they would not normally consume, or that having made that purchase that customers would then consume more of the product in question than they normally would. This would be akin to a claim that a promotional offer on Corn Flakes would cause purchasers to consume two bowls of breakfast rather than their normal one."

From the Liquor Stores Association: "There is no evidence to suggest that discounts of 'greater than 50 per cent' or promotions running for a very short period lead to excessive or rapid consumption. Does a promotion heavily discounting breakfast cereal or toilet paper result in consumers using more toilet paper at home?"

These arguments are gibberish. [...]

Look at the form of Coles' argument. [...]

It could even come with a template: "There is no conclusive evidence linking [insert product] and [insert problem here]."

[...] Then look at the arguments used by Woolworths and the liquor stores. They've used the same logical fallacy, a "false analogy".
('Liquor logic might as well be written on toilet paper', Gareth Hutchens, *The Sydney Morning Herald*, 17 July 2013)

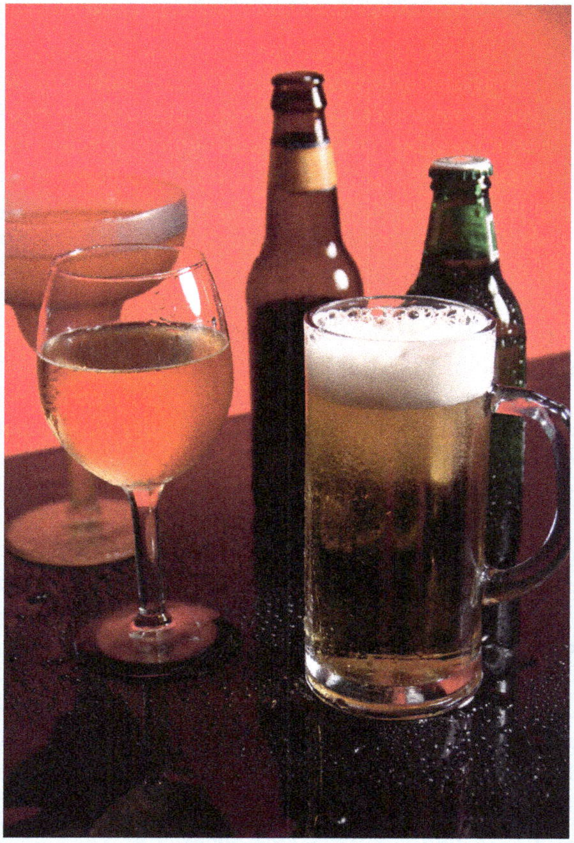

Fig. 6.3 Heavily discounted alcohol has been credited with increasing alcohol consumption (Photo by Debora Cartagena is reproduced courtesy of the CDC, 2012)

Questions

(a) Hutchens criticizes the liquor industry for using claims of the form "There is no conclusive evidence linking [insert product] and [insert problem here]". What type of informal fallacy takes this claim as a premise?

(b) Hutchens argues that Woolworths and the Liquor Stores Association use the same logical fallacy, a false analogy. Describe the form that this fallacious argument takes.

(c) What attributes do Woolworths and the Liquor Stores Association use to ground their analogy between liquor and toilet paper?

(d) What property are the liquor industry representatives using the attributes in (c) to support? Are these attributes relevant to this property?

(e) Are there any dissimilarities between liquor and toilet paper that suggests an analogy between them is not warranted?

6.6 Experimental Studies of Analogical Reasoning

The ability to reason by analogy has attracted the attention of a range of psychologists. Developmental psychologists are interested in establishing when children first acquire the ability to use analogies in reasoning. Cognitive psychologists examine the relationship between analogical reasoning and cognitive abilities in working memory and **executive function**. Clinical psychologists want to understand how analogical reasoning is impaired in people with conditions like schizophrenia and autism spectrum disorder, and what implications this impairment has for their cognitive functioning and behaviour. While these different branches of psychology can shed light on the psychological processes by means of which we engage in analogical reasoning, none has examined these processes in the context of medicine and health. It was for this reason that I undertook some years ago a public health study of analogical reasoning in 879 members of the public (Cummings 2014a, b, 2015). The aim of the study was to establish if adults are able to assess the conditions under which analogical arguments are more or less rationally warranted. Although detailed results are reported elsewhere and will not be repeated here, some comments about the findings of this study are in order. There then follows a discussion of some other findings that have emerged from psychological experiments of analogical reasoning in children and adults.

The public health study of analogical reasoning that I undertook was novel in a further respect. Psychological experiments of analogical reasoning almost invariably present participants with premises that are abstracted from context. The expectation on the part of experimenters is that the information contained in these premises, and only this information, should be used as a basis for drawing an inference. In my public health study, participants were not presented with a fixed argument—premises and conclusion—which they had to evaluate. Instead, they were presented with short, written public health scenarios where they had to select the information that would form the premises in their reasoning. It was argued that this alternative methodology is typical of naturalistic reasoning, where information that functions as premises is selected by a participant rather than determined in advance by an experimenter. Using this methodology, I was able to demonstrate that the adults in the study were highly skilled in analogical reasoning across a range of public health scenarios. What was particularly revealing during open-ended comments on each scenario was the extent to which participants interrogated the grounds of their analogical judgements. For the most part, participants were discerning about the types of similarities that could be used as a basis for inference. A scenario about BSE and scrapie prompted the following comment from a 32-year-old female participant. The analogy between these diseases was a 'flawed' basis on which to conclude that BSE would not transmit to humans, according to this participant:

> At this time it was not conclusive that BSE and scrapie were related diseases – it was only a suggestion, therefore the reasoning behind the suggestion that BSE would not transmit to humans was flawed.

Participants also interrogated the relevance of similarities to a new target property. The same analogy between BSE and scrapie prompted this comment from a 62-year-old male participant. The purported similarities between BSE and scrapie had limited relevance to the property of disease transmission to humans for this particular participant:

> It doesn't seem to me a safe assumption that because two diseases are 'related' they will necessarily act in the same way as far as transmission to humans is concerned.

Participants also commented on the probabilistic nature of argument from analogy. It was acknowledged that a conclusion based on analogy, even a strong analogy, is not certain. The following remark about the analogy between AIDS and hepatitis B was produced by a 46-year-old male participant:

> Comparison with hepatitis B is only an analogy – therefore there must be a degree of uncertainty about the conclusion drawn.

In summary, this study demonstrated that adults of both genders, and diverse ages, educational backgrounds, and ethnic identities exercised considerable judgement during the rational evaluation of analogical arguments. For further discussion of the findings, readers are referred to Cummings (2014a, b, 2015).

The age at which young children first begin to use analogies in reasoning is an issue of interest to developmental psychologists. It used to be thought that children could not reason analogically prior to Piaget's formal operations stage in cognitive development at approximately 13 or 14 years of age. However, Goswami and Brown (1990) showed that children as young as 3 years of age could solve classical analogies (*a* is to *b* what *c* is to *d*) if they understood the causal relations on which they were based. One causal relation examined by Goswami and Brown was 'melting'. However, not all developmental changes in analogical reasoning can be explained by increasing domain knowledge of the type that is needed to understand causal relations. There is considerable evidence that cognitive maturation of working memory and executive functions also explains developmental gains in children's analogical reasoning. Simms et al. (2018) assessed analogical reasoning, and working memory, inhibitory control, and cognitive flexibility in 5- to 11-year-old children. Performance on an analogical mapping task was best predicted by individual differences in children's working memory, even when controlling for age. This finding, Simms et al. argued, suggests a strong interrelationship between analogical reasoning and working memory development. That increased knowledge *and* cognitive development contribute to children's analogical reasoning is demonstrated in a study by Richland and Burchinal (2013). These investigators found that children with greater executive function skills and vocabulary knowledge in early elementary school displayed higher scores on a verbal analogies task, even after adjusting for key covariates like gender and mother's education.

Impairment of analogical reasoning in children and adults with clinical disorders has also been investigated in psychological experiments. Analogical reasoning has been found to contribute to the language difficulties of children with specific language impairment (SLI). Krzemien et al. (2017) used a scene analogy task to evaluate the analogical performance of children with SLI. They found that the analogical reasoning of these children was similar to that of language-matched peers, but was worse than that of age-matched peers, a finding which the investigators took to confirm an association between language disorders and analogical reasoning. Analogical reasoning is impaired in people with schizophrenia. Simpson and Done (2004) reported reduced performance on an analogical reasoning task in people with schizophrenic delusions relative to a group of depressed subjects and non-psychiatric control subjects. Krawczyk et al. (2014) also found reduced performance on an analogical reasoning task in the subjects with schizophrenia in their study. Additionally, social cognitive ability and analogical reasoning were significantly correlated. Perhaps surprisingly, analogical reasoning in children with autism spectrum disorder (ASD) appears to be intact for the most part. Although Tan et al. (2018) found that children with ASD were less competent solving analogical problems than typically developing children, their inferior performance was related to general cognitive impairments. Children with ASD can undertake analogical reasoning tasks based on social content and perform abstract analogical reasoning (Green et al. 2014, 2017).

EXERCISE 6.3: Analogies for depression

Simpson and Done (2004) used individuals with depression as a control group in their study of analogical reasoning in people with schizophrenia. The experience of suffering depression, and treatment of the condition have always been rich sources of analogies. The following extracts from articles that appeared in *The Guardian* are cases in point. Read each extract carefully, and then answer the questions that follow:

Extract A

> Magic mushrooms may effectively "reset" the activity of key brain circuits known to play a role in depression, the latest study to highlight the therapeutic benefits of psychedelics suggests.
>
> Psychedelics have shown promising results in the treatment of depression and addictions in a number of clinical trials over the last decade. Imperial College London researchers used psilocybin – the psychoactive compound that occurs naturally in magic mushrooms – to treat a small number of patients with depression, monitoring their brain function, before and after. [...]
>
> Dr Robin Carhart-Harris, head of psychedelic research at Imperial, who led the study, said: "We have shown for the first time clear changes in brain activity in depressed people treated with psilocybin after failing to respond to conventional treatments."
>
> "Several of our patients described feeling 'reset' after the treatment and often used computer analogies. For example, one said he felt like his brain had been 'defragged' like a computer hard drive, and another said he felt 'rebooted'."
>
> "Psilocybin may be giving these individuals the temporary 'kick start' they need to break out of their depressive states and these imaging results do tentatively support a 'reset' analogy. Similar brain effects to these have been seen with electroconvulsive therapy."
>
> ('Magic mushrooms 'reboot' brain in depressed people – study', Haroon Siddique, *The Guardian*, 13 October 2017)

Extract B

» [T]he monoamine theory of depression [...] argues that, because most antidepressants increase levels of neurotransmitters of the monoamine class, depression is caused by depletion of monoamines in the brain.

Except, the monoamine hypothesis is increasingly seen as insufficient. It's part of what's going on, sure, but not the whole story. For one, antidepressants boost neurotransmitter activity pretty much immediately, but therapeutic effects usually take weeks to kick in. Why? It's like filling your car's empty tank with petrol and it only starting to run again a month later; it means no fuel may have been *a* problem, but it's clearly not the *only* problem.

There are other possible explanations. Neuroplasticity, the ability to form new connections between neurons, has been shown to be impaired in depressed patients. The theory is that this prevents the brain from responding "correctly" to aversive stimuli and stress. Something bad happens, and the impaired plasticity means the brain is more 'fixed' as is, like a cake left out too long, preventing moving on, adapting, or escaping the negative mindset, and thus depression. Antidepressants also gradually increase neuroplasticity, so this may be actually why they work as they do, long after the transmitter levels are raised. It's not like putting fuel in a car, it's more like fertilising a plant; it takes time for the helpful elements to be absorbed into the system.
('How do antidepressants actually work?', Dean Burnett, *The Guardian*, 10 July 2017)

Questions

(a) In extract A, an analogy is used to describe patients' experiences of being treated with psilocybin, the psychoactive agent found naturally in magic mushrooms. What is this analogy?
(b) Has the analogy that you identified in your response to (a) a logical or a non-logical function in this extract? Justify your response.
(c) In extract B, no fewer than three analogies are used to characterise depression and its treatment. What are these analogies?
(d) Do the analogies that you identified in your response to (c) have a logical or a non-logical function?
(e) In what way does the 'fertilising a plant' analogy in extract B differ from the computer analogy in extract A?

6.7 Analogies as a Cognitive Heuristic

We began this chapter by describing how there is a strong tendency on the part of humans to find similarities between entities and people in their environment. It was argued that this tendency has considerable survival value in that it allows humans to conserve their cognitive resources and avoid physical harm. The avoidance of harm can be easily explained. It is rational to avoid a person, entity, or situation that is similar to one that caused us harm. The conservation of cognitive resources is less intuitive and requires some explanation.

In any analogical argument, we draw a conclusion about a property of an unfamiliar person or thing based on the features of a person or thing that is more familiar to us. When scientists concluded that BSE would not transmit to humans, they based this conclusion on what was known about the host range of scrapie. Scrapie is a transmissible spongiform encephalopathy (TSE) that had been endemic in the sheep population of Britain for some 250 years when BSE first emerged in cattle. Scrapie had also been extensively investigated by scientists. These studies included epidemiological investigations that sought to establish if there was any link between scrapie and Creutzfeldt-Jakob disease, a TSE in humans. One study of particular significance, a 15-year-investigation of scrapie and CJD in France and review of the world literature undertaken by Brown et al. (1987), concluded that scrapie had not transmitted to humans. In short, scrapie provided a well-developed analogical template onto which the new disease of BSE could be mapped. Having mapped BSE onto this template, scientists were able to draw tentative conclusions about the way in which BSE would likely behave. All manner of conclusions, from the species that would be susceptible to BSE to the efficiency of different routes of transmission, then ensued.

This example illustrates an important characteristic of all analogical arguments. These arguments encourage us to draw conclusions about features of new situations and things based on the attributes of situations and things that are already familiar to us. The analogical mapping from something that is less familiar or less well known onto something that is more familiar or better known, is the basis of any analogical argument. Where this mapping does not occur, or the direction of the mapping is reversed, an analogy is certain to fail. The transfer of features along an epistemic gradient from low familiarity (new phenomenon) to high familiarity (known phenomenon) achieves a number of cognitive gains for us. We can avoid the need to conduct extensive investigations into a new situation or entity if we can simply map it onto a similar one that is already familiar to us. While the mapping inevitably incurs some expenditure of cognitive resources, the effort required to conduct this mapping is substantially less than that needed to investigate a new phenomenon. On the assumption that the mapping is conducted correctly, and there is a high degree of similarity between an analogical template and a new phenomenon, the template can then be used to generate conclusions about the features of the new phenomenon. In some cases, the template can be a highly productive resource. For example, the analogical template based on scrapie supported a wide range of claims about BSE, including its host range, routes of transmission, dose of infective agent required for transmission, and infectivity of bovine tissues.

It can be seen that argument from analogy has all the hallmarks of a cognitive heuristic. If we can avoid the need to undertake lengthy investigations into a new phenomenon, the speed of reasoning is increased. By using an analogical template in our deliberations, time-consuming literature searches and experiments can be effectively bypassed. We can also conserve important cognitive resources such as working memory by using an analogical template in reasoning. The memory storage that is needed to map a novel situation or phenomenon onto a pre-existing analogical template is much less than that which is required to store information from a literature search or other form of evidence gathering. Argument from analogy can achieve considerable cognitive efficiencies for those agents who attend to the various logical conditions on its use. This chapter illustrated these conditions using actual examples of analogical arguments in medicine and health. When these conditions are not observed, or are observed only partially, the argument confers no advantage or benefit on reasoning. It is an instance of fallacious reasoning that can subvert cognitive inquiry and other deliberations of which it is a part. This chapter has also been at pains to emphasize the different ways in which analogical argument can fall short of standards of reasonable argumentation. These discussions have broadened our understanding of this important argument. However, it remains to be seen if informal logicians can develop a psychologically plausible analogical heuristic that is relevant to reasoning in medicine and health.

DISCUSSION POINT: Health analogies in other disciplines

Health analogies are used extensively in a broad range of fields including economics, law, and politics. In this way, *The Telegraph* reported on 16 May 2018 that the deputy governor of the Bank of England, Ben Broadbent, had described Britain's economy as entering a "menopausal" phase after passing peak productivity. On 25 September 2016, *The Guardian* compared Donald J. Trump to an autoimmune disease. Meanwhile, cancer has been used as an analogue for everything from terrorism to poverty. In a small group, list as many examples as you can of how health analogies are used to shed light on problems and issues in fields beyond medicine and health. Which features of these analogies are particularly strong in your opinion? Are there any examples of health analogies that do not work so well? Which features of these analogies do you not find convincing?

Chapter Summary

Key points

- Analogies have a logical purpose when they are used to support a claim in argument. But there are also many non-logical uses of analogies. Analogies may be used to illuminate an issue or explain a problem. Descriptive and explanatory uses of analogy are common in different types of discourse, including argumentation.
- Analogies are common in medicine and health. Doctors can make extensive use of analogies to help patients understand illnesses and their treatment. Analogies may also be used to guide medical decision-making and perform scientific risk assessments.
- Logic textbooks variously represent the logical structure of argument from analogy. One premise of this argument states that two entities *A* and *B* are similar in respects *x*, *y*, and *z*. A second premise states that *A* has property *P*. The conclusion states that *B* also has property *P*.
- Argument from analogy is rationally warranted when the number and type of similarities between *A* and *B* are carefully interrogated, these similarities are

relevant to a new property *P*, and there are no significant dissimilarities between the analogues. The conclusion must also be expressed as a probabilistic consequence of the premises.

- Logical errors occur in the use of argument from analogy when a proponent attempts to overstate the similarities between *A* and *B*, ignores or suppresses significant dissimilarities between *A* and *B*, or uses similarities that have little relevance to a new property *P*. The strength of the warrant for the conclusion based on the premises may also be exaggerated.
- Analogical reasoning has been the focus of many experiments. This has generated a large body of findings about how young children acquire the ability to use analogies in reasoning, and how analogical reasoning is impaired in the presence of clinical disorders. It has also resulted in different methodological approaches to the study of analogical reasoning.
- Analogies have a vital heuristic function during reasoning. By mapping a new situation or entity onto a more familiar situation or entity, a cognitive agent can increase the speed of processing and conserve important resources such as memory.

Suggestions for Further Reading

(1) Cummings, L. (2015). *Reasoning and public health: New ways of coping with uncertainty*. Cham, Switzerland: Springer.

Chapter 5 in this volume examines the use of argument from analogy in public health. The argument is analysed in dialectical and epistemic perspectives. The chapter considers empirical findings of a study of analogical reasoning in 879 members of the public. The role of analogical argument in heuristic reasoning is addressed. A wide range of actual analogical arguments in public health is used to illustrate features of this argument throughout the chapter.

(2) Ribeiro, H. J. (Ed.). (2014). *Systematic approaches to argument from analogy*. Heidelberg: Springer.

This edited volume contains 16 chapters that are organised in two parts: theoretical and applied approaches to argument from analogy. In theoretical approaches, Douglas Walton examines in his chapter two different argumentation schemes for argument from analogy. One of these schemes is based on reasoning from a source case to a target case, while the other scheme compares factors in two cases. In applied approaches, argument from analogy is examined across a range of contexts, including legal argumentation, TV election night specials, and clinical practice.

(3) Walton, D., & Hyra, C. (2018). Analogical arguments in persuasive and deliberative contexts. *Informal Logic, 38*(2), 213–261.

In this article, the authors emphasize that context relating to dialogue type (in this case, persuasion dialogue and deliberation dialogue) is an important factor to consider when evaluating analogical arguments. A survey of literature on analogical argument considers different classifications of the argument and terminological distinctions drawn by analysts. Three examples of analogical argument are analysed. These examples relate to a legal trial around an event at a baseball game, a news article that characterized Barack Obama as an appeaser, and civil rights protests in Saudi Arabia.

Questions

(1) In ► Sect. 6.3, we examined an analogy between smoking tobacco and sugar consumption that was used by doctors in a public health campaign. The following extract is taken from an article that appeared in the Scottish newspaper *The Herald*. Journalist Judith Duffy is reporting a health warning issued by Geoff Ogle, the chief executive of Food Standards Scotland. Mr Ogle is using tobacco in an analogy about obesity rather than sugar consumption (Fig. 6.4). Read the extract carefully and then answer the questions below:

Food chief warns obesity health threat equivalent to tobacco

» THE head of Scotland's food watchdog agency has issued a stark warning that the obesity crisis will be this generation's equivalent of tobacco in causing disease and premature deaths.

Geoff Ogle, chief executive of Food Standards Scotland (FSS), said shocking statistics which predict 40% obesity levels in Scotland in just 15 years' time should be a wake-up call for everyone to get serious about tackling the problem.

He said it is possible to reverse the trend like smoking - but warned there was no single solution and everyone from individuals and parents to retailers and government had to take action now.

Ogle said tobacco was a good analogy of the health consequences this generation is facing due to obesity. Poor diet is linked to an increased risk of a range of health problems including diabetes, heart disease, stroke and certain cancers.

He said: "If you look at where tobacco was in the 1940s and 1950s, it was cool and 'chic' then to smoke. I don't think anyone would argue it is cool and 'chic' to smoke now."

"In the 1940s and 1950s, you didn't really have much understanding of the health consequences of smoking, it was starting to emerge."

"Now everyone clearly understands the health consequences of smoking. I think there are analogies where you can show that society's attitude will change over time." ('Food chief warns obesity health threat equivalent to tobacco', Judith Duffy, *The Herald*, 5 June 2016)

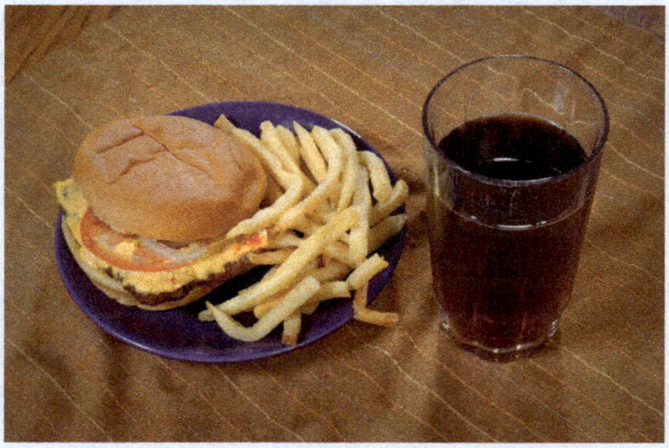

Fig. 6.4 Poor diet is linked to obesity. But is smoking really a good analogy for the adverse health effects of obesity? (Photo by James Gathany is reproduced courtesy of CDC/ Mary Anne Fenley, 2007)

Questions

(a) Mr Ogle describes tobacco as a 'good analogy' of the health consequences that today's generation is facing due to obesity. State what this analogy is. How does Mr Ogle's view of this analogy compare to the views of the different actors described in ► Sect. 6.3?

(b) Mr Ogle uses the tobacco analogy to emphasize two temporal dimensions of tobacco smoking which he believes are relevant to obesity. What are these temporal dimensions?

(c) Construct an argument from analogy for each of the two temporal dimensions that you have identified in response to (b).

(d) Mr Ogle observes that society's attitude to smoking has changed over time. A once 'cool' and 'chic' behaviour, smoking is no longer perceived in those terms, he claims. To what extent is this true? Is the comparison of obesity to changing societal attitudes to smoking a valid one?

(e) Mr Ogle is claiming that people's understanding of the adverse health consequences of smoking has improved over time, and with this improved understanding there has been a consequent reduction of smoking. It is clear that he expects the same will happen to obesity. In your view, is this a valid assessment of what will happen with obesity?

(2) On 9 September 2005, Science Editor for *The Telegraph*, Roger Highfield, reported a controversial decision by the Human Fertilisation and Embryology Authority in the UK. The decision gave scientists permission to alter for the first time the mitochondria in the cells of an embryo. So-called mitochondrial-replacement procedures (see ► Sect. 3.1) could be used to treat a group of serious mitochondrial genetic disorders that can result in premature death and reduced

quality of life. The article described how a team of researchers at the University of Newcastle hoped to be able to conduct the procedure in as little as three years. The extract begins with the response to the decision of Professor Doug Turnbull, the leader of the Newcastle team. Read the extract carefully and then answer the questions below:

Designer babies to wipe out diseases

» Prof Doug Turnbull [...] told The Daily Telegraph last night that he was "delighted" by the authority's decision.

When considering the application twice before, the authority cited the Human Fertilisation and Embryology Act 1990, which prohibits "altering the genetic structure of any cell while it forms part of an embryo". However, its appeal committee heard that the phrase "genetic structure" had no precise scientific meaning.

Another objection rested on the ban on any proposal to change the nuclei of cells, the technique used to clone Dolly the sheep. But the Newcastle method is significantly different from cloning.

Prof Azim Surani, professor of physiology and reproduction at Cambridge University, said: "It does not involve making a copy of an existing adult."

"I also see few ethical problems, as we are dealing with the embryo at a very early stage when the cells have not even started to divide yet."

Prof John Burn, of the department of clinical medical sciences at Newcastle University, said the decision would not lead to designer babies.

"I would use the analogy of simply replacing the battery in a pocket radio to explain what we are doing," he said. "You are not altering the radio at all, just giving it a new power source."

Prof Peter Braude, of King's College London, welcomed the authority's decision.

"If [the technique] works and is safe it will be the answer to the prayers of those people afflicted by these awful mitochondrial genetic disorders, for which there is no treatment."
('Designer babies to wipe out diseases approved', Roger Highfield, *The Telegraph*, 9 September 2005)

Questions

(a) In this extract, Professor John Burn draws an analogy between the mitochondria in cells and the battery in a pocket radio. What attribute or feature is the basis of this analogy?

(b) When Professor Burn uses this analogy, he intends it to function as a premise in an analogical argument. What is this analogical argument?

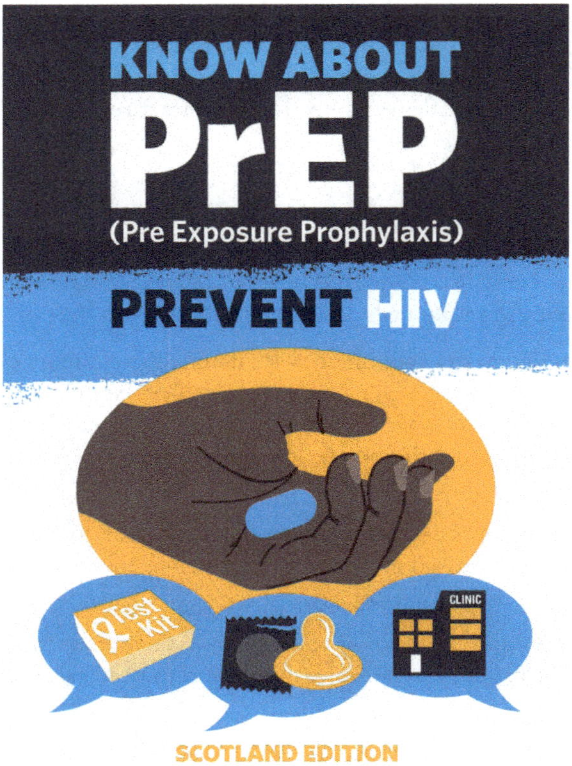

Fig. 6.5 Pre-exposure prophylaxis (PrEP) is effective in the prevention of HIV infection (©HIV Scotland, the University of Edinburgh and PrEPster)

(c) In the analogical argument that you have reconstructed in response to (b), is there a high degree of relevance between the attribute or feature that is the basis of the analogical premise and the new property that is expressed in the second premise?
(d) Opponents of the decision taken by the Human Fertilisation and Embryology Authority might reject Professor Burn's analogy by arguing that batteries and mitochondria are dissimilar in a significant respect. In what respect might it be argued that batteries and mitochondria are dissimilar?
(e) Is the dissimilarity that you identified in your response to (d) relevant to the new property expressed in the second premise of Professor Burn's analogical argument?

(3) On 12 September 2018, Brett Campbell of the *Belfast Telegraph* reported on the introduction of a scheme at the city's Royal Victoria Hospital that would see individuals at high risk of contracting HIV offered a drug called PrEP (pre-exposure prophylaxis). Mr Wells, a former health minister and member of the Democratic Unionist Party (DUP), is opposed to the introduction of the scheme. He uses an analogy with smoking to express his disagreement towards the use of PrEP (Fig. 6.5). Read the following extract and then answer the questions below:

Ex-DUP minister Wells has 'grave concerns' over pill that can prevent HIV

» A former DUP Health Minister has criticised the introduction to the Northern Ireland Health Service of a pill that can prevent people contracting HIV.

The drug known as PrEP, which can reduce the chance of high risk individuals contracting the virus by up to 86%, will be administered by clinicians at the Belfast Trust's new HIV Prevention Clinic as part of a £450,000 drive aimed at revolutionising sexual health services.

However, former DUP Minister said he had "grave concerns" about the scheme when he led the Department of Health.

The specialist pilot scheme, based at the Royal Victoria Hospital's GUM clinic and funded by the Health and Social Care Board's Transformation Fund, will run for an initial two years. [...]

But speaking on BBC Radio Ulster's Talkback programme, Mr Wells said: "Can you imagine a drug company came up with a cure for lung cancer as a result of smoking? Would we make that drug universally available to all smokers or would we urge smokers to give up?"

"The whole premise of public health is to urge people to make wise lifestyle choices, not to make unwise choices." [...]

LGBT campaigner Greg Owen branded Mr Wells' comments "homophobic" because they suggested gay sex was detrimental to an individual's health.

"Are we seriously going to have a person who was formerly in office as a health minister compare sex, which is one of the driving forces of life, to a smoking analogy?" he asked.
('Ex-DUP minister Wells has 'grave concerns' over pill that can prevent HIV', Brett Campbell, *Belfast Telegraph*, 12 September 2018)

Questions

(a) How would you characterise the analogy that Mr Wells is drawing between smoking and homosexuality? What *two* similarities does Mr Wells use to support his analogy?
(b) Which of the similarities that you have identified in your response to (a) is challenged by LGBT campaigner Greg Owen?
(c) Use the analogy that you identified in your response to (a) to reconstruct the argument from analogy that Mr Wells is advancing. How does the conclusion of this argument differ from the conclusions of the other analogical arguments that we have examined in this chapter?
(d) Mr Wells asked listeners to the radio programme to imagine a drug company developing "a cure for lung cancer as a result of smoking". In what way does this scenario differ from the proposals to use PrEP?
(e) How might public health agencies use smoking to develop a counter-analogy to Mr Wells' argument from analogy?

Answers

Exercise 6.1

(a) Argument 2 contains an explicit analogy premise. Argument 2 is similar in structure to the argument used by Munson and Black.

(b) Argument 1

(c) Analogical premise: Object *A* is similar to object *B* in respect of features *v*, *w*, *x*, and *y*.

(d) The first premise of argument 2 does not state the attributes or features that *A* and *B* are taken to share. In the absence of these features, it is difficult to determine if the new property *P* will also be a feature of *A*. This is because property *P* must have some relevance to the shared attributes of *A* and *B* in order for it to be a likely attribute of *A*.

(e) Argument 2

Exercise 6.2

(a) The informal fallacy is the argument from ignorance.

(b) Analogical argument:
Liquor and toilet paper are similar in certain respects.
Discounting toilet paper does not lead to increased consumption.
Therefore, discounting liquor will not lead to increased consumption.

(c) Attributes shared by liquor and toilet paper are that they are both consumer products and are sold in shops.

(d) The property is <*does not lead to increased consumption*>. The shared attributes of liquor and toilet paper (both consumer products, etc.) only have general relevance to this property.

(e) A significant dissimilarity between liquor and toilet paper is that consumption of liquor can be addictive or habit-forming while this is not the case for the consumption of toilet paper. This dissimilarity is highly relevant to the property at the centre of this analogical argument, as an addiction will lead to increased consumption of liquor.

Exercise 6.3

(a) A computer analogy is used to describe patients' experiences of being treated with psilocybin. The analogy can be captured as follows: The physiological effects of taking psilocybin for the treatment of depression are similar to the performance-enhancing effects of defragging or rebooting a computer.

(b) The analogy identified in response to (a) has a non-logical function in that it is used to *describe* the effects of treatment with psilocybin.

(c) The taking of anti-depressants is like putting *fuel into a car* or *fertilising a plant*. The depressed brain is like *a cake that is left out too long*.

(d) All three analogies identified in response to (c) have a non-logical function in extract B.

(e) The computer analogy in extract A is serving a *descriptive* function. It allows patients to describe or characterise their subjective experience of being treated with psilocybin. The 'fertilising a plant' analogy in extract B is serving an *explanatory* function. It allows the author of the article to explain why the effects of drug treatment for depression are not immediate. It takes time for "helpful elements to be absorbed into the system" (drugs, in this case) in the same way that it takes time for fertiliser to be absorbed by a plant.

End-of-chapter questions

(1)

(a) Analogy = Smoking tobacco and obesity cause disease and premature death.
Mr Ogle believes tobacco smoking is a good analogy for how obesity will affect people's health. His view is similar to that of the doctors in ► Sect. 6.3, who believe the analogy between smoking tobacco and sugar consumption is also warranted.

(b) The two temporal dimensions of tobacco smoking that Mr Ogle believes are relevant to obesity are that (i) smoking has become more negatively evaluated over time (it is no longer 'cool' and 'chic'), and (ii) people's understanding of the adverse health consequences of smoking has increased over time.

(c) *Analogy 1*
Obesity is similar to tobacco smoking.
Tobacco smoking has become more negatively evaluated over time.
Obesity will become more negatively evaluated over time.

Analogy 2
Obesity is similar to tobacco smoking.
The adverse health consequences of smoking have become better understood over time.
The adverse health consequences of obesity will become better understood over time.

(d) It is not entirely true to claim that smoking is no longer perceived to be a 'cool' and 'chic' behaviour. For many young people who start smoking, they do so in order to appear cool and chic. This feature of smoking does not relate particularly well to obesity. It is not true to say that obesity used to be positively evaluated like smoking and is less positively evaluated today.

(e) This is a valid assessment of what will happen with obesity. Extensive public health education about smoking has improved the public's understanding of the adverse health effects of smoking and contributed *in part* to a reduction in smoking. Similar education efforts can be expected to improve the public's understanding of obesity and the factors that contribute to it. This might be expected to achieve the behaviour modification that could reduce rates of obesity. But the qualification *in part* applies with equal force to smoking and obesity. There are large numbers of smokers and obese people who are very well informed about the adverse health consequences of smoking and obesity, and who do not desist from the behaviours that are damaging their health. Improved understanding does not always lead to positive behaviour modification in either smoking or obesity.

(2)

(a) The attribute or feature that is the basis of the analogy is that mitochondria provide power to the cell in the same way that a battery provides power to a pocket radio.

(b) Analogical argument:
A battery in a pocket radio and mitochondria in a cell are both sources of power.
A battery can be removed without altering a pocket radio.
Therefore, mitochondria can be removed without altering a cell.

(c) The attribute *<source of power>* has moderate relevance to the property *<can be removed without altering the essence of X>*.
(d) Batteries and mitochondria are dissimilar in that only mitochondria contain genetic material that, if removed, significantly changes the essence of the cell. A battery can be removed from a pocket radio without altering it in any significant way.
(e) The dissimilarity between batteries and mitochondria, namely, the presence of genetic material in mitochondria, is highly relevant to the property expressed in the second premise of Professor Burn's analogical argument. If mitochondria and the genetic material they contain are removed from a cell, the essence of the cell is changed.

(3)
(a) The analogy is: Smoking and homosexuality are similar in that they are lifestyle choices and can place a person at risk of serious disease. The similarities are (i) both activities are lifestyle choices, and (ii) both activities place a person at risk of serious disease.
(b) Greg Owen challenges both of the similarities identified in response to (a). He takes issue with the suggestion that gay sex is detrimental to an individual's health. He also denies that homosexuality is a lifestyle choice when he describes sex as one of the 'driving forces of life'. Presumably, Owen intends by this remark that people do not *choose* their sexual orientation.
(c) Argument from analogy:
Smoking and homosexuality are similar in that they are lifestyle choices and can place a person at risk of serious disease.
A drug to prevent or cure lung cancer should not be universally available to all smokers.
A drug to prevent or cure HIV should not be universally available to homosexual people.

The conclusion of this argument contains a deontic 'should'. The conclusions of the other analogical arguments examined in this chapter have expressed what 'will' happen, not what should or should not happen.

(d) PrEP is not intended to 'cure' HIV once it has been contracted. Rather, it is designed to prevent a person contracting HIV in the first place. Prevention of HIV is more cost effective than attempting to treat it. This aspect of PrEP should be acceptable to Mr Wells who is also concerned at the cost of this drug.
(e) Public health agencies could develop a counter-analogy to Mr Wells as follows:
Smoking and homosexuality can place individuals at risk of developing serious illnesses.
Smokers can reduce the risk of serious illness by practicing risk minimization (e.g. vaping).
Homosexuals can reduce the risk of serious illness by practicing risk minimization (e.g. PrEP).

References

Baronett, S. (2008). *Logic*. Upper Saddle River, NJ: Pearson Prentice Hall.

Brown, P., Cathala, F., Raubertas, R. F., Gajdusek, D. C., & Castaigne, P. (1987). The epidemiology of Creutzfeldt-Jakob disease: Conclusion of a 15-year investigation in France and review of the world literature. *Neurology, 37*(6), 895–904.

Cummings, L. (2010). *Rethinking the BSE crisis: A study of scientific reasoning under uncertainty*. Dordrecht: Springer.

Cummings, L. (2014a). Circles and analogies in public health reasoning. *Inquiry, 29*(2), 35–59.

Cummings, L. (2014b). Analogical reasoning in public health. *Journal of Argumentation in Context, 3*(2), 169–197.

Cummings, L. (2015). *Reasoning and public health: New ways of coping with uncertainty*. Cham, Switzerland: Springer.

Dancygier, B., & Sweetser, E. (2014). *Figurative language*. New York: Cambridge University Press.

Goswami, U., & Brown, A. L. (1990). Melting chocolate and melting snowmen: Analogical reasoning and causal relations. *Cognition, 35*(1), 69–95.

Green, A. E., Kenworthy, L., Gallagher, N. M., Antezana, L., Mosner, M. G., Krieg, S., et al. (2017). Social analogical reasoning in school-aged children with autism spectrum disorder and typically developing peers. *Autism, 21*(4), 403–411.

Green, A. E., Kenworthy, L., Mosner, M. G., Gallagher, N. M., Fearon, E. W., Balhana, C. D., et al. (2014). Abstract analogical reasoning in high-functioning children with autism spectrum disorders. *Autism Research, 7*(6), 677–686.

Guarini, M., Butchart, A., Smith, P. S., & Moldovan, A. (2009). Resources for research on analogy: A multi-disciplinary guide. *Informal Logic, 29*(2), 84–197.

Howard-Snyder, F., Howard-Snyder, D., & Wasserman, R. (2009). *The power of logic* (4th ed.). New York: McGraw Hill.

Hurley, P. J. (2015). *A concise introduction to logic* (12th ed.). Stamford, CT: Cengage Learning.

Krawczyk, D. C., Kandalaft, M. R., Didehbani, N., Allen, T. T., McClelland, M. M., Tamminga, C. A., et al. (2014). An investigation of reasoning by analogy in schizophrenia and autism spectrum disorders. *Frontiers in Human Neuroscience, 8*, 517.

Krzemien, M., Jemel, B., & Maillart, C. (2017). Analogical reasoning in children with specific language impairment: Evidence from a scene analogy task. *Clinical Linguistics & Phonetics, 31*(7–9), 573–588.

Munson, R., & Black, A. (2017). *The elements of reasoning* (7th ed.). Boston, MA: Cengage Learning.

Richland, L. E., & Burchinal, M. R. (2013). Early executive function predicts reasoning development. *Psychological Science, 24*(1), 87–92.

Simms, N. K., Frausel, R. R., & Richard, L. E. (2018). Working memory predicts children's analogical reasoning. *Journal of Experimental Child Psychology, 166*, 160–177.

Simpson, J., & Done, D. J. (2004). Analogical reasoning in schizophrenic delusions. *European Psychiatry, 19*(6), 344–348.

Steen, G., & Gibbs, R. (2004). Questions about metaphor in literature. *European Journal of English Studies, 8*(3), 337–354.

Tan, E., Wu, X., Nishida, T., Huang, D., Chen, Z., & Yi, L. (2018). Analogical reasoning in children with autism spectrum disorder: Evidence from an eye-tracking approach. *Frontiers in Psychology, 9*, 847.

Watson, J. C., & Arp, R. (2015). *Critical thinking: An introduction to reasoning well*. London and New York: Bloomsbury Academic.

Post Hoc, Ergo Propter Hoc

L. Cummings, *Fallacies in Medicine and Health*,
https://doi.org/10.1007/978-3-030-28513-5_7

LEARNING OBJECTIVES: Readers of this chapter will

- be able to explain why *post hoc* reasoning is a common occurrence in medicine and health where false or erroneous claims of causation can have particularly serious consequences.
- be able to identify different forms of the fallacy of false cause, including *post hoc ergo propter hoc*, a variant of *post hoc* where a causal conclusion is based on multiple occurrences of one event followed by multiple occurrences of another event, *non causa pro causa*, and oversimplified cause.
- be able to articulate a more nuanced understanding of *post hoc* reasoning that does not assume that *post hoc* argument is inherently fallacious.
- be able to recognise the logical conditions under which it is rationally warranted to base a claim of causation on temporal succession between two events.
- be able to identify the conditions under which the logical significance of temporal succession between events is overstated and is a weak basis for a claim of causation in consequence.
- be able to appreciate that even when *post hoc* reasoning is rationally warranted that it marks the start of a more extensive process of investigation in which a causal claim is rigorously tested.

7.1 Introduction

The desire to explain events in the natural world is one of our strongest intellectual drives. Throughout history, humans have attempted to explain weather phenomena, the diseases that people experience, the behaviour of those who harm others, and much else besides. Many of these explanations are not acceptable by today's scientific standards. None of us would appeal to vengeful gods to explain natural disasters such as earthquakes and tsunamis, even though such explanations were commonplace in ancient civilisations. The purpose of any explanation is to identify the *cause* of an event. This is not as straightforward as it sounds. For many events, there is no single cause but a number of factors that contribute to causation. If I develop a disease like cancer, a positive family history of the disease suggests that genetic factors may have caused my cancer. But if I am also obese, smoke 60 cigarettes a day, and take no exercise, genetic factors may not be the only, or even the most significant, cause of my cancer. Sometimes, what appears to be a cause of an event is not a cause. I may assume that my gastrointestinal symptoms are caused by work-related stress. However, stress may play no part in causing these symptoms. Instead, certain foods that I consume while I am at work may be the cause of my symptoms. Also, correlations between two events may be misconstrued as causation. A study may demonstrate a correlation between coffee consumption and reduced heart disease. But if it can be shown that people who take more exercise also drink more coffee, then it may be exercise and not coffee that is a cause of good heart health. Causation, it can be seen, is a very complex concept.

The type of causal reasoning that will be examined in this chapter has the Latin name *post hoc, ergo propter hoc* (literally, 'after this, therefore because of this'). This form of reasoning leads us to conclude that because *B follows A*, *A* must be the *cause* of *B*. The temporal sequence between two events is sometimes a basis for concluding that the earlier event is the cause of the later event. If I receive a vaccination for hepatitis B and a month later have a blood test that reveals a high level of hepatitis B antibodies, I can reasonably conclude that the vaccination is the cause of those antibodies. The temporal sequence between the administration of the vaccine (event *A*) and the presence of antibodies in the blood (event *B*) is significant in establishing causation in this case as the immune system requires a period of time in which to mount a response to the administered vaccine. In medicine and health, there are many occasions in which it is appropriate to base a conclusion about the causation of an event on a temporal sequence between two events. However, there are also many occasions in which a temporal sequence between two events has no bearing on causation and yet it is used to warrant the claim that *A* causes *B*. I may develop headache and a fever after receiving a vaccination for hepatitis B. But the vaccination may not be the cause of these symptoms and may simply have been coincidental in its timing to my exposure to salmonella food poisoning. The term *post hoc, ergo propter hoc* has generally been reserved for the unwarranted support of a claim about causation based on temporal sequence. We will see in this chapter that the *post hoc* fallacy has been responsible for some significant failures in public health.

The chapter unfolds as follows. In ▸ Sect. 7.2, we examine why *post hoc* reasoning is commonly found in medical and health contexts. This is despite the fact that many medical commentators are aware of the logical flaw in this form of reasoning and even actively caution against it. In ▸ Sect. 7.3, we discuss how *post hoc* reasoning is only one form of the **fallacy of false cause**. The logical features of *post hoc* argument and other forms of this fallacy are examined in this section. In ▸ Sect. 7.4, we consider the conditions under which it is rationally warranted to base a claim of causation on temporal succession between two events. This dispels the commonly held view that *post hoc* is an inherently fallacious form of argument. In ▸ Sect. 7.5, we discuss the different traps or pitfalls that we can fall into when using causal reasoning of the *post hoc* type. These pitfalls include a failure to consider other causes of an event, and to interrogate the plausibility of the purported causal relationship between events *A* and *B*. It is argued that when these pitfalls occur, temporal succession between events is a decidedly weak basis on which to base any claim of causation.

7.2 *Post Hoc* in Medicine and Health

On reading medical literature, one is struck by the number of occasions on which medical experts challenge the use of *post hoc* reasoning. This error in reasoning, it seems, is not only common in the representation of medical studies and their findings to the public, but also in the reasoning of medical disciplines. Grouse (2016) is in no doubt about the cause of misunderstanding of the results of medical studies. *Post hoc* reasoning, he claims, is the "most common" error in the reporting of medical news:

> The Greeks and Romans recognized this fallacy in argument thousands of years ago. Because one event follows another event does not mean that the first event caused the second (*post hoc ergo propter hoc*). However, in contemporary medical news this logic is not understood. This faulty reasoning is the most common cause of false and misleading conclusions of research results that are presented as medical news. (p. E511)

Commentators in a wide range of medical disciplines have remarked on the presence of *post hoc* reasoning in their respective fields. Traumatic events in particular are often implicated in this type of reasoning. In ophthalmology, Bullock (2001) describes how *post hoc* reasoning can lead to an erroneous diagnosis of traumatic retinal detachment for no other reason than the detachment occurred *after* a traumatic event:

> I have recently reviewed three legal cases involving "traumatic" retinal detachments, all of which originated from illogical post hoc reasoning. (p. 356)

In obstetrics, Rowe (2015) argues that traumatic events are falsely believed by many women to be the cause of complications in pregnancy such as miscarriage. Like Bullock, Rowe attributes this type of thinking to *post hoc* reasoning:

> The state of being pregnant carries its own stresses and anxieties, specifically about the outcome of the pregnancy. Most of us have patients who have been convinced that a specific event triggered a complication of pregnancy. Post hoc, ergo propter hoc. The most prominent of these associations is likely between a sudden shocking or traumatic event and miscarriage. (p. 393)

Traumatic medical events like a heart attack are often falsely assumed to be a cause of depression, Freedland and Carney (2009) argue. The *post hoc* error in this reasoning becomes apparent, these authors claim, when we consider that the onset of depression often pre-dates the 'causal' medical event:

> It is often simply assumed that medical illness causes depression. This may be due in part to the logical fallacy *post hoc, ergo propter hoc*. A patient has a heart attack, undergoes further evaluation, and is found to be depressed. The depression is assumed, with little or no evidence, to have been *caused* by the heart attack, simply because the depression was discovered after the medical condition. Causality seems plausible because heart attacks are aversive, stressful, "depressing" experiences. However, many patients who are depressed after a serious medical event were depressed before the event; many have had histories of depression that began years or even decades before any physical health problems; and many other patients who have the same kind of medical event do not become depressed. (p. 116)

It is no coincidence that traumatic events like heart attacks appear to be implicated so often in *post hoc* reasoning. We aim for plausibility in our causal explanations and, as Freedland and Carney remarked, stressful events like a heart attack appear to fit the bill perfectly. We will return to this issue in later sections, when we come to consider why certain types of causal reasoning appear to be more rationally warranted than they actually are.

Post hoc reasoning is clearly a well-recognized phenomenon in medicine. Its presence can be explained by a couple of factors. First, medical therapies will only be effective in the treatment of disease if the cause of a disease can be accurately identified. Some causes are more amenable to direct investigation than others. If I am a physician and I suspect one of my patients has hepatitis B infection, I can perform serological testing to establish if this is the case. If this testing identifies certain hepatitis B virus-specific antigens and antibodies, then I can be certain that infection with the hepatitis B virus is the cause of my patient's illness. Many causes of disease in patients can be identified in this way—symptoms suggest a certain pathogen or other cause of a disease and investigations can indicate if this cause actually exists. But there are also many occasions in medicine when the identification of the cause of a disease or medical event is not a straightforward matter. If I have a patient who has experienced recurrent miscarriages, I can investigate prenatal infections, uterine anomalies, and chromosomal abnormalities as potential causes of these events. But imagine I conduct extensive investigations and no cause of my patient's recurrent miscarriages can be identified.[1] It is easy to see how traumatic events that precede miscarriages may end up occupying this explanatory void, even when there is no evidence to support them as a cause of my patient's recurrent miscarriages. *Post hoc* reasoning fulfils the understandable human need to have *some* explanation of a distressing event like miscarriage when no cause can be identified. But while human psychology makes the logical error explicable, it does not negate the fact that we have fallen back on fallacious *post hoc* reasoning.

A second reason why *post hoc* reasoning is a common occurrence in medicine is that it mimics the temporal development of human disease. For most diseases that we experience, it can appear reasonable to conclude that an event *A* is the cause of *B* exactly because *B* follows *A*. Event *A* may be a spontaneous mutation in my DNA that leads to the replication of cells in an organ of my body and eventually the formation of a tumour. Event *A* may also be my exposure to a pathogen that causes severe respiratory illness after a two-week incubation period. Often, the events that trigger pathological processes lie beyond our awareness. I will not know, for example, if a particular gene in one of my chromosomes has mutated, or if I contracted the virus that is causing my respiratory illness from the man who sat beside me on the bus. But the point is that it is plausible for me to posit these events as causes of my cancer or of my respiratory illness exactly because this is how pathogenesis works. *Post hoc* reasoning arises when the temporal dimension of pathogenesis is emphasized in the absence of a pathological process that might connect an initial trigger event to the disease or illness that someone develops. If I posit that the measles, mumps, and rubella (MMR) vaccine is the cause of my child's autism exactly because my child developed autism *after* receiving the vaccine, then I have allowed the temporal properties of pathogenesis to weigh heavily in my reasoning—my child is exposed to a supposed trigger event (vaccination) and some weeks or months later develops autism. But temporal properties are all that I have considered. I have no pathological process that can link vaccination to the onset of this neurodevelopmental disorder.

CASE STUDY: Traumatic retinal detachment or *post hoc* reasoning?

One of the three legal cases that Bullock (2001) assessed is presented below. All three cases were instances of *post hoc* reasoning—there were no grounds in Bullock's view for attributing a detached retina to a preceding 'traumatic' event in each case. When we look at the details of this case, we can probably see how Bullock arrived at this conclusion, even as we lack his expertise in ophthalmology. The accident was a particularly minor one which left only a faint scratch on the rear bumper of the patient's car. The patient reported that he did not hit his eye or orbital area, and there was no evidence of a head, eye, or orbital injury to any extent. In the emergency room, no ocular signs or symptoms were observed. In attempting to explain his retinal detachment, the patient falsely attributed causation to his earlier, minor car accident:

> A 60-year-old male was involved in a motor vehicle accident. He was sitting in his car at a stop light when the car behind him was struck by a third car, which caused the car behind him to strike his car. Photographs of the rear portion of his car revealed a faint scratch on the rear bumper, adjacent to the license plate. The patient stated that he did not hit his eye or orbital area, and there was no evidence of a head, eye, or orbital injury, to any extent. Right after the accident the patient was taken to a local emergency room; no ocular signs or symptoms were noted. Ten days later the patient complained of floaters in the left eye. He was seen by an optometrist who noted bilateral myopia measuring -7.00 sphere in the right eye and -6.25 sphere in the left eye. The corrected visual acuity measured 20/20 in each eye. A retinal detachment was suspected, and he was referred to a vitreoretinal surgeon, who saw the patient the following day. A superotemporal (macula on) retinal detachment of the left eye was described along with a superotemporal horseshoe tear. The following day the patient underwent a left scleral buckling procedure with a vitrectomy. This procedure re-attached the retina. Post-operatively the visual acuity measured 20/20 in the right eye and 20/30 in the left eye. The patient then filed a lawsuit against the driver of the car that struck the car behind him. (p. 356)

7.3 Logical Features of the Fallacy of False Cause

Causal reasoning can go awry for reasons that are unrelated to the temporal succession of events. Consequently, *post hoc* reasoning is only one type of error in a wider group of logical errors known as the fallacy of false cause. In this fallacy, a proponent uses a false or weak causal connection to support the inference from the premises to the conclusion of an argument. Hurley (2015) identifies three variants of the fallacy of false cause: *post hoc ergo propter hoc*; *non causa pro causa*; and oversimplified cause. *Post hoc* is the only form of the fallacy where temporal sequence is integral to the logical flaw in the argument. But where *post hoc* has been characterized so far as a temporal relationship between a single occurrence of *A* and a single occurrence of *B*, where

A and *B* are temporally sequenced events, some authors describe the relationship in terms of a correlation between multiple occurrences of *A* and multiple occurrences of *B*. One such author is Douglas Walton (2008), who describes *post hoc* as an "argument from a correlation to a causal connection":

> The traditional *post hoc* fallacy was said to be the unjustified argument that concludes that one event causes another event simply because there is a positive correlation between the two events. Let *A* and *B* stand for events, or states of affairs that may obtain at a certain time. Then the *post hoc* fallacy was said to occur where it is concluded that *A* causes *B* simply because one or more occurrences of *A* are correlated with one or more occurrences of *B*. (pp. 259–260)

This alternative characterization of the fallacy is not without consequence. For while it may never seem to be rationally justified to conclude that *A* is the cause of *B* based on a single occurrence of *B* coming after a single occurrence of *A*, the same cannot be said if multiple occurrences of each event are considered. If many occurrences of *B* follow many occurrences of *A*, then the grounds for claiming that *A* causes *B* are certainly strengthened. If I have an asthma attack every time I visit the house of a friend who owns a cat, then I have reasonable grounds for claiming that hair from her cat is causing my attacks. My grounds for making this causal claim are much stronger than if I had one asthma attack after one visit to my friend's house. But my grounds for this causal connection are still not conclusive. This is because it may be pollen from my friend's indoor plants, and not her cat's hair, that may be causing my asthma attacks. Even a correlation is no guarantee of causation in the end.

In his chapter on *post hoc ergo propter hoc*, Pinto (1995) identifies a third conception of the *post hoc* fallacy. This is a type of faulty generalization, in which it is concluded that there is a causal relation between two event types, *A* and *B*, based on the fact that a single instance of *B* follows a single instance of *A*. In logical terms, this appears to be the weakest of all three conceptions of *post hoc* reasoning. For not only is a claim of causation based on a single instance of *B* coming after a single instance of *A*, but this single temporal sequence is then used to support a causal generalization. If I drink a certain cocktail drink and some hours later I am violently ill, I may conclude based solely on the temporal sequence between these events that the cocktail drink has caused my illness. I may then refuse all future offers of this same cocktail in the belief that they all will cause illness, or I may avoid all cocktails of any type because I believe cocktails in general induce violent illness. I may uphold this misguided reasoning even though I can see many instances that serve to falsify these causal generalizations. For example, I may know that my friends are able to consume the same cocktails without experiencing adverse health consequences. Also, I may have attended a dinner party where one of my friends served me a cocktail disguised as a non-alcoholic fruit juice. I may have consumed the drink and experienced no illness. But even knowing this, I may continue to maintain my causal generalization based on a single occurrence of illness that developed after I consumed the cocktail in question. If this type of reasoning strikes readers as strange, they should note that it is not dissimilar from the many superstitions that can hold sway in our thinking.

Hurley's second variant of the fallacy of false cause is ***non causa pro causa*** (literally, 'not the cause for the cause'). This form of the fallacy arises when we identify something to be a cause of an event when it is not the cause. But on this occasion, temporal succession plays no part in the false cause that we identify. If I observe that people who smoke have more respiratory illness than those who do not smoke, I may conclude that having respiratory illness causes people to smoke. Not only have I falsely identified respiratory illness as a cause of smoking, but I have confused an effect of smoking—respiratory illness—as a cause of smoking. If I identify that people who develop diabetes are often overweight, I may falsely conclude that diabetes is the cause of their obesity. Once again, I have confused the cause of diabetes, namely obesity, with the effect of diabetes. Other false causes that are unrelated to temporal succession arise when the occurrence of two events is merely coincidental. It may be observed that there is an increase in the use of crystal meth and in the rate of suicide in men under 30 years of age. However, there may be no causal connection between these increases, and to identify either one as the cause of the other is to commit false cause reasoning of the *non causa pro causa type*. Also, an increase in the rate of female depression may co-occur with an increase in the rate of teenage pregnancies in a city or country. But once again, these may be purely coincidental events, with neither event a true cause of the other event. In both scenarios, no temporal sequence is involved as the increases occur simultaneously and not sequentially.

Hurley calls his third and final form of the false cause fallacy **oversimplified cause**. This form of the fallacy arises when an event has a number of different causes, but a proponent of an argument emphasizes just one of these causes to the exclusion of the others. Oversimplified cause is a particularly common logical error in medicine. This is because most human diseases and medical events do not have a single cause. Instead, multiple factors contribute to their causation. It was described in ▶ Sect. 7.1 how genetic factors may play a role in the development of my cancer. If several of my relatives have developed cancer before the age of 55 years, then I have a positive family history of the disease. However, we now understand how carcinogenesis operates, and genetic factors are merely one causal factor, albeit a particularly important one. If I smoke heavily, am obese, and do not engage in exercise, the combined effect of these additional factors may be an even more important cause of my cancer than genetic factors. The same is true of medical events. If a patient undergoes abdominal surgery and then dies in the early post-operative period, the hospital may explain this death by saying that it was caused by a haemorrhage during surgery. However, if the patient experienced minimal blood loss as a result of the haemorrhage, but then went on to contract MRSA in the intensive care unit, a unit in which he was also administered incorrect medication, then it seems reasonable to conclude that the haemorrhage was not the only or even the most important cause of the patient's premature death. Any hospital that suppressed these other causal factors could be said to have oversimplified the cause of the patient's death as a means of avoiding culpability.

EXERCISE 7.1: The fallacy of false cause

As the above discussion demonstrates, it is not always easy to identify the true cause of an event. Even when there is no intention to perpetrate a deception, we can fall into the error of committing the fallacy of false cause. In the following extract, Baffy (2010) is considering factors that affect the outcome of patients with advanced cirrhosis who require intra-operative blood transfusion. Read the extract carefully, and then answer the questions that follow:

> Major haemorrhage during abdominal surgery has repeatedly been found to correlate with poor prognosis of cirrhotic patients, and this notion is now corroborated by Telem et al. who found that intraoperative blood loss and transfusion requirement is a significant predictor of adverse outcome [...] Surprisingly, the authors recommend limiting packed red blood cell transfusion during surgery as a possible method of reducing postoperative mortality in this clinical scenario. While it is easy to accept that the extent of intraoperative bleeding forebodes poor surgical outcome, administering blood transfusion is not necessarily a cause of higher mortality rates, and a proposal to limit this form of support in the hope of improving mortality may send the wrong message. (p. 996)

Questions

(a) Douglas Walton (2008) characterizes *post hoc* as an "argument from a correlation to a causal connection". Does this characterization apply to the scenario that Baffy is addressing?

(b) Baffy reports the work of Telem et al. who examined the outcome of cirrhotic patients who had intraoperative blood loss and blood transfusions during abdominal surgery. What do Telem et al. identify as the cause of the poor prognosis of these patients? Is this the actual cause of their poor prognosis?

(c) Baffy clearly believes that Telem et al. have attributed the poor prognosis of cirrhotic patients to a false cause. What statement in this extract suggests this is the case?

(d) Is there any causal relationship between major haemorrhage and blood transfusion in this scenario? If there is such a relationship, explain what it is.

(e) Based on your response to (d), how would you characterize the fallacy of false cause committed by Telem et al.?

7.4 Rationally Warranted *Post Hoc* Reasoning

It was described in ▸ Sect. 7.3 how *post hoc* reasoning does not always use temporal succession between two events to warrant a claim of causation. For some authors, the argument uses a correlation between events to support a causal conclusion. However we decide to conceive of *post hoc* reasoning, one thing is clear. There are many occasions in medicine and health when it is rationally warranted to argue that *A* causes *B* based on temporal succession and/or correlation between events. *Post hoc* is no more inherently fallacious than any of the other arguments that we have examined in this volume. In arriving at a logical characterization of this argument, we need to examine the contexts in which *post hoc* can support a claim of causation and is a rationally warranted argument in consequence. We will discover certain commonalities among these contexts. When *post hoc* is used in a rationally warranted way, a strong case for causation is usually made. Temporal sequence and correlation are the starting points for investigative processes that rigorously interrogate the basis of causal claims. When these processes are circumvented or bypassed, a causal claim that is based on *post hoc* reasoning can appear very shaky indeed. If our logical guard is down, these investigative shortcuts can pass undetected, and we accept the proponent's false cause as the true cause of the event in question. But if we ask searching questions of those who would have us accept a claim of causation, we can often expose critical weaknesses. This section illustrates how this can best be achieved without offering a guarantee of reader infallibility in causal reasoning.

To begin our discussion, let us consider a public health issue that caused considerable concern to medical authorities in the United States in the 1970s and 1980s. Reye syndrome is a rare, acute, life-threatening condition that is characterized by vomiting and lethargy and may progress to delirium and coma. Children with this condition experience acute encephalopathy and fatty infiltration of the liver (see ◘ Fig. 7.1). In the US, the condition was the focus of national surveillance between 1973–1974 and 1976–1977 by the Centers for Disease Control (CDC). In its third national surveillance period between 1 December 1980 and 31 October 1981, the CDC received written reports of 221 cases of Reye syndrome (CDC 1982a). Some background information about these cases is required in order to understand the public health challenge that was posed by this illness:

- Where the age of patients was known, 35% were less than or equal to 4 years of age and 59% were 5–14 years.
- An antecedent illness was reported in 203 cases. This illness took the form of respiratory symptoms in 121 (60%) cases, varicella (chicken pox) in 60 (30%) cases, and diarrhoea in 22 (10%) cases.

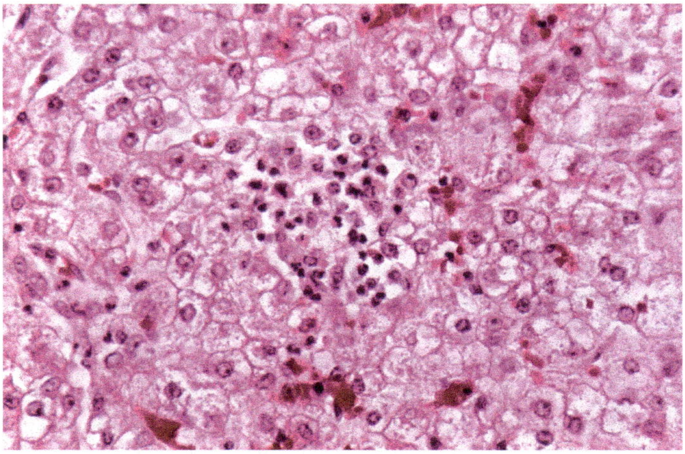

◘ **Fig. 7.1** This photomicrograph revealed histopathological changes found in a liver tissue autopsy specimen from a child who died of Reye syndrome. The hepatocytes, or liver cells, are seen as pale staining due to the accumulation of intracellular fat droplets (Photo reproduced courtesy of CDC/Dr. Edwin P. Ewing, Jr., 1972)

- Most patients (77%) were hospitalized from 5 December 1980 to 27 March 1981, a period that was coincident with reports of increased influenza A virus activity in the US.
- Of the 208 cases in which an outcome was reported, there were 58 deaths, resulting in a case fatality ratio of 28%.

A link between Reye syndrome and use of the salicylate aspirin to control fever was suggested by earlier studies in Arizona, Michigan, and Ohio. A fourth study reported to the CDC also suggested a link between aspirin use and Reye syndrome. This study was conducted by the Michigan Department of Public Health which had also completed the earlier investigation in Michigan. It found that all 12 of its patients with Reye syndrome had used medications containing salicylates during the prodromal illness. Only 12 of 29 (41.4%) controls had used these same medications. None of the 12 patients with Reye syndrome versus 16 of 29 (55.2%) controls had been administered a product containing acetaminophen (a nonsalicylate that is used to treat fever in children).

The CDC asked eight outside consultants to review data from all four studies. The consultants concluded that the strength and consistency of the observed association between Reye syndrome and salicylates were such that the relationship could not be explained by the limitations of the studies. They concluded that there was "sufficient evidence to support the cautionary statements on salicylate usage that had been published previously by the Centers for Disease Control and the National Institutes of Health Consensus Development Conference", and that "until the nature of the association between salicylates and Reye syndrome is clarified, the use of salicylates should be avoided, when possible, for children with varicella infections and during presumed influenza outbreaks". Based on the CDC data and reviews by other agencies (e.g. the Food and Drug Administration), the Surgeon General in June 1982 advised against the use of salicylates and salicylate-containing medications for children with influenza and chicken pox. An advisory published in the *Mortality and Morbidity Weekly Report* stated:

> The association of salicylates with Reye syndrome is based upon evidence from epidemiologic studies that are sufficiently strong to justify this warning to parents and health care personnel. (CDC 1982b)

This episode in US public health illustrates how scientists can draw valid conclusions about causal relationships between events without succumbing to fallacious *post hoc* reasoning. At the time the CDC was conducting national surveillance of Reye syndrome, each year in the US between 600 and 1200 children developed Reye syndrome *after* taking salicylates like aspirin to control fever during influenza and chicken pox (CDC 1982b). That there was temporal succession between the taking of aspirin and the development of Reye syndrome is beyond doubt—typically, a 5–7 day interval occurred between the antecedent illness that prompted the use of aspirin and hospitalization of patients with Reye syndrome (CDC 1982a). For the proponent of fallacious *post hoc* reasoning, this temporal sequence is enough to draw the conclusion that aspirin *causes* Reye syndrome. But to arrive at this conclusion so early into an investigation of what was causing Reye syndrome would have been a monumental scientific error for a number of reasons. First, the number of Reye syndrome cases was relatively small in comparison to the many thousands of children who used aspirin safely to control fever during viral illnesses. Second, it is possible that Reye syndrome was caused by the viral illnesses that prompted the use of aspirin rather than by aspirin itself. Third, some other factor in a child's environment or genes could have caused susceptibility to Reye syndrome, with aspirin playing little or no role in causation. It was with a view to excluding these other possibilities that the CDC and other public health agencies undertook several epidemiological studies. Some information about the design of the second study conducted by the Michigan Department of Public Health is shown below:

- All medications taken during the preceding illness were examined. This included their dosage and frequency of administration.
- For each child with Reye syndrome in the study, 1–3 controls were used.
- Controls were matched for year in school (plus or minus 1), race, febrile response (100F, 100F-102.9F, and greater than or equal to 103F), and nature of prodromal illness (i.e. chickenpox or respiratory or gastrointestinal illness).
- Interviews were conducted with the parents of children with Reye syndrome as soon as possible (mean 5.5 days) after each case was reported.

The scientific rigour of this study and other epidemiological investigations allowed investigators to control for factors that may have been playing a role in the causation of Reye syndrome. These factors had to be excluded if investigators were to claim a role for salicylate medications like aspirin in the causation of Reye syndrome. But even then, investigators proceeded with caution. It was possible that the correlation between aspirin and Reye syndrome identified by the Michigan Department of Public Health would not be found in other epidemiological studies. To ensure that as complete a review as possible of all relevant data was undertaken, the CDC enlisted the assistance of eight external consultants. It was only when these consultants reviewed all the evidence and confirmed the association between aspirin and Reye syndrome that the CDC drew its own conclusion about the likely cause of Reye syndrome. But here again, caution was exercised. The CDC stated that salicylates *may* be a factor in the pathogenesis of Reye syndrome, and that the observed association *did not prove causality*. They also stated that *additional well-controlled studies* were needed:

> In summary, these studies indicate to CDC that salicylates may be a factor in the pathogenesis of Reye syndrome, although the observed epidemiologic association does not prove causality. The exact pathogenesis of this disease and the possible role of salicylates in its pathogenesis remain to be determined. Additional well-controlled studies are also needed. Until definitive information is available, CDC advises physicians and parents of the possible increased risk of Reye syndrome associated with the use of salicylates for children with chickenpox or influenza-like illness. (CDC 1982a)

What we have described here is a scientifically rigorous approach to the investigation of the cause of Reye syndrome. It started with simple observations. It was observed that certain children who took aspirin to control fever during viral illnesses developed some 5–7 days later a serious, life-threatening condition called Reye syndrome. For the parents of these children, it must have seemed certain that the viral illness was causing their children's life-threatening condition. These children were, after all, well up until the point of contracting chicken pox or influenza and only after this developed Reye syndrome. However, the mind of the scientist is trained not to succumb to intuitive judgements of causation based on temporal succession. The scientist observes temporal succession between the onset of viral illness and the development of Reye syndrome, but knows that this is not an adequate basis on which to claim causation. Instead, this observation marks the start of a process of rigorous scientific inquiry into the likely cause of Reye syndrome. This inquiry should be comprehensive in that not just a single viral illness or a single medication that was administered prior to the development of Reye syndrome should be investigated. It should use control subjects that are matched on a range of variables that might explain the onset of Reye syndrome. It should consider the results of more than one epidemiological study in order to ensure that findings are reproducible. In other words, it should adhere closely to the principles of sound scientific methodology. Even when this is achieved, it should avoid strong claims of causation in favour of a more tentatively worded association between the events of interest. This exacting standard of scientific inquiry is not easily attained. But it was exemplified by the work of the CDC on Reye syndrome.

It emerges that *post hoc* reasoning, when used fallaciously, is a subversion of the scientific processes by means of which causation between events is established. The proponent who engages in fallacious *post hoc* reasoning attempts to foreclose inquiry into the cause of an event on the basis of temporal succession between events. In so doing, the investigations that scientists embark on to interrogate the basis of causal claims are effectively bypassed. *Post hoc* reasoning might have led some parents and doctors to conclude that the viral illness was the cause of Reye syndrome, while others may have attributed a causal role to aspirin. But even in the latter case, the conclusion, albeit correct, would have been established by means of flawed logic that could not withstand rational scrutiny. These parents and doctors would simply have been fortuitous in attributing a causal role to aspirin use—their reasoning could so easily have led to a mistaken conclusion about the probable cause of Reye syndrome, with disastrous consequences for child health. In the next section, we will examine an episode in UK public health where just such a scenario came about. But before doing so, we will examine further the logical conditions under which *post hoc* reasoning can be rationally warranted.

The central objection to *post hoc* reasoning is that temporal succession between events is an inadequate basis on which to conclude that one event caused another event. And to some extent this is true. If the epidemiologists who were charged with investigating Reye syndrome had only used temporal succession between events to guide their judgements about the cause of the condition, they would have expended considerable time and resources investigating all manner of things that we would not consider to be causes of human diseases. They might have explored visits to theme parks, trips to the beach, and time spent with grandparents as potential causes of Reye syndrome in children, simply because these events preceded the onset of the condition. What this demonstrates is that even when we are guided during causal reasoning by temporal succession between events, these events must be *of the right type*.

Scientists who were charged with investigating Reye syndrome had to decide to examine certain events and leave other events aside. Events that were explored further as possible causes of Reye syndrome were those which had disease-bearing properties such as the toxic effects of medication and exposure to viral pathogens. Where the proponent of a causal relationship between two events appeals to events that have low plausibility as causes (in this case, of human disease), then we may expect the rational standing of temporal succession based on these events to be diminished in consequence. When events of high plausibility underpin temporal succession, then succession between events has greater rational warrant as a basis for a claim of causation. This gives rise to the first logical feature of the rationally warranted use of *post hoc* reasoning:

Logical feature 1: Proposed causes must be plausible for causation

Of the potential causes of an event such as the onset of human disease, some causes have greater plausibility than other causes. When temporal succession between events involves plausible causes, *a claim of causation based on temporal succession is more rationally warranted in consequence.*

It is instructive at this point to think about the words in italics above. Temporal succession between events can confer rational warrant on a claim of causation, but only under certain conditions. One such condition is that it is possible to identify plausible events as potential causes of a disease or other phenomenon. When this condition is satisfied, temporal succession is not such a spurious basis after all on which to base a claim of causation. But neither is it a failsafe guarantee that two events are causally related. Instead, there begins a process of inquiry into the exact nature of the association between two events. This inquiry may validate one of these events as a probable cause of the other event. When this occurs, a claim of causation is more strongly rationally warranted as a result. But it is still not definitively established and can be overturned with the emergence of new evidence. Openness to revision must be ever present in causal reasoning as in science in general. This was a feature of the CDC's investigation into Reye syndrome. Although the investigation suggested that aspirin was a likely cause of this life-threatening condition, the CDC emphasized that it did not prove causality and recommended that additional, well-controlled studies be undertaken. But it is important to remember where this causal relationship between aspirin use and Reye syndrome began its journey. It started with temporal succession between two events, one of which—the ingestion of aspirin—had disease-bearing properties that satisfied the requirement of plausible cause.

It emerges that temporal succession between events is not as misguided a route into causal reasoning as it might at first appear. When a plausible cause is identified, temporal succession is a rational initial basis on which to explore causation between events. But temporal succession also has other features that make it a sound starting point for an investigation of causation between events. Temporal succession is typically defined in terms of *order* between two events, *A* and *B*, with *A* the presumed cause of *B* because *A* precedes *B* in time. Another important dimension of this temporal relationship is the *amount of time* that elapses between the occurrence of *A* and the occurrence of *B*. It must also satisfy a requirement of plausibility in *post hoc* reasoning. Given the acute onset of Reye syndrome, it was unlikely to be explained by events that occurred six months earlier in the lives of affected children. But it could be plausibly explained by the onset of viral illnesses or the use of medication in the days immediately preceding the admission of these children to hospital with Reye syndrome. These latter events would take days rather than weeks or months to have their serious effects on the health of these children. It was for this reason that epidemiologists focussed their efforts on examining antecedent illnesses and medication use in their investigation into the likely cause of Reye syndrome. Once again, temporal succession has much greater significance to causation than is generally acknowledged to be the case, with the amount of time between events and not just the order of events providing rational warrant for claims of causation. This gives rise to the second logical feature of the rationally warranted use of *post hoc* reasoning:

Logical feature 2: Duration between events must be plausible for causation

In any temporal succession, the duration between events must form a plausible basis for a claim of causation. If there is not adequate time for a proposed cause to take effect, then any temporal succession of which this proposed cause is a part is a weak basis for a claim of causation. Temporal succession that includes an event that is too temporally remote from the event that it is presumed to cause is also a weak basis for a claim of causation.

The reason that duration between events in temporal succession also has logical bearing on a claim of causation is that it takes time for processes that give effect to a cause to be realized. We do not display the symptoms of an infectious disease as soon as we are exposed to the pathogen that causes the disease. Instead, the pathogen requires an incubation period of several days or weeks during which it invades cells in our body, undergoes replication, and produces the toxins that eventually make us ill. We must have reasonable grounds for believing that this pathogenesis can be achieved in the time that elapses between the events in a temporal succession. The events that lead to the development of cancer (e.g. exposure to ionizing radiation) may be temporally remote from the symptoms that are the first signs that a person has developed the disease. Given what we know about carcinogenesis, it makes very little sense to base a claim about the cause of a person's cancer on temporal succession between two events that are separated by just one month. By the same token, a person may develop iatrogenic Creutzfeldt-Jakob disease. But the medical intervention that causes this disease—a neurosurgical procedure or use of human derived growth hormone—may have occurred decades earlier. What these examples demonstrate is that when we use temporal succession between two events as a starting point in causal reasoning, we must be prepared to consider some very extended time periods between the events in question. Whether or not a certain amount of time is plausible depends on the event that we are attempting to explain, and the likely mechanism of pathogenesis between exposure to a disease-causing agent or situation and the onset of symptoms.

This discussion demonstrates that temporal succession between events is not such a weak basis after all for a claim of causation. Temporal succession that involves a plausible cause and sufficient time between events during which pathogenesis may occur is a rational starting point for an investigation into causation. What makes it appear otherwise is an interpretation of *post hoc* reasoning that has fallaciousness built into the very conception of the argument. Clearly, if all we consider during *post hoc* reasoning is mere temporal order between events, then there are grounds for saying that temporal succession is an inadequate basis upon which to base a claim of causation. Such a narrowly understood notion of temporal succession would lead us to conclude that completely irrelevant events—a child's birthday party or a new family pet—could be a cause of Reye syndrome simply because these events preceded the onset of the disease. But when we look to temporal succession between events as a basis for causal reasoning, we are not appealing to such a narrow conception of temporal succession. Temporal succession brings with it all sorts of assumptions about what constitutes a plausible cause of an event, and the length of time that it might take for a disease to develop to the point where symptoms become evident or for the toxic effects of a drug to become apparent. When this richer conception of temporal succession is considered, what we have is a valuable rational resource that can become the basis of further causal reasoning. This is not to say, however, that even when we adopt this richer conception of temporal succession that we cannot run into error. Temporal succession between events may ultimately be shown to lead to a false cause. But it is at least a rational starting point in an inquiry into causation.

It is now time for you to get some practice in evaluating causal reasoning by attempting Exercise 7.2.

EXERCISE 7.2: Child victimization and cognitive functioning

Psychologists, psychiatrists, and educationalists have a professional interest in investigating the effect of abuse and victimization on the cognitive functioning of children. However, as Costello (2017) observes, it is easy to commit *post hoc* reasoning when we consider the relationship between victimization and cognitive functioning. It can somehow seem inevitable that a victimized child will suffer some sort of serious consequence as a result of its abuse, and that cognitive problems are a highly plausible contender for such a consequence. Examine Costello's views in the following extract, and then answer the questions below:

> "Post hoc, ergo propter hoc" ("After this, therefore because of it") is a very common way of thinking. Sometimes it is true, but often it is a logical fallacy. There is abundant evidence that victimized children have poorer cognitive functioning than other children, and not surprisingly plenty of research papers link the two causally. What's wrong with that? Child victimization is wrong, and suboptimal cognitive functioning is a waste of human resources, so why not go ahead and work to reduce both? Well, for one thing, it is not good science. The most valuable, and practical, scientific explanation of a causal process is the one that is still standing when all others have been knocked down. (p. 305)

Questions

(a) Costello describes how research papers draw a causal relationship between child victimization and poor cognitive functioning. Which type of *post hoc* reasoning discussed in ▶ Sect. 7.3 best describes what these research papers are doing?

(b) The research papers appear to assume that child victimization is the cause of poor cognitive functioning. What other interpretation of the relationship between these variables is possible?

(c) There may be no cause-effect relationship between child victimization and poor cognitive functioning. Instead, these variables may appear to be related because of the influence of a third variable. Give an example of this variable and explain its interaction with victimization and poor cognitive functioning.

(d) *Post hoc* reasoning involves a temporal sequence between event *A* and event *B*, or multiple occurrences of *A* and multiple occurrences of *B*. Imagine that event *A* is child victimization. How might a research study characterize this temporal sequence between child victimization and cognitive functioning?

(e) Costello believes that causal reasoning should involve a process in which contenders for a causal explanation of an event are actively rejected and the 'correct' causal explanation is the one that is 'still standing' after all others have been overturned or defeated. A causal explanation has the same status for Costello as another important scientific construct. What is that construct?

DISCUSSION POINT: Stroke, depression and *post hoc* reasoning

In an article in the journal *Neurology*, Amy Brodtmann (2014) poses the question "Why do patients with stroke get depression?" A strong association between stroke and depression, she writes, has been described for many decades. Brodtmann then considers if we should not be asking the reverse question "Why do patients with depression get stroke?" The article continues:

> An association between late-life depression (LLD) as a risk factor for stroke has also been proposed for some time. Controversy remains as to whether the risk of depression on incident stroke is causal or whether it is conditional on other underlying factors, including pre-existing personality. Many researchers now believe that LLD is an indicator of vascular burden, and that it is this incipient cerebrovascular disease and ischemic change that damages pathways in the brain and increases the risk of associated depression. (p. 1688)

Clearly, whatever relationship exists between stroke and depression, it is unlikely to be a simple cause-effect relationship. In a group with other students, you should discuss the different permutations of the relationship between stroke and depression that are considered by Brodtmann.

SPECIAL TOPIC: Implied causation and *post hoc* reasoning

Post hoc arguments are most pernicious when they are difficult to detect. Often, a perpetrator of such an argument will avoid explicit causal claims and assertions in the knowledge that they will be easily uncovered and found to be lacking. A more successful strategy from the proponent's perspective is to create the impression in the mind of the reader or hearer that two events are causally related without making an explicit claim to this effect. If the proponent can create the conditions for such an impression to take root, then he or she can leave it to the reader or hearer to draw the desired causal inference. This occurs quite commonly in public discourse, and is a significant cause of *post hoc* errors in reasoning.

In an article in *The Guardian* on 17 March 2015, Ann Waters—cabinet member for children and families in Haringey council—described how the North London borough achieved a 37% drop in teenage pregnancies between 2012 and 2013. Waters described how the issue of teenage pregnancy was prioritised at the highest level in Haringey. Measures taken by the council and others included improved sexual and relationship advice, increased access to contraception, and efforts to raise young people's aspirations and educational attainment (◘ Fig. 7.2). Waters claimed that a key factor in Haringey's approach was the involvement of young people and the wider community in the design of materials that promote local contraception and sexual health services. Although Waters acknowledges that Haringey's reduction in teenage pregnancy "cannot be attributed to a single, silver bullet intervention", she encourages readers to draw a causal connection between the reduction and the council's interventions in remarks such as the following:

> It is no coincidence that in Haringey the reduction took place at a time when performance in schools increased. Between 2010 and 2014 Haringey saw the second highest improvement in GCSE results of any local authority. ('How we halved teenage pregnancy rates in Haringey', Ann Waters, *The Guardian*, 17 March 2015)

If, as Waters is claiming, it is "no coincidence" that the reduction occurred at a time of improved academic attainment in Haringey, then readers are encouraged to conclude that the reduction in teenage pregnancy was *caused* by improved academic achievement in the borough. Waters has very skilfully planted this causal relationship in the minds of readers without making any direct claim or assertion to this effect. That not all readers of the article are prepared to accept Waters' implied causation between the council's interventions and the reduction in teenage pregnancy is evident in one of the comments posted below the article. Whilst welcoming the changes implemented by Haringey, Alan Stanton, a former Haringey councillor, urged caution about drawing the causal relationships implied by the article and its headline. He stated:

> Plainly we need to acknowledge and welcome the changes in Haringey, and the valuable work which agencies there have been doing.
>
> But I wonder if Haringey Council is rather too ready to claim credit for causing a change which is actually a national and international trend. In some countries a quite startling change. [...]
>
> I'd [...] feel more confident if the article included what they are unsure about and need to learn. And was less about selling the "How we did it" story signalled by the headline.

To be fair, Ann Waters' closing paragraphs make sensible points about the complexities of the issue; and the need for: *"a well-thought out and collaboratively produced prevention strategy"*. So I was surprised at the apparently confident claim that the Council's actions had led to the improvements shown. That may indeed be wholly accurate. But do they actually know this? It may also be wholly or partly the *post hoc ergo propter hoc* logical fallacy. The claim that: 'X happened after Haringey did Y; and therefore that Y caused X.

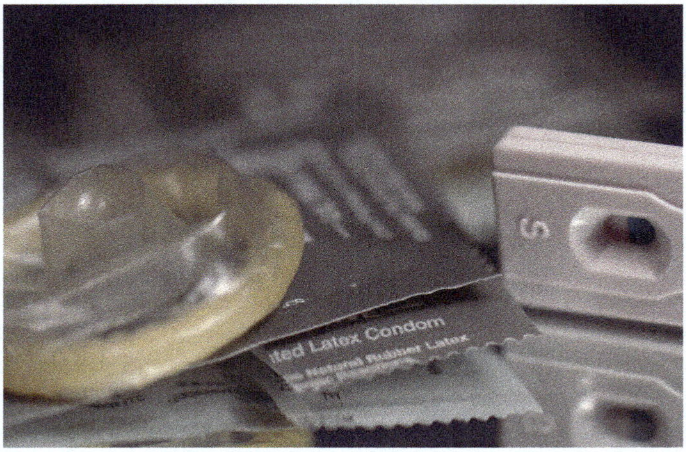

Fig. 7.2 Improved access to contraception and sexual health services was part of Haringey's strategy to achieve a reduction in teenage pregnancy (Photo by Debora Cartagena is reproduced courtesy of CDC/Debora Cartagena, 2012)

7.5 Fallacious *Post Hoc* Reasoning

Temporal succession between events is not always a productive resource during reasoning. Scientists and others can make fallacious use of temporal succession during reasoning, sometimes with disastrous consequences for human health. In this section, we examine a health scare that occurred in the UK in the late 1990s and which continues to have wide-reaching implications for public health in the UK and beyond (see Discussion Point below). The event concerns claims made by Dr Andrew Wakefield about the safety of the measles, mumps, and rubella (MMR) vaccine. In an article published in *The Lancet* in February 1998, Dr Wakefield and his colleagues claimed to have examined a consecutive series of 12 children with chronic enterocolitis and pervasive developmental disorder (or autism). The article stated that the onset of the behavioural symptoms of autism was associated by the parents with MMR vaccination in eight of the 12 children investigated. On 6 February 2010, *The Lancet* retracted Wakefield's article. The retraction followed the judgement of the UK General Medical Council's Fitness to Practise Panel on 28 January 2010 that Dr Wakefield had, among other things, performed unnecessary invasive procedures on the children and had not revealed conflicts of interest in his conduct of the study. Wakefield and his colleagues did not assert that the MMR vaccination caused autism. They stated in their article that "[w]e did not prove an association between measles, mumps, and rubella vaccine and the syndrome described" (1998: 641). However, it is clear from comments Wakefield made at a press conference after the publication of his article that he believed the vaccine was responsible for the behavioural and gastrointestinal anomalies of the children in his study. He remarked:

> For the vast majority of children the MMR vaccine is fine, but I believe there are sufficient anxieties for a case to be made to administer the three vaccinations separately. I do not think that the long-term safety trials of MMR are sufficient for giving the three vaccines together. ('Andrew Wakefield—the man behind the MMR controversy', Rebecca Smith, *The Telegraph*, 29 January 2010).

The public anxiety that ensued about the safety of the MMR vaccine led to a dramatic reduction in the number of parents who brought their children forward to be vaccinated for measles, mumps, and rubella. MMR uptake in 1997–1998 prior to the publication of Wakefield's article was 90.8%. In the wake of the MMR safety scare, MMR coverage dropped to a low of 79.9% in 2003–2004. This resulted in measles outbreaks in a susceptible population of children aged 10 to 16 years who had not been vaccinated some years earlier against these infectious diseases, and the announcement in April 2013 of a national catch-up vaccination programme (see ▶ Sect. 4.4). With so much unnecessary distress and suffering arising out of Wakefield's work, we must consider the following question: How did the destruction of this safe and effective vaccination programme come about? For some commentators, the answer to this question is clear. Wakefield and his colleagues were engaging in *post hoc* reasoning when they considered the MMR vaccine to be a likely cause of these children's behavioural symptoms:

> Because vaccinations are universally applied and (distinctly) memorable, they are frequently implicated as the cause by some parents and clinicians for unexplained illnesses. With post hoc ergo propter hoc, however, the ancient logicians have cautioned us to the danger of assessing causality based on human observations alone. As requested by *The Lancet*, our commentary applied the principles of causal inference in vaccine safety to the report by Andrew Wakefield and colleagues—and found it wanting. (Chen and DeStefano 1998: 63)

In the eight children whose parents believed the onset of behavioural problems was linked to the MMR vaccination, the average interval from exposure to first behavioural symptoms was 6.3 days (range 1–14) (Wakefield et al. 1998). Temporal succession between vaccination and the onset of behavioural symptoms seemed to provide reasonably strong grounds for the claim that the MMR vaccine was *causing* the symptoms of these children. But when we consider the timing of the MMR vaccination schedule in children and the age at which young children first display the symptoms of autism, temporal succession between vaccination and symptom onset no longer appears so causally significant after all. In the UK, MMR vaccine is administered to children on the National Health Service in two doses. The first dose is usually administered to babies within a month of their first birthday. The second dose is administered before starting school, usually at 3 years and 4 months. The timing of these vaccinations is largely consistent with the ages at which children first exhibit the behavioural symptoms of autism (Ozonoff et al. 2008). The children in Wakefield's study displayed onset of behavioural symptoms between 12 months and 4.5 years. This suggests that rather than *causing* autism, MMR vaccination is *coincidental with* the emergence of this neurodevelopmental disorder in children. What appeared to be a cause-effect relationship between MMR vaccination and autism is, in fact, two unrelated events that simply happened to occur around the same time in the lives of young children.

It may seem facile to declare that Wakefield and his colleagues were engaging in fallacious *post hoc* reasoning. After all, today we have the benefit of hindsight, and the results of many other investigations completed since Wakefield's study that have disproved a link between MMR vaccination and autism. But signs that Wakefield and his colleagues were using fallacious *post hoc* reasoning were apparent even in 1998. The first sign that temporal succession was an unreliable basis for causal reasoning in this case was that Wakefield only examined 12 children. The onset of behavioural symptoms occurred *after* MMR vaccination in all 12 children. But in the absence of a much larger sample of children, this finding had no true causal import. The second investigation into Reye syndrome conducted by the Michigan Department of Public Health also had only 12 patients. However, this study was only one of several reviewed by the CDC, and so a much larger sample of children was examined by investigators. The study conducted by the Ohio State Department of Health alone examined 159 children with Reye syndrome. In an addendum to their article, Wakefield and his colleagues stated that up until 28 January 1998—their article was published in *The Lancet* on 28 February 1998—a further 39 patients with the 'syndrome' had been identified. This would still only have brought the total number of children investigated to just 51. Given the small number of identified cases, a more cautious strategy for Wakefield and his colleagues might have been to delay publication of their findings until a larger sample of children could be examined. At a minimum, Wakefield should have avoided any suggestion of a causal association between MMR vaccination and autism based on this insufficient sample.

It emerges that Wakefield and his colleagues attributed causal significance to MMR vaccination which was not warranted given the small number of children in their study. With only 12 children involved in this investigation, we could conclude nothing about the cause of autism from the fact that behavioural symptoms emerged after the MMR vaccination was administered. The timing of these events in all 12 children may simply have been a coincidence. With no other studies or data to corroborate their findings, Wakefield and his colleagues attributed unwarranted causal significance to the fact that these children had all received MMR vaccination prior to the onset of symptoms. But why did such a small sample lead these investigators to conclude that the vaccination was likely to be responsible for these children's symptoms? The fervent conviction of parents that the MMR vaccination had caused their children's illness may well have influenced Wakefield and his colleagues more than they were prepared to admit. We tend to assume that medical professionals are dispassionate and can take a detached, objective stance towards the events that they are attempting to explain.[2] But when your informants are distressed parents who are wholly convinced that vaccination is responsible for their children's autism, it is easy for the judgement of even medical professionals to become clouded. It can seem that no other explanation of these children's symptoms is possible—MMR vaccination *must* be the cause of these symptoms. When this occurs, temporal succession between events is made to carry logical weight that is not justified by the small sample involved in the study. This gives rise to the first logical pitfall in the use of *post hoc* reasoning:

> ***Logical pitfall 1*: Overstating the causal significance of temporal succession**
>
> Temporal succession between events has little logical weight when it is based on a small number of cases. The fact that one event precedes another event in these cases may simply be a matter of coincidence. If a proponent overstates the logical (and causal) significance of temporal succession, then the result is a causal fallacy.

Temporal succession between MMR vaccination and the onset of behavioural symptoms was a weak basis for causal inference in a further respect that should also have been apparent to Wakefield and his colleagues. The average interval between vaccination and behavioural symptoms was 6.3 days. One child developed behavioural symptoms 24 hours after vaccination, another after 48 hours. Still other children displayed symptoms after just 1 or 2 weeks. For the vaccination to have been responsible for these symptoms, a very fast-acting pathological process would need to occur. But this was not the type of pathogenesis that Wakefield and his colleagues proposed. They described a pattern of colitis and ileal-lymphoid-nodular hyperplasia in the children in their study. In these inflammatory bowel diseases, there is increased intestinal permeability related to the disruption of the normally sulphated glycoprotein matrix of the gut wall which regulates cell and molecular trafficking. The disruption of this glycoprotein matrix and increased intestinal permeability were posited to cause neuropsychiatric dysfunction. Wakefield and his colleagues considered that these intestinal pathological processes provided the most plausible explanation of the brain dysfunction in the children in their study:

> Both the presence of intestinal inflammation and absence of detectable neurological abnormality in our children are consistent with an exogenous influence upon cerebral function. (1998: 640)

That MMR vaccination could have triggered these intestinal histopathological changes to occur with subsequent disruption of cerebral function all within a 24-hour or 48-hour period scarcely seems plausible. It is also possible, and much more likely, that the onset of these inflammatory bowel diseases predated MMR vaccination of these children. Wakefield and his colleagues acknowledged in their article that the parents of the children were not clear about the timing of onset of abdominal symptoms because the children were not toilet trained at the time, or their behavioural problems meant they were unable to communicate their symptoms (1998: 638). What we are left with is a pathological process of uncertain onset that, if Wakefield and his colleagues are to be believed, was able to exert its destructive effects in just 24 hours on both the intestinal health and cerebral function of at least some of the children in Wakefield's study. Wakefield did not address this important temporal dimension of his proposed mechanism of pathogenesis. But its lack of plausibility certainly weakened the claim that MMR vaccination may be responsible for these children's autism. This error in Wakefield's thinking is the basis of the second logical pitfall in *post hoc* reasoning:

Logical pitfall 2: Duration between events in temporal succession is implausible

When a proponent advances a causal mechanism that cannot be plausibly executed in the time between events in temporal succession, but still uses the order of these events to warrant a causal claim, then fallacious *post hoc* reasoning has been committed.

The key issue of how long it might plausibly take for the type of pathogenesis that Wakefield and his colleagues had in mind to unfold appeared not to trouble these investigators. But it was another early sign that the logical direction taken by Wakefield was mistaken. How did this implausibly short period of time for pathogenesis evade detection by Wakefield and his colleagues? According to some commentators, Wakefield was so convinced that his 'theory' about the cause of these children's behavioural symptoms and intestinal abnormalities was correct that he was blinded by this conviction. Wakefield has even described himself as under a moral duty to parents to establish a cause of their children's unexplained illness.[3] For other commentators, such as the editors of the *British Medical Journal*, Wakefield was perpetrating a deliberate fraud when he attempted to draw a link between MMR vaccination and autism (Godlee et al. 2011). Whatever ultimately motivated Wakefield's logical lapse—unintentional error or deliberate deception—it was clear that temporal succession between MMR vaccination and the onset of symptoms of autism was a very weak basis for further causal reasoning. Nothing could be concluded about the cause of autism from the fact that only 12 children displayed behavioural symptoms of autism after MMR vaccination, particularly when the proposed mechanism of pathogenesis was incomplete and implausible. That Wakefield and his colleagues were engaging in fallacious *post hoc* reasoning did not need to await the results of further studies. It was apparent even in 1998 when Wakefield first advanced his ideas about MMR and autism.

To get further practice in evaluating causal reasoning, you should now attempt Exercise 7.3.

EXERCISE 7.3: Identifying the effect in causation

This chapter has focussed on the *causes* of events. But it is at least as important to causation that we are able to identify with accuracy the *effects* of an event. In the extract below, Finucane (2012) is making the point that it is very difficult to identify post-operative events that are caused by gastrostomy placement and are thus a complication of the procedure. He wonders how many of the events identified as post-operative complications are true complications of gastrostomy placements and how many are examples of *post hoc* reasoning. Read the extract carefully, and then answer the questions that follow:

» Analyzing events after a procedure or surgery can be heavily fraught. Semantics are important. "Postoperative mortality" is scarcely controversial. Define some interval after the surgery as "postoperative" and deaths occurring in that interval are "postoperative." "Postoperative complication," however, is complicated. Postoperative wound infection could reasonably be seen as a complication, and carries a subtle suggestion of fault. But what about a fall the night after surgery, a paroxysm of atrial fibrillation, a pulmonary embolism, or a myocardial infarction? What adverse postoperative events can reasonably be considered complications of surgery? These questions are not yet resolved, and their resolution is likely to be problematic. Is a periprosthetic femur fracture 10 days after hip replacement a postoperative complication? Suppose it happened when the patient was struck by a car? Stepped off the curb and tripped? Walked down the stairs to the street? (p. 197)

Questions

(a) Finucane emphasizes the importance of semantics in defining terms like *postoperative mortality* and *postoperative complication*. Why does semantics make the scope of the former term easy to identify but not the scope of the latter term?

(b) It can be useful to distinguish between *distal* and *proximal* causes of an event. For example, if I develop lung cancer, my smoking may be a proximal cause of my cancer and genetic factors may be a distal cause. How might this distinction be usefully applied to some of the events that follow gastrostomy placement?

(c) Many events in medicine and elsewhere have more than one cause. When we focus on one of these causes to the exclusion of others, we commit a particular fallacy of false cause. What is this fallacy? Is there a need for a counterpart fallacy that relates to the effects of an event?

(d) Finucane presents a reason why it is important to have a clear understanding of what counts as a postoperative complication of gastrostomy placement. What is that reason? Can you think of another reason why it is important to understand the effects of this surgical procedure?

(e) Finucane argues that just because an event occurs *after* gastrostomy placement that it should not be considered an *effect* of this procedure. One reason why this would be an invalid conclusion to draw is that both gastrostomy placement and what appears to be a postoperative complication may both be effects of a third variable. Give *one* example of such a variable and explain how it might operate.

DISCUSSION POINT: Parental fears about vaccine safety

In a Retro Report in *The New York Times*, Clyde Haberman describes the impact that the scare about MMR vaccine safety continues to have on parents' willingness to vaccinate their children against infectious diseases. In order to address parental concerns, health professionals need to have a sound understanding of the psychological factors that lead many parents to reject vaccination of their children and to disregard the advice of doctors and health

professionals. Read the following extract from Haberman's article, and then watch his full video documentary at: ► https://www.nytimes.com/2015/02/02/us/a-discredited-vaccine-studys-continuing-impact-on-public-health.html. In a group with other students, discuss what psychological factors lead parents to reject vaccination, and explain why these factors are more compelling to parents than the expert advice offered by medical and health professionals (◘ Fig. 7.3).

» **A discredited vaccine study's continuing impact on public health**

In the churning over the refusal of some parents to immunize their children against certain diseases, a venerable Latin phrase may prove useful: Post hoc, ergo propter hoc. It means, "After this, therefore because of this." In plainer language: Event B follows Event A, so B must be the direct result of A. It is a classic fallacy in logic.

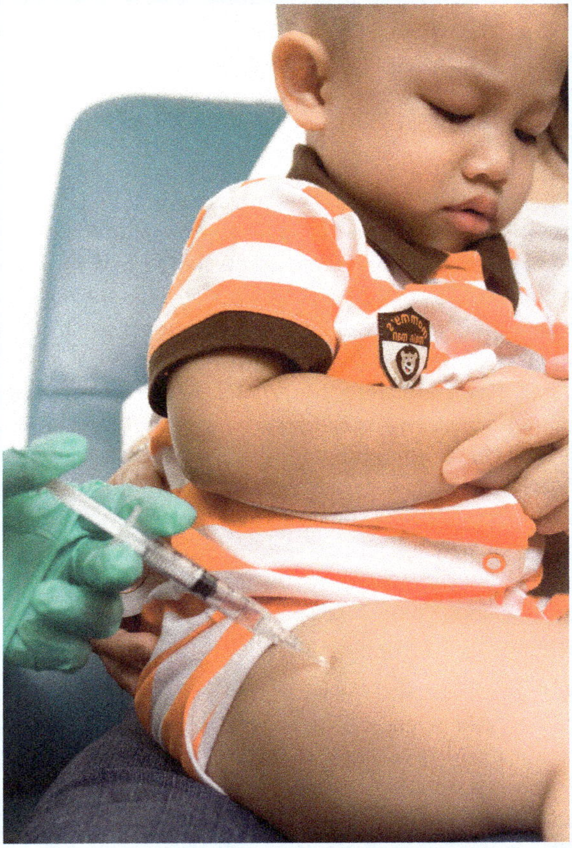

◘ **Fig. 7.3** Childhood vaccinations are vital in the fight against infectious diseases. Their uptake has been compromised in recent years by unfounded parental concerns about vaccine safety (Photo by Amanda Mills is reproduced courtesy of CDC/Amanda Mills, 2011)

It is also a trap into which many Americans have fallen. That is the consensus among health professionals trying to contain recent spurts of infectious diseases that they had believed were forever in the country's rearview mirror. They worry that too many people are not getting their children vaccinated, out of a conviction that inoculations are risky.

Some parents feel certain that vaccines can lead to autism, if only because there have been instances when a child got a shot and then became autistic. Post hoc, ergo propter hoc. Making that connection between the two events, most health experts say, is as fallacious in the world of medicine as it is in the field of logic. [...]

What motivates vaccine-averse parents? One factor may be the very success of the vaccines. Several generations of Americans lack their parents' and grandparents' visceral fear of polio [...]. For those people, "you might as well be protecting against aliens — these are things they've never seen," said Seth Mnookin, who teaches science writing at the Massachusetts Institute of Technology and is the author of "The Panic Virus," a 2011 book on vaccinations and their opponents.

('A discredited vaccine study's continuing impact on public health', Clyde Haberman, *The New York Times*, 1 February 2015)

SPECIAL TOPIC: The public and *post hoc* reasoning

The public is often better equipped to evaluate reasoning than many logicians and argumentation theorists are prepared to acknowledge. In an article in *The Guardian* on 12 December 2016, Alison Moodie discussed the different ways in which the food industry funds scientific research. Industry involvement in scientific research, she argued, is a significant source of bias, with many studies producing findings that are favourable to their funders. In response to Moodie's article, several readers posted comments and opinions. Two readers exchanged views with each other about what they believed was causing the obesity epidemic—an issue that was related to Moodie's article. The exchange begins with one of the contributors, Contributor 1, remarking on how the sugar industry and the meat and dairy industry like to blame each other for the obesity epidemic. Contributor 1 then stated: "In actual fact, we know that both refined carbs/sugar and saturated fats are bad for our health". The second contributor, Contributor 2, took issue with this statement, describing it as a myth that saturated fats are bad for our health:

» It is a myth that saturated fats are bad for our health. (That myth was a combination of bad science compounded by political interference). There is plenty of science to the contrary. In fact, the obesity and then type-2 diabetes epidemics began soon after the "low fat" guidelines were published in the USA and UK. But, yes, sugar and refined carbohydrates are the killers. So typically the ideal food-lifestyle is "low carbohydrate high fat".

Contributor 1 made the following response to this post:

» We should be wary of committing the fallacy of *post hoc ergo propter hoc*. The strongest case that can be made is that obesity was contributed to due to people replacing saturated fat with refined carbohydrates/sugars, instead of with healthy monounsaturated and polyunsaturated fats and plant proteins.

Contributor 1 has correctly observed that the mere fact that the obesity epidemic began "soon after" the publication of the low-fat guidelines is not valid grounds for concluding that reduced consumption of saturated fats *caused* the epidemic. Instead, Contributor 1 claims that the true cause of the obesity problem is that people replaced saturated fats in their diet with refined carbohydrates and sugars. It is these carbohydrates and sugars, and not reduced consumption of saturated fats, that caused an increase in cases of obesity.

Comments posted in response to a Leader in *The Guardian* also suggest that readers are adept at identifying *post hoc* errors in reasoning. The Leader reports that the number of cannabis users has declined since cannabis laws were liberalized in 2004. It also speculates on why government ministers have been reluctant to admit the success of their policy on cannabis. The following extract appears at the beginning of the Leader:

» When evidence crops up to support a controversial policy, ministers normally shout about it. But there was no megaphone announcement of last week's figures revealing that since the 2004 liberalisation of the cannabis laws the proportion of young people using the drug had fallen from 25% to 21%. The British Crime Survey also showed the number of youngsters smoking regularly was down almost a third, and that there were fewer users across the population as a whole. Ministers are coy about the success of their policy because they are preparing to ditch it. ('Disowning success', Leader, *The Guardian*, 29 October 2007)

In comments posted in response to the article, one contributor asked if we might not be engaging in *post hoc* reasoning when we discuss the relationship between the liberalization of cannabis laws and reduced rates of cannabis use. It might simply be a coincidence that the number of users fell following liberalization of the laws on the use of cannabis, or another factor altogether may be responsible for the decrease. One mother remarked that what had dissuaded her teenager from using cannabis were all the warnings about its association with mental health problems: "How it looks from where I stand - parent of a teenager who is open to persuasion - the reason usage has dropped is not because of the change in law, but precisely because of the increased media coverage of its potentially destructive effects. Threats to your sanity are more scary to the kids I know, than the threat of a policeman." Whatever is the true cause of the decrease in cannabis use, it is fallacious to argue that this decrease has been caused by the liberalization of the cannabis laws simply because it followed changes to these laws.

A further respondent to the Leader wondered if the purported link between cannabis use and mental health problems might not also be an instance of *post hoc* reasoning. Often, severe mental health problems have their onset when many young people are beginning to use drugs for the first time. It is all too easy for parents to look back upon events that preceded the onset of conditions like schizophrenia in their children and conclude that prior cannabis use must have *caused* these conditions:

» It's impossible, as a parent myself of two children, not to read X's post and not feel compassion and a sense of "there but for the grace of God"... However - paranoid schizophrenia does appear to occur to people in this age range of late teens /early twenties. It is something one is either pre-disposed to, or one is not. Taking cannabis may exacerbate the predisposition, it may not. The fact that this is the age range when illegal drugs are initially taken - if they are taken at all - naturally leads parents and some doctors to extrapolate that without the drug use, the mental illness would not have struck.

These comments by readers in response to online news articles demonstrate clearly that the public is well versed in matters of logic and causal reasoning. *Post hoc* errors do not always pass undetected, as many logical commentators would have us believe.

NOTES

1. This scenario is highly plausible. In a retrospective review of 301 couples attending the recurrent miscarriage clinic at two tertiary teaching hospitals in the UK, Dobson and Jayaprakasan (2018) reported that only 26% of women had explained recurrent miscarriage. 74% had unexplained recurrent miscarriage.
2. Emotional or psychological factors may have had much less influence on Dr Wakefield's objectivity than an apparent conflict of interest. One of the charges levelled against Dr Wakefield is that he did not declare to *The Lancet* that he received funding from the Legal Aid Board, a body that was representing parents of children who were possibly injured by the MMR vaccine. Dr Wakefield denied that there was any conflict of interest because his funding from the Legal Aid Board was for a separate scientific study, and not for the 1998 study that was published in *The Lancet*.
3. Jeremy Laurance described how in an interview conducted with Wakefield and published in *The Independent* in 1998, Wakefield remarked: "If I am wrong, I will be a bad person because I will have raised this spectre. But I have to address the questions my patients put to me. My duty is to investigate their stories. It is a moral issue with me." ('Andrew Wakefield's MMR vaccine theory has been discredited for years, but he just won't go away', Jeremy Laurance, *The Independent*, 5 May 2018.)

Chapter Summary

Key points

- A key driver of human behaviour is the need to understand why the events around us occur. The identification of causes of events requires that we engage in causal reasoning.
- A form of causal reasoning that has invariably been characterized as a fallacy is *post hoc ergo propter hoc*. This is where we argue that event *B* is caused by event *A* simply because *B* occurs after *A*. Temporal succession between events, it is argued, is not a valid basis on which to claim causation.
- There are other forms of causal fallacy besides *post hoc* reasoning. *Post hoc* is usually reasoning based on single occurrences of *A* and *B*. We can also base causal claims on multiple occurrences of *A* and *B*. Walton calls this an argument from a correlation to a causal connection.
- Two other forms of causal fallacy are *non causa pro causa* where we argue that one event caused another event without there being any temporal succession between events, and oversimplified cause where we focus on only one factor as a cause of an event and suppress or overlook other factors. Oversimplified cause is common in medicine and health, because most illnesses and injuries do not have a single causal factor.
- *Post hoc* reasoning is not inherently fallacious. There are conditions under which it is rationally warranted to use temporal succession between events as a basis for a claim of causation. These conditions are that a posited cause is of the right type, and that the duration between events is adequate for causal processes to take effect.
- Temporal succession between events may also be a weak basis for further causal reasoning. If temporal succession is only identified in a small number of cases, or if the time that elapses between events is inadequate for a causal process to take effect, then *post hoc* reasoning is fallacious.
- Even when rationally warranted, *post hoc* reasoning should mark the start of a process of inquiry or investigation in which causal claims are rigorously tested.

Suggestions for Further Reading

(1) Walton, D. (2016). *Argument evaluation and evidence*. Cham, Switzerland: Springer.

In ▶ Chapter 6 of this volume, Walton examines three examples of arguing from correlation to causation that relate to health issues: the question of whether eating chocolate makes people smarter; a correlation between weather patterns in the southern Pacific and flu pandemics; and the question of whether ingestion of copper causes Alzheimer's disease. Arguments from correlation to causation are evaluated by means of critical questions that require us to interrogate the nature of correlations between events, and whether they can support claims of causation.

(2) Govier, T. (2010). *A practical study of argument* (7th ed.). Belmont, CA: Wadsworth: Cengage Learning.

In ► Chapter 10 of this volume, Govier examines causal inductive arguments. There is a dedicated section on errors in causal reasoning which includes among other causal errors the *post hoc* fallacy and confusing correlation with cause. There is an opportunity to get practice at identifying fallacious causal arguments in exercises at the end of the chapter, and Govier includes a helpful glossary of terms that she has used. This is an accessible introduction to causal reasoning for readers of all backgrounds.

(3) Damer, T. E. (2013). *Attacking faulty reasoning* (7th ed.). Boston, MA: Wadsworth.

Damer examines a wide range of causal fallacies in ► Chapter 8 of this book. Arguers may confuse a necessary with a sufficient condition, engage in causal oversimplification, commit a *post hoc* fallacy, confuse cause and effect, and neglect a common cause. Readers can get practice at identifying these errors in causal reasoning by completing the assignments at the end of the chapter.

Questions

(1) We each harbour between 10 and 100 trillion symbiotic microbial cells in our bodies. These cells are primarily bacteria in the gut. The human microbiome consists of the genes in these microbial cells (Ursell et al. 2012). There is considerable interest in the role of the microbiome in the development of human disease. Among the conditions which appear to be linked to the microbiome are obesity and type 2 diabetes (Aydin et al. 2018) and autism spectrum disorder (Hughes et al. 2018). In the extract below, Roeselers et al. (2016) describe how we can commit the error of *post hoc* reasoning when we discuss the relationship between the gut microbiome and human health. Examine the extract from their article, and then answer the questions below.

The gut microbiome, human health, and *post hoc* reasoning

> Many studies that report on the composition of the gut microbiome in association with human health fail to exclude underlying factors (e.g. genetic, dietary or biogeographic) that may affect both microbiome composition and health proxies. As always with observational human studies (be they retrospective or prospective), special care must be taken to avoid "post hoc, *ergo propter hoc*" reasoning, translated as "*after this, therefore because of this.*" (p. 303) (◘ Fig. 7.4)

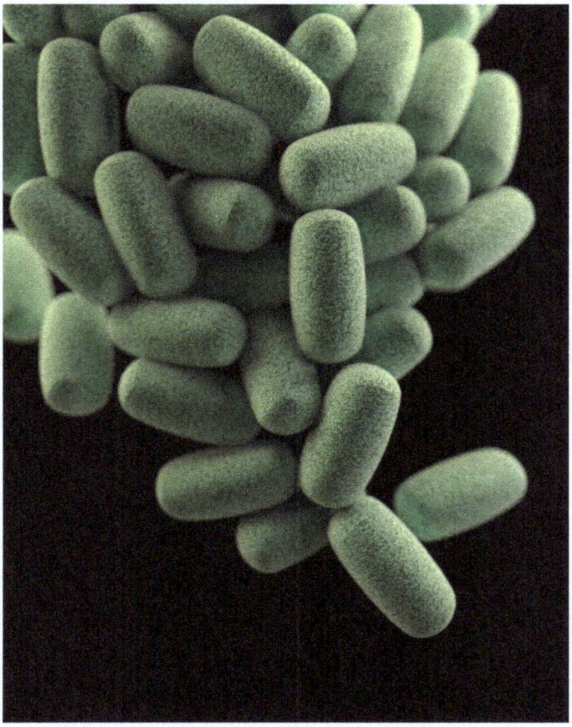

Fig. 7.4 A three-dimensional, computer-generated image of a cluster of barrel-shaped *Clostridium perfringens* bacteria. *C. perfringens* is common in the normal intestinal microbiota and is the most frequently isolated form of *Clostridium* from clinical specimens (Bien et al. 2013) (Illustration by Jennifer Oosthuizen is reproduced courtesy of CDC/James Archer, 2016)

Questions

(a) *Post hoc* is defined in this chapter as a form of reasoning in which a claim of causation is based on temporal succession between event *A* and event *B*. Does temporal succession apply to the case of the gut microbiome and its effects on human health?

(b) *Post hoc* reasoning is just one fallacy of false cause. Is there another form of this fallacy that might better characterize the relationship between the gut microbiome and human health?

(c) Roeselers et al. do not believe that there is a simple cause-effect relationship between the gut microbiome on the one hand and human health on the other hand. What is their alternative interpretation of the relationship between these variables?

(d) Explain how dietary factors may play an independent causal role in both the gut microbiome and human health.

(e) The use of antibiotics can alter the gut microbiome. The proliferation of *Clostridium difficile* accounts for 10–20% of cases of antibiotic-associated diarrhoea (AAD), and the majority of cases of colitis associated with antibiotic therapy (Bartlett 2002). When discussing causation in AAD and colitis, it makes sense to distinguish between a distal cause of these events and a proximal cause. How would you characterize this distinction?

(2) In an Op-Ed in *The New York Times* on 23 January 2018, Jeremy Samuel Faust and Edward W. Boyer—two emergency physicians who also hold positions at Harvard Medical School—criticized the decision by the state of Massachusetts to ban opioids such as fentanyl and carfentanil from its courtrooms. The state's decision, these authors argue, is based on a mistaken belief that passive exposure to these drugs poses a serious risk to human health. Whilst acknowledging the significant dangers associated with synthetic opioids—"when abused they can kill"—Faust and Boyer are concerned that the hysteria surrounding these drugs will deter emergency medical workers from performing their normal lifesaving duties. Read the following extract from the article, and then answer the questions below:

Opioid hysteria comes to Massachusetts courts

» This month, Massachusetts became the first state to ban fentanyl and carfentanil from being brought into courthouses as exhibits, out of concern that these substances are simply too dangerous to be in public places. The policy is based in part on the idea that even minuscule amounts of skin exposure to these drugs can be life-threatening. This is patently false — and we fear that it will worsen what is already a public health crisis.

This false belief about the danger of these drugs seems to stem from several unsubstantiated — though widely disseminated — media reports over the past year. In one such story, a drug patrolman became ill after brushing some powder off his uniform that he picked up while searching a suspect's car. [...] In another case, also in Ohio, three nurses went from cleaning a patient's room to waking up in hospital beds of their own. [...] In both cases, the victims were given naloxone, the highly effective opioid reversal agent, and ultimately recovered.

But the damage was done. Both stories are examples of the post hoc ergo propter hoc fallacy: Just because somebody received naloxone and later recovered is not by itself proof that the medication had any more effect than that other tried-and-true antidote for what are likely to have been severe panic attacks: time. Indeed, given the tall-tales circulating in the press and in law enforcement circles about the supposed hazard of passive fentanyl exposure, one can hardly blame them for panicking.

('Opioid hysteria comes to Massachusetts courts', Jeremy Samuel Faust and Edward W. Boyer, *The New York Times*, 23 January 2018)

Questions

(a) What is the *post hoc* argument identified by Faust and Boyer in this extract?
(b) Does the *post hoc* argument that you have identified in your response to (a) support the conclusion that passive exposure to synthetic opioids caused the illnesses of the patrolman and nurses? If not, what other *post hoc* argument is implied by the above extract?
(c) Opioid use was addressed in ► Sect. 4.2 in a discussion of fear appeal argument. It could be argued that a fear appeal argument has motivated the decision by the state of Massachusetts to ban synthetic opioids from its courtrooms. To the extent that this is the case, what form might this fear appeal argument take?
(d) Often in *post hoc* reasoning in health, the time that elapses between event *A* and event *B* is the time that it takes for an infectious disease to complete its incubation period, or for a cancer to progress to the point where clinical symptoms become evident. Faust and Boyer explain the lapse of time between the administration of naloxone and the recovery of the patrolman and nurses from illness in quite different terms. What do they believe is happening during this time period?
(e) Faust and Boyer claim that the media has widely promulgated reports about medical and law enforcement personnel becoming ill following exposure to unidentified substances. But these authors are actually making a much stronger claim, possibly even an accusation, against the media. What is that claim?

(3) Environmental tobacco smoke (ETS) is associated with disease and premature deaths in non-smokers (◘ Fig. 7.5). It is with a view to reducing the harms associated with ETS that many countries around the world have introduced a smoking ban policy in public places and the workplace (McNabola and Gill 2009). This has led to the publication of studies that have examined the effectiveness of these bans. In 2008, a report by the Associated Press that appeared in various media outlets described the findings of one such study. This study reported that the number of heart attack hospitalizations in Pueblo, Colorado had decreased by 41% in the three-year period following the introduction of a workplace smoking ban on 1 July 2003. The study was the ninth investigation to link smoking bans to decreased heart attacks, but the first one to examine rates over an extended period of three years. One of the study's authors, Terry Pechacek of the Centers for Disease Control and Prevention, is reported to have remarked that the study suggests that secondhand smoke is an under-recognized cause of heart attacks in the United States. However, not everyone was convinced that it is possible to claim that the smoking ban *caused* the reduction of heart attack hospitalizations in Pueblo, Colorado. Examine the following extract from the report and then answer the questions below.

Study reveals secondhand smoke hazard: Smoking ban good for heart health

> In the new study, researchers reviewed hospital admissions for heart attacks in Pueblo. Patients were classified by ZIP codes. They then looked at the same data for two nearby areas that did not have bans—the area of Pueblo County outside the city and for El Paso County.

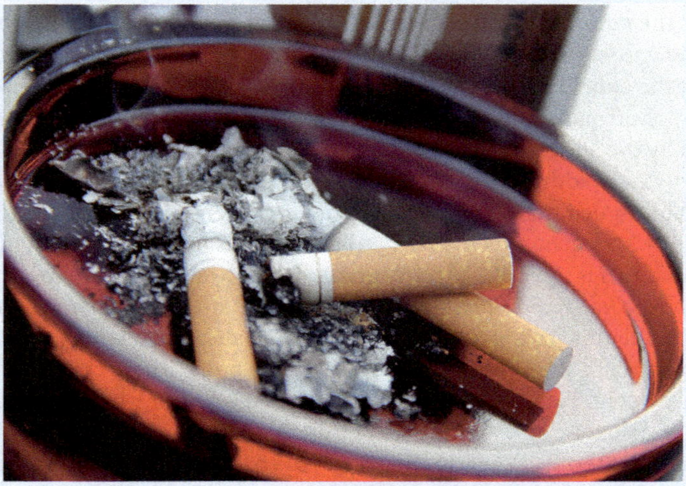

Fig. 7.5 Environmental tobacco smoke causes serious illness and premature death and is the target of smoking bans around the world (Photo by Debora Cartagena is reproduced courtesy of CDC/Debora Cartagena, 2012)

In Pueblo, the rate of heart attacks dropped from 257 per 100,000 people before the ban to 152 per 100,000 in the three years afterward. There were no significant changes in the two other areas. [...]

But the study had limitations: It assumed declines in the amount of secondhand smoke in Pueblo buildings after the ban, but did not try to measure that. The researchers also did not sort out which heart attack patients were smokers and which were not, so it's unclear how much of the decline can be attributed to reduced secondhand smoke.

One academic argued there's not enough evidence to conclude the smoking ban was the cause of Pueblo's heart attack decline.

The decline could have had more to do with a general decline in smoking in Pueblo County, from about 26% in 2002–2003 to less than 21% in 2004–2005. If there were stepped-up efforts to treat or prevent heart disease in the Pueblo area, that too could have played a role, said Dr. Michael Siegel, a professor of social and behavioral sciences at the Boston University School of Public Health. "I don't think it's as clear as they're making it out to be," Siegel said.

Questions:

(a) What aspects of the new study and its findings suggest there may be a causal link between the introduction of a smoking ban in Pueblo and a reduction of heart attack hospitalizations?

(b) Causation between events is usually established incrementally on the basis of more than one piece of evidence. What feature of Dr Siegel's contribution to the debate suggests that he holds this view of causation?

(c) The claim that event *A* causes event *B* can be overturned if it can be shown that an event other than *A* could be a plausible cause of *B*. Dr Siegel clearly believes he has identified two such events. What are they?
(d) The general decline in smoking in Pueblo County occurred around the same time as the reduction of heart attack hospitalizations. What third variable may be an independent cause of both of these events?
(e) The study had a number of limitations. It did not measure the amount of second-hand smoke in Pueblo buildings after the ban. It also did not distinguish between heart attack patients who were smokers and those who were non-smokers. How might these limitations have affected the presumed cause of reduced heart attacks in Pueblo County?

Answers

Exercise 7.1

(a) Walton's characterization of *post hoc* as an "argument from a correlation to a causal connection" does apply to the scenario Baffy is addressing. The passage describes how major haemorrhage during abdominal surgery has "repeatedly been found to correlate with" poor prognosis of cirrhotic patients. From this correlation the conclusion is drawn that major haemorrhage in these patients *causes* a poor prognosis.
(b) Telem et al. identify blood transfusions as the cause of the poor prognosis of cirrhotic patients who have intraoperative blood loss during abdominal surgery. The actual cause of their poor prognosis is the fact that they have experienced a major haemorrhage.
(c) Baffy reports how Telem et al. recommend limiting packed red blood cell transfusion during surgery as a means of reducing postoperative mortality. This is described as surprising by Baffy who clearly takes this recommendation to indicate that Telem et al. believe that transfusion is the cause of postoperative mortality.
(d) There is a causal relationship between major haemorrhage and blood transfusion. A major haemorrhage is the reason why someone needs a blood transfusion. A haemorrhage is the event that precipitates or causes a blood transfusion.
(e) Blood transfusion and postoperative mortality are both effects of a major haemorrhage. Telem et al. incorrectly frame one of these effects, namely blood transfusion, as a cause of postoperative mortality.

Exercise 7.2

(a) The research papers are arguing from a correlation between victimization and poor cognitive functioning to a causal connection between these variables. This is the form of *post hoc* reasoning that was attributed to Douglas Walton in ► Sect. 7.3.

(b) It may be that poor cognitive functioning is the cause of victimization. Cognitive weaknesses may mark a child out as vulnerable and place it at risk of victimization by others. So the cause-effect relationship that seems to be assumed by research papers may actually operate in the opposite direction.
(c) A third variable may be maternal education. Poor maternal education may cause child victimization and may also cause poor cognitive functioning in children. So what appears to be a causal relationship between victimization and poor cognitive functioning may, in fact, indicate the independent influence of maternal education on victimization on the one hand and poor cognitive functioning on the other hand.
(d) A research study might hypothesize that early child victimization leads to poor cognitive test scores at 8 or 10 years of age. In this case, there is an early trigger event (victimization) that presses into action a series of academic and social processes that result in compromised cognitive functioning in a child at 8 or 10 years of age.
(e) The attempt to overturn or defeat contenders for a causal explanation of an event is founded on the scientific principle that we are more likely to approximate truth if we set out in the spirit of disconfirmation rather than if we seek to confirm causal explanations. If we try to overturn a causal explanation and it remains standing, then it grows in epistemic stature. This is the same as a hypothesis in science. A hypothesis that can withstand attempts to reject it becomes stronger as a consequence.

Exercise 7.3

(a) The scope of *mortality* is more easily identified than the scope of *complication*. This is because mortality involves a binary concept, namely, someone is *either* dead *or* alive in a certain period of time after surgery has occurred. There is no such binary concept that we can use to fix the scope of complication.
(b) Events that occur after gastrostomy placement can be usefully distinguished as proximal and distal effects of surgery. Infections and thromboembolic events (e.g. pulmonary embolism) are well-recognized complications of all forms of surgery and can be conceived of as *proximal* effects of gastrostomy placement. Myocardial infarction (a heart attack) two months after gastrostomy placement may be conceived of as a *distal* effect of the procedure if a patient's recovery has been compromised by infections, malnutrition, and other adverse circumstances that make a heart attack more likely to occur.
(c) When one cause of an event is emphasized to the exclusion of other causes, the proponent has committed a fallacy of false cause called *oversimplified cause*. There is a need for a counterpart fallacy called *oversimplified effect*. This is because the effects of an event are complex, with one effect leading to another effect. Gastrostomy placement may cause a patient to develop a postoperative infection. This infection may have to be treated with antibiotics, which leads to the proliferation of intestinal *Clostridium difficile*. In an elderly or frail patient, *C. difficile* infection may lead to heart failure. In attempting to reduce these different effects of gastrostomy placement to a single effect, we are committing a fallacy of oversimplified effect.

(d) Finucane states that certain postoperative complications carry "a subtle suggestion of fault". Accordingly, it is important to understand what does and does not constitute a postoperative complication of gastrostomy placement in order to judge accusations of medical liability. Another reason it is important to understand the complications of gastrostomy placement is that it can lead physicians to revise the procedure in order to make it safer. For example, if a particular model of gastrostomy tube is associated with a high rate of postoperative infection, it may be necessary to discontinue use of that tube.

(e) In patients with advanced HIV infection, there may be significant weight loss because of reduced energy intake. The latter may necessitate the placement of a gastrostomy tube. However, patients with advanced HIV infection are also more susceptible to infection on account of their compromised immune systems. So HIV infection may be an independent cause of gastrostomy placement and the development of a postoperative infection. There may be no cause-effect relationship between gastrostomy placement and the development of a postoperative infection.

End-of-chapter questions

(1)

(a) It is difficult to characterize the relationship between the gut microbiome and human health in terms of temporal sequence. The microbiome is present from the time of birth and operates in parallel to human health. It does not precede health in time. However, if there are specific events that change the composition of the microbiome such as the use of antibiotics (see (e) below), then these events do precede health consequences such as colitis and diarrhoea in time, and a temporal sequence for *post hoc* reasoning can be identified.

(b) *Non causa pro causa* is used to capture a false cause of an event when there is no temporal succession between event *A* and event *B*. This form of the fallacy may better capture the relationship between the gut microbiome and human health which, as we saw in the response to (a), can only be characterized in terms of a temporal sequence under specific circumstances.

(c) Roeselers et al. believe that the gut microbiome and human health can each be independently caused by a third variable such as genetic or dietary factors. What appears to be a cause-effect relationship between the gut microbiome and human health may instead reflect the independent causal effects of this third variable.

(d) Diet has an independent causal role to play in human health and the gut microbiome. A diet that is rich in saturated fats can lead to the development of coronary heart disease, for example. Diet can also directly affect the composition of the gut microbiome. The consumption of probiotic drinks containing *Lactobacillus casei* can alter the gut microbiome.

(e) Antibiotic therapy is the distal cause of antibiotic-associated diarrhoea (AAD) and colitis. Proliferation of *Clostridium difficile* is the proximal cause of these illnesses. So the causal chain can be represented as follows: antibiotic therapy (distal cause) → proliferation of *Clostridium difficile* (proximal cause) → colitis and AAD (effect).

(2)

(a) The *post hoc* argument identified by Faust and Boyer is that the patrolman and nurses recovered *after* the administration of naloxone and so their recovery must have been *caused* by this opioid reversal agent.

(b) The *post hoc* argument identified in response to (a) does not support the conclusion that passive exposure to synthetic opioids caused the illnesses of the patrolman and nurses. A different *post hoc* argument is required in order to arrive at this conclusion. It can be formulated as follows: The patrolman and nurses became unwell after exposure to an unidentified substance, so the unidentified substance (presumably, synthetic opioids) must have caused their illnesses.

(c) The fear appeal argument that might have motivated the decision of the state of Massachusetts to ban synthetic opioids from its courtrooms can be reconstructed as follows:
If the state of Massachusetts permits synthetic opioids into its courtrooms, then members of the public will be passively exposed to these drugs.
Passive exposure to synthetic opioids will result in a very serious outcome, namely, the illness and death of people who are exposed to these drugs.
Therefore, the state of Massachusetts should ensure that it does not permit synthetic opioids into its courtrooms.

(d) The lapse of time between the administration of naloxone and the recovery from illness is explained by Faust and Boyer as the time that is needed to recover from a panic attack. They argue that a panic attack, rather than passive exposure to synthetic opioids, is the likely cause of the illnesses experienced by the patrolman and nurses.

(e) Faust and Boyer are effectively accusing the media of encouraging the public to engage in *post hoc* reasoning by drawing the false conclusion that illness in medical and law enforcement personnel has been caused by passive exposure to synthetic opioids.

(3)

(a) There are three features of the new study and its findings that suggest there may be a causal link between the introduction of a smoking ban and a reduction of heart attack hospitalizations:
   (i) the new study's findings are consistent with the findings of eight earlier studies, all of which have linked smoking bans to reductions of heart attacks;
   (ii) unlike these earlier studies, the new study examined heart attacks over a long period of time (3 years), reducing the likelihood that any decrease was only a temporary occurrence;
   (iii) the study compared its findings in Pueblo to those in two other areas that had not introduced smoking bans; neither of these areas had seen a reduction of heart attack hospitalizations.

(b) Dr Siegel is reported to have said that there is not *enough evidence* to conclude that the smoking ban was the cause of Pueblo's heart attack decline.

(c) The two events that Dr Siegel believes could be plausible causes of reduced heart attack hospitalizations in Pueblo are a general decline is smoking in Pueblo County, and increased efforts to treat or prevent heart disease in the county.

(d) The introduction of a smoking ban may be a third variable that independently caused a general decline in smoking and a reduction of heart attack hospitalizations in Pueblo County. A smoking ban made it illegal for smokers to smoke tobacco in any public place. The inconvenience that this would have caused to smokers might have served as a powerful incentive for them to stop smoking. Reduced exposure to secondhand smoke as a result of the smoking ban might also have resulted in a reduction of heart attack hospitalizations.
(e) There may have been no difference in the amount of secondhand smoke in Pueblo buildings after the ban if employees and other members of the public disregarded the ban and/or there was no attempt to enforce the ban. In such a case, it would not be possible to attribute a reduction of heart attacks to reduced exposure to secondhand smoke as a result of the ban. The study also failed to distinguish between heart attack patients who are smokers and those who are non-smokers. If the rate of heart attacks in non-smokers remained unchanged following the introduction of the smoking ban, then there was no significant effect of reduced exposure to secondhand smoke (assuming this actually occurred) on the rate of heart attacks.

References

Aydin, Ö., Nieuwdorp, M., & Gerdes, V. (2018). The gut microbiome as a target for the treatment of type 2 diabetes. *Current Diabetes Reports, 18*(8), 55.
Baffy, G. (2010). Negative outcomes for intraoperative blood transfusion in patients with advanced cirrhosis: Post hoc ergo propter hoc? *Clinical Gastroenterology and Hepatology, 8*(11), 996.
Bartlett, J. G. (2002). Antibiotic-associated diarrhea. *New England Journal of Medicine, 346,* 334–339.
Bien, J., Palagani, V., & Bozko, P. (2013). The intestinal microbiota dysbiosis and *Clostridium difficile* infection: Is there a relationship with inflammatory bowel disease? *Therapeutic Advances in Gastroenterology, 6*(1), 53–68.
Brodtmann, A. (2014). Vascular risk, depression, and stroke: Post hoc ergo propter hoc…or not. *Neurology, 83,* 1688–1689.
Bullock, J. D. (2001). Post hoc, ergo propter hoc. *Survey of Opthalmology, 45*(4), 355–357.
Centers for Disease Control. (1982a). National surveillance for Reye syndrome, 1981: Update, Reye syndrome and salicylate usage. *Morbidity and Mortality Weekly Report, 31*(5), 53–56, 61.
Centers for Disease Control. (1982b). Surgeon General's advisory on the use of salicylates and Reye syndrome. *Morbidity and Mortality Weekly Report, 31*(22), 289–290.
Chen, R. T., & DeStefano, F. (1998). Vaccine safety. *The Lancet, 352,* 63–64.
Costello, E. J. (2017). Post hoc, ergo propter hoc. *American Journal of Psychiatry, 174*(4), 305–306.
Dobson, S. J. A., & Jayaprakasan, K. M. (2018). Aetiology of recurrent miscarriage and the role of adjuvant treatment in its management: A retrospective cohort review. *Journal of Obstetrics and Gynaecology, 38*(7), 967–974.
Finucane, T. E. (2012). Post hoc ergo propter hoc: Complications and death after gastrostomy placement. *Journal of the American Medical Directors Association, 13*(3), 197–198.
Freedland, K. E., & Carney, R. M. (2009). Depression and medical illness. In I. H. Gotlib & C. L. Hammen (Eds.), *Handbook of depression* (2nd ed., pp. 113–141). New York and London: Guilford.
Godlee, F., Smith, J., & Marcovitch, H. (2011). Wakefield's article linking MMR vaccine and autism was fraudulent. *BMJ, 342,* c7452.
Grouse, L. (2016). Post hoc ergo propter hoc. *Journal of Thoracic Disease, 8*(7), E511–E512.
Hughes, H. K., Rose, D., & Ashwood, P. (2018). The gut microbiota and dysbiosis in autism spectrum disorders. *Current Neurology and Neuroscience Reports, 18*(11), 81.

Hurley, P. J. (2015). *A concise introduction to logic* (12th ed.). Stamford, CT: Cengage Learning.
McNabola, A., & Gill, L. W. (2009). The control of environmental tobacco smoke: A policy review. *International Journal of Environmental Research and Public Health, 6*(2), 741–758.
Ozonoff, S., Heung, K., Byrd, R., Hansen, R., & Hertz-Picciotto, I. (2008). The onset of autism: Patterns of symptom emergence in the first years of life. *Autism Research, 1*(6), 320–328.
Pinto, R. C. (1995). Post hoc ergo propter hoc. In H. V. Hansen & R. C. Pinto (Eds.), *Fallacies: Classical and contemporary readings* (pp. 302–314). University Park: The Pennsylvania State University Press.
Roeselers, G., Bouwman, J., & Levin, E. (2016). The human gut microbiome, diet, and health: *"Post hoc non ergo propter hoc". Trends in Food Science & Technology, 57,* 302–305.
Rowe, T. (2015). The stress of pregnancy. *Journal of Obstetrics and Gynaecology Canada, 37*(5), 393–394.
Ursell, L. K., Metcalf, J. L., Parfrey, L. W., & Knight, R. (2012). Defining the human microbiome. *Nutrition Reviews, 70*(Suppl. 1), S38–S44.
Wakefield, A. J., Murch, S. H., Anthony, A., Linnell, J., Casson, D. M., Malik, M., et al. (1998). Ileal-lymphoid-nodular hyperplasia, non-specific colitis, and pervasive developmental disorder in children. *The Lancet, 351*(9103), 637–641.
Walton, D. (2008). *Informal logic: A pragmatic approach* (2nd ed.). New York: Cambridge University Press.

Supplementary Information

L. Cummings, *Fallacies in Medicine and Health*,
https://doi.org/10.1007/978-3-030-28513-5

Glossary

Ad baculum argument: see *fear appeal*

Amphiboly: One of a group of fallacies that is dependent on language, according to Aristotle. Amphiboly occurs when a sentence can be understood in two ways due to its grammatical construction rather than to any ambiguity in the component words or phrases. Although amphiboly is often discussed in the fallacy literature, there are few convincing examples of its use.

Analogical argument: see *argument from analogy*

Analogical reasoning: see *argument from analogy*

Analogue: The term used to describe the two items that are compared in an argument from analogy. The items may be people, entities, processes, situations, or events.

Analogy: A similarity between two or more people, entities, or situations. The similarity may be used to support a claim in argument (logical analogy), or it may be used to describe or explain an issue or problem (non-logical analogy).

Argument: A set of propositions in which one or more propositions (so-called premises) provide grounds or reasons to support another proposition (the conclusion).

Argumentation: A type of discourse in which an arguer uses certain propositions (premises) as grounds or reasons to accept other propositions (conclusions) in a process of reasoning. Argumentation can contain several arguments of different types (deductive and inductive arguments, for example), or it may contain just a single argument.

Argumentation scheme: A template that is used to represent the inferential structure of different types of arguments that are used in everyday discourse and in special contexts such as science and law.

Argument evaluation: After an argument has been fully reconstructed, the process of its evaluation begins. This is where an argument is assessed against certain normative criteria that vary with the type of argument under consideration (e.g. deductive, inductive, plausible argument). If an argument does not conform to these criteria, it is judged to be invalid or fallacious.

Argument from analogy: Use of an analogy consisting of one of more similarities between *A* and *B* to argue that if *A* has property *P* then *B* will also have property *P*.

Argument from authority: Also known as the appeal to expertise or *argumentum ad verecundiam*. In an argument from authority, a claim is argued to be true because it is advanced by an expert or authority. If the authority has extensive expertise in the domain to which the claim belongs, the appeal may be rationally warranted. In fallacious appeals to authority, an individual may not have genuine expertise or his expertise may be in an area that is unrelated to the claim he is advancing.

Argument from expert opinion: see *argument from authority*

Argument from ignorance: An informal fallacy in which an arguer draws a conclusion from a single premise. The premise states that there is no evidence or knowledge that *X* is true (*X* is false). From this premise the conclusion is drawn that *X* is false (*X* is true). The argument from ignorance is non-fallacious in certain contexts. It is the basis of the presumption of innocence in the law, e.g. There is *no evidence* that *X* is guilty, therefore *X* is innocent.

Argument from negative consequences: A single-premise argument in which a proponent argues from the negative consequence(s) of an action to the conclusion that the action should not be taken.

Argument reconstruction: Before an argument can be evaluated, it must be reconstructed. During reconstruction, the analyst must decide what propositions are the premises and conclusion of an argument. Any implicit premises (enthymemes) must be made explicit in this process.

Argument schema: Also known as argumentation schemes, these devices are explicit representations of the inferential structure of arguments used in everyday discourse such as legal and scientific argumentation. Most students of logic are familiar with the argumentation schemes of deductive inferences like *modus ponens*. They are less familiar with the schemes for presumptive, defeasible arguments such as fear appeal argument or the argument from expertise.

Argumentum ad hominem: An informal fallacy in which an opponent uses a proponent's character, circumstances, or principles to invalidate his thesis or claim. Many fallacious *ad hominem* arguments are little more than abusive personal attacks such as when an arguer's previous conviction for drink driving is used to undermine his claim that high inflation is bad for the economy.

Argumentum ad populum: An appeal to popular opinion and belief in argument as a reason to accept that a claim is true. An *ad populum* argument might take this form: Most people believe that there is life after death; therefore, it is true that there is life after death.

Argumentum ad verecundiam: see *argument from authority*

Assertion: A speech act that entails the truth of the proposition that is asserted. Assertion is a central concept in the philosophy of language where it has traditionally assumed a key role in linguistic meaning.

Availability: A heuristic in which the probability of an event is estimated according to the ease with which instances of the event can be conceived. Applied to medical diagnosis, availability leads clinicians to attribute a presentation to a particular diagnosis based on how recent or salient this diagnosis has been.

Begging the question: An arguer 'begs' the question when he assumes as part of the premises the conclusion that he is attempting to prove. Normally in argument, we attempt to prove a conclusion through premises that are more certain than, or better known than, the conclusion. But this condition cannot be satisfied in the case where the premise *is* the conclusion. This is why begging the question, *petitio principii*, or circular argument is an informal fallacy.

Bovine spongiform encephalopathy: A degenerative brain disease that first emerged in British cattle in November 1986. BSE belongs to the group of transmissible spongiform encephalopathies that affect mammalian vertebrates, including humans. They are caused by an infectious protein called a 'prion'.

Burden of proof: A dialectical move between a proponent and an opponent in a critical discussion. The burden of proof rests on the proponent who advances a claim. If the proponent brings forward sufficient evidence to support the claim, he succeeds in shifting the burden of proof onto his opponent in argument. If the opponent does not accept the proponent's claim, then there is a burden of proof on him to bring forward evidence to support his counter-claim.

Circular reasoning: see *begging the question*

Cognitive bias: Humans deviate from rational norms in their thinking in certain predictable ways or according to systematic patterns. These deviations are given names such as 'availability', 'anchoring' and 'representativeness'.

Cognitive heuristic: A mental shortcut that allows us to bypass information and arrive at a quick decision or solution to a problem.

Cognitive salience: A property of information and knowledge that makes it obvious, unique, and distinctive. Cognitively salient information is more readily attended to and recalled than other information and knowledge.

Composition: A fallacy in which it is argued that a composite has a particular property because each of its parts has this property. For example, it is not the case that a football team is high performing because each member of the team is high performing.

Conclusion: The proposition in an argument that makes explicit content that is implied by the premise(s). The conclusion may be a deductive consequence of the premises or it may be inductively supported by the premises.

Confounding variable: A variable other than the independent variable that may affect the dependent variable. A confounding variable can result in erroneous conclusions about the relationship between the independent and dependent variables. For example, we may conclude that weight gain (dependent variable) is related to a lack of exercise (independent variable). A confounding variable might be the amount of food consumption as this can also affect weight gain.

Counter-analogy: In argument, a proponent may use an analogy to support a conclusion in argument. If an opponent then brings forward an analogy that supports an opposing conclusion, the opponent is said to have used a counter-analogy.

Creutzfeldt-Jakob disease: A transmissible spongiform encephalopathy that is found in humans. CJD has an estimated prevalence rate of approximately 1 per one million population. It typically affects individuals in the sixth and seventh decades of life. There are sporadic, familial, and iatrogenic (medical treatment-related) forms of the disease.

Critical thinking: The ability to engage in an evaluation of claims, beliefs, and arguments with a view to deciding their logical or rational merits. Critical thinking is encouraged in schools, universities, and professional contexts as a means of improving decision-making and other forms of judgement.

Deduction: see *deductive logic*

Deductive logic: The study of truth relations between propositions in an argument. Deductive logicians are interested in deductive validity. In a deductively valid argument, if the premises are true, then the conclusion must also be true. Deductive arguments are valid by virtue of their formal or logical structure. The content or meaning of the propositions that form the premises and conclusions of these arguments is not of interest to deductive logic.

Deductively valid argument: An argument in which there is no logically possible situation where all the premises are true and the conclusion is false. If the premises are true, then it necessarily follows that the conclusion must also be true.

Deductivism: An often latent bias or prejudice towards deductive logic as the standard of good or correct argument and reasoning. Deductivism is embodied in the soundness doctrine, the idea that a good argument is one that is deductively valid and has true premises.

Defeasibility: A property of non-deductive arguments whereby they can be defeated or overturned as new evidence emerges. The premises in a defeasible argument provide support for the conclusion. However, unlike valid deductive arguments, it is possible for the premises to be true and the conclusion false in a defeasible argument.

Discourse: In terms of linguistic analysis, discourse is the level of language above individual sentences. The focus of study is on extended extracts of language in spoken and written texts. Discourse can exhibit different linguistic features depending on the context in which it is used, purpose for which it is advanced, and the number of participants involved in its production.

Division: A fallacy in which it is argued that a part has a particular property because the composite or whole has this property. For example, it is not the case because a speech is long-winded that every sentence in the speech is also long-winded.

Emotionality: The emotional content of a health message. Emotionality includes positive emotions (e.g. happiness, joy) as well as negative emotions (e.g. fear, anger, regret). The emotional content of health messages can be effectively manipulated in order to achieve audience persuasion (e.g. fear appeal argument).

Executive function: A group of cognitive skills that is essential to goal-directed behaviour. Executive functions include planning ability, mental flexibility, and inhibitory control. These cognitive abilities can be impaired in a range of clinical disorders (e.g. schizophrenia).

Fallacy: An argument that subverts or falls short of standards of valid reasoning. Fallacies may be deductive or inductive in nature. Arguments may also fall short for reasons that are unrelated to deductive and inductive logic. These arguments are called 'informal fallacies'.

Fallacy of false cause: Any error or fallacy in causal reasoning and inference. There are several ways in which causal reasoning can go awry. Temporal succession between two events, *A* and *B*, can be used to conclude that *B* was caused by *A* because *B* comes after *A*. This is the form of the fallacy known as *post hoc ergo propter hoc*. A variant of *post hoc* involves an inference that *A* caused *B* because multiple occurrences of *B* come after multiple occurrences of *A* (the so-called argument from a correlation to a causal connection). In the form of the fallacy known as *non causa pro causa*, one event is mistakenly taken to be a cause of another event but temporal succession is not involved in the identification of a false cause. An event may have more than one cause but only one of these causes is identified. This form of the fallacy is known as oversimplified cause.

False analogy: A fallacy in which two entities, *A* and *B*, are insufficiently similar to draw inferences about the properties or features of *B* from the properties or features of *A*. A false analogy between BSE and scrapie early in the BSE epidemic led health officials to conclude erroneously that BSE would not transmit to humans because scrapie had not transmitted to humans. This conclusion was based on a false analogy that BSE was bovine scrapie. BSE was subsequently shown to be a novel disease that was unrelated to scrapie.

Fear appeal: An argument that uses the emotion of fear rather than grounds or reasons to secure an opponent's acceptance of a conclusion. Some fear appeal arguments are rationally warranted, while others are little more than scaremongering.

Formal logic: see *deductive logic*

Halo effect: An effect in which one positive attribute or feature of a person or institution results in a positive evaluation of other attributes or features, even in the case where the latter is not warranted. The authority and respect that we have for a doctor's medical knowledge and expertise, for example, may lead us to defer to him or her on all sorts of issues that are unrelated to medicine. In effect, one positive attribute creates something of a warm, positive glow on other attributes.

Hepatitis A: Inflammation of the liver that is caused by the hepatitis A virus. This disease can be contracted through ingestion of contaminated food and water and through direct contact with an infectious person.

Heuristic reasoning: A type of reasoning that is based on heuristics, which are a set of mental shortcuts through more complex modes of reasoning (e.g. systematic reasoning). Heuristic reasoning is considered to be part of an older (in evolutionary terms) cognitive system that prioritised survival and that only later came to be supplemented by systematic reasoning.

Ignoratio elenchi: The fallacy of arguing to a conclusion that does not bear on the issue at hand, and is therefore irrelevant. An *ignoratio elenchi* is committed, for example, when an arguer attempts to defeat the claim that Calgary is Canada's fastest growing city by using a sound argument to the effect that Calgary is not Canada's biggest city.

Inference: A conclusion that is drawn from evidence in the form of premises on the basis of reasoning.

Informal fallacy: An argument that contains a logical flaw or error. The error may be perpetrated intentionally as a deceptive tactic during argumentation or committed unintentionally when an arguer is unaware that he has made a logical error. Informal fallacies can be rationally warranted arguments within certain contexts of use.

Informal logic: An approach to logic that emerged in the second half of the 20th century, largely in response to dissatisfaction with standard (usually deductive) techniques of argument analysis and evaluation. The emphasis of informal logic is on the analysis and evaluation of real arguments in the actual contexts in which they occur.

Logic: Logic can be variously defined as the study of truth relations between propositions and the study of principles of correct or valid reasoning. There are many different types of logic, including deductive and inductive logic, and deontic and epistemic logic.

Logical connector: In argumentation, conjunction words like 'so' and 'therefore' explicitly signal that we are drawing or inferring a conclusion from one or more premises. Because they connect the conclusion to the premises via inference, these words are known as logical connectors.

Message frame: Message framing is a common health communication technique in which behaviour change messages are focused on the potential outcomes of proposed health behaviours. For example, in relation to smoking, the message "If you quit smoking you will be less likely to get lung cancer" is a gain-framed message as it emphasizes the avoidance of an undesirable outcome.

Metaphor: A pragmatic phenomenon in which a speaker intends to describe an attribute of X by relating X to prominent features or characteristics of Y. For example, in the utterance *The rugby players were lions on the field*, a speaker does not intend to say that the players were actual lions, merely that the players were courageous, strong and fearless during a game of rugby.

Modus tollens inference: In propositional logic a deductively valid inference of the following form: *If P then Q; not-Q; therefore, not-P*.

Non causa pro causa: see *fallacy of false cause*

Oversimplified cause: see *fallacy of false cause*

Petitio principii: see *begging the question*

Post hoc ergo propter hoc: The fallacy known as *post hoc ergo propter hoc* (literally: after this, therefore because of this) occurs when it is argued that event *B* is caused by event *A* by virtue of the fact that *B* occurred *after A*. The temporal order between events is not always a reliable basis upon which to draw a causal inference. See also *fallacy of false cause*.

Premise: The proposition in an argument that states reasons or grounds for acceptance of the conclusion. Arguments can contain one or more premises.

Presumption: An epistemic concept in which we have a tentative commitment to the truth of a proposition. Presumptions are defeasible in the presence of contrary evidence. In a dialectical framework, there is a presumption in favour of the truth of a contested claim when the proponent of the claim succeeds in shifting his or her burden of proof. A well-known presumption is the presumption of innocence in law.

Presumptive reasoning: A type of plausible, tentative reasoning that guides practical actions and decision-making. A claim that is presumptively true can be easily overturned but has some rational purchase nonetheless.

Proposition: A unit of meaning that can be true or false. The premises and conclusions of arguments consist of propositions. In the modus ponens inference (*If P then Q; P; therefore, Q*) the major premise (*If P then Q*) contains two propositions that are conjoined by the connective *If…then*.

Psychologism: Many philosophers argue that logical laws are not psychological laws, and that it is a mistake (so-called psychologism) to identify the former with the latter. For other philosophers, 'psychologism' is a neutral or even positive term, meaning the application of psychological techniques to problems in philosophy.

Rationality: A mental faculty that allows us to think and engage in action and decision-making according to principles of reason or logic.

Reasoning: A higher-order cognitive function in which individuals draw specific conclusions from general principles or premises (deductive reasoning) or general principles from specific instances (inductive reasoning). Aside from deduction and induction, there are also presumptive or plausible forms of reasoning.

Response efficacy: A concept employed in social science to describe an individual's belief that a recommended protective action will be successful in averting a negative outcome or consequence. A fear appeal argument is likely to be effective if the recipient of the argument perceives the recommended actions to have high response efficacy.

Scrapie: A transmissible spongiform encephalopathy that is endemic in many sheep populations around the world. The disease derives its name from an intense itching sensation that is one of its symptoms. This causes the animal to engage in rubbing, scraping or chewing behaviour with resulting deterioration of the fleece.

Secundum quid: The fallacy of neglecting qualification. The arguer who commits this fallacy is mistakenly treating what is true with certain qualifications as also true without them. It is a fallacy to argue, for example, that because it is always permissible to kill *in war* that it is always permissible to kill.

Self-efficacy: A concept employed in social science to describe an individual's belief that he or she is able to undertake recommended protective actions that will avert a negative outcome or consequence. Self-efficacy can explain why some fear appeal arguments are effective while others fail. A fear appeal argument is more likely to succeed if the person to whom it is directed has high self-efficacy.

Slippery slope argument: An argument that uses a negative (usually, disastrous or catastrophic) consequence of an action to argue that the action that leads to this consequence should not be taken. The slippery slope argument is a type of argument from negative consequences, but has additional logical features. The disastrous consequence in a slippery slope argument, for example, is usually arrived at by a series of interrelated actions rather than by just one action.

Soundness: A property of deductive arguments in which an argument is valid and has all true premises. See also *deductivism*.

Speech act: A term used by John Austin and later John Searle to describe utterances which perform acts or actions. Both Austin and Searle recognised different types of speech acts such as assertives (e.g. statements) and directives (e.g. requests). Common speech acts include promises, apologies, threats and warnings.

Systematic reasoning: A type of reasoning in which extensive evidence is gathered and its implications for a claim are carefully evaluated. The emphasis of systematic reasoning is on a detailed consideration of all the evidence in an area regardless of the time and cognitive resources that are used in deliberation. Legal deliberation and scientific inquiry both involve systematic reasoning.

Transmissible spongiform encephalopathy: A group of invariably fatal neurodegenerative diseases in animals and humans. TSEs are distinguished by their long incubation periods and the characteristic spongiform changes that occur in the brain as a result of loss of neurones.

Trust: A feature of transactional and other relationships between people. Trust is forged on cognitive and affective factors. These factors typically give rise to two main dimensions of trust, namely, competence and expertise, and personal integrity and trustworthiness.

Validity: see *deductive logic*

Bibliography

Albano, J. D., Ward, E., Jemal, A., Anderson, R., Cokkinides, V. E., Murray, T., et al. (2007). Cancer mortality in the United States by education level and race. *Journal of the National Cancer Institute, 99*(18), 1384–1394.

Alderson, P., & Roberts, I. (2000). Should journals publish systematic reviews that find no evidence to guide practice? Examples from injury research. *British Medical Journal, 320,* 376.

Allum, N. (2007). An empirical test of competing theories of hazard-related trust: The case of GM food. *Risk Analysis, 27*(4), 935–946.

Aristotle. *On sophistical refutations* (W. A. Pickard-Cambridge, Trans.). Available online at: ▶ http://classics.mit.edu//Aristotle/sophist_refut.html.

Armstrong, K., Ravenell, K. L., McMurphy, S., & Putt, M. (2007). Racial/ethnic differences in physician distrust in the United States. *American Journal of Public Health, 97*(7), 1283–1289.

Arnauld, A., & Nicole, P. (1850). *Logic, or the art of thinking: Being the port-royal logic* (T. S. Baynes, Trans.). Edinburgh: Sutherland and Knox.

Aydin, Ö., Nieuwdorp, M., & Gerdes, V. (2018). The gut microbiome as a target for the treatment of type 2 diabetes. *Current Diabetes Reports, 18*(8), 55.

Baffy, G. (2010). Negative outcomes for intraoperative blood transfusion in patients with advanced cirrhosis: Post hoc ergo propter hoc? *Clinical Gastroenterology and Hepatology, 8*(11), 996.

Bagnall, G. (2004). MMR and conflicts of interest. *BMJ, 328,* 483.

Baronett, S. (2008). *Logic*. Upper Saddle River, NJ: Pearson Prentice Hall.

Bartlett, J. G. (2002). Antibiotic-associated diarrhea. *New England Journal of Medicine, 346,* 334–339.

Bastien, S. (2011). Fear appeals in HIV-prevention messages: Young people's perceptions in northern Tanzania. *African Journal of AIDS Research, 10*(4), 435–449.

Bien, J., Palagani, V., & Bozko, P. (2013). The intestinal microbiota dysbiosis and *Clostridium difficile* infection: Is there a relationship with inflammatory bowel disease? *Therapeutic Advances in Gastroenterology, 6*(1), 53–68.

Bleich, S., Blendon, R., & Adams, A. (2007). Trust in scientific experts on obesity: Implications for awareness and behavior change. *Obesity, 15*(8), 2145–2156.

Boer, T. A. (2003). After the slippery slope: Dutch experiences on regulating active euthanasia. *Journal of the Society of Christian Ethics, 23*(2), 225–242.

Brodtmann, A. (2014). Vascular risk, depression, and stroke: Post hoc ergo propter hoc…or not. *Neurology, 83,* 1688–1689.

Brown, P., Cathala, F., Raubertas, R. F., Gajdusek, D. C., & Castaigne, P. (1987). The epidemiology of Creutzfeldt-Jakob disease: Conclusion of a 15-year investigation in France and review of the world literature. *Neurology, 37*(6), 895–904.

Brown-Johnson, C. G., Boeckman, L. M., White, A. H., Burbank, A. D., Paulson, S., & Beebe, L. A. (2018). Trust in health information sources: Survey analysis of variation by sociodemographic and tobacco use status in Oklahoma. *JMIR Public Health Surveillance, 4*(1), e8.

Bullock, J. D. (2001). Post hoc, ergo propter hoc. *Survey of Opthalmology, 45*(4), 355–357.

Burgess, J. A. (1993). The great slippery-slope argument. *Journal of Medical Ethics, 19*(3), 169–174.

Carcioppolo, N., Jensen, J. D., Wilson, S. R., Collins, W. B., Carrion, M., & Linnemeier, G. (2013). Examining HPV threat-to-efficacy ratios in the Extended Parallel Process Model. *Health Communication, 28*(1), 20–28.

Carcioppolo, N., John, K. K., Jensen, J. D., & King, A. J. (2019). Joking about cancer as an avoidance strategy among US adults. *Health Promotion International, 34*(3), 420–428.

Centers for Disease Control. (1982a). National surveillance for Reye syndrome, 1981: Update, Reye syndrome and salicylate usage. *Morbidity and Mortality Weekly Report, 31*(5), 53–56, 61.

Centers for Disease Control. (1982b). Surgeon General's advisory on the use of salicylates and Reye syndrome. *Morbidity and Mortality Weekly Report, 31*(22), 289–290.

Centers for Disease Control and Prevention. (2016). *Wide-ranging online data for epidemiologic research (WONDER)*. Atlanta, GA: National Center for Health Statistics. ▶ http://wonder.cdc.gov. Accessed December 2016.

Centers for Disease Control and Prevention. (2017). *Prevent childhood lead poisoning*. Available online: ▶ www.cdc.gov/nceh/lead/infographic.htm. Accessed 15 May 2018.

Chen, R. T., & DeStefano, F. (1998). Vaccine safety. *The Lancet, 352,* 63–64.

Choi, H. J., Krieger, J. L., & Hecht, M. L. (2013). Reconceptualizing efficacy in substance use prevention research: Refusal response efficacy and drug resistance self-efficacy in adolescent substance use. *Health Communication, 28*(1), 40–52.

Costello, E. J. (2017). Post hoc, ergo propter hoc. *American Journal of Psychiatry, 174*(4), 305–306.

Coxon, J., & Rees, J. (2015). Avoiding medical errors in general practice. *Trends in Urology & Men's Health, 6*(4), 13–17.

Croskerry, P. (2003). The importance of cognitive errors in diagnosis and strategies to minimize them. *Academic Medicine, 78*(8), 775–780.

Cummings, L. (2002). Reasoning under uncertainty: The role of two informal fallacies in an emerging scientific inquiry. *Informal Logic, 22*(2), 113–136.

Cummings, L. (2004). Analogical reasoning as a tool of epidemiological investigation. *Argumentation, 18*(4), 427–444.

Cummings, L. (2009). Emerging infectious diseases: Coping with uncertainty. *Argumentation, 23*(2), 171–188.

Cummings, L. (2010). *Rethinking the BSE crisis: A study of scientific reasoning under uncertainty*. Dordrecht: Springer.

Cummings, L. (2011). Considering risk assessment up close: The case of bovine spongiform encephalopathy. *Health, Risk & Society, 13*(3), 255–275.

Cummings, L. (2012a). Scaring the public: Fear appeal arguments in public health reasoning. *Informal Logic, 32*(1), 25–50.

Cummings, L. (2012b). The public health scientist as informal logician. *International Journal of Public Health, 57*(3), 649–650.

Cummings, L. (2013a). Public health reasoning: Much more than deduction. *Archives of Public Health, 71*(1), 25.

Cummings, L. (2013b). Circular reasoning in public health. *Cogency, 5*(2), 35–76.

Cummings, L. (2014a). Informal fallacies as cognitive heuristics in public health reasoning. *Informal Logic, 34*(1), 1–37.

Cummings, L. (2014b). The 'trust' heuristic: Arguments from authority in public health. *Health Communication, 29*(10), 1043–1056.

Cummings, L. (2014c). Coping with uncertainty in public health: The use of heuristics. *Public Health, 128*(4), 391–394.

Cummings, L. (2014d). Circles and analogies in public health reasoning. *Inquiry, 29*(2), 35–59.

Cummings, L. (2014e). Analogical reasoning in public health. *Journal of Argumentation in Context, 3*(2), 169–197.

Cummings, L. (2015). *Reasoning and public health: New ways of coping with uncertainty*. Cham, Switzerland: Springer.

Dancygier, B., & Sweetser, E. (2014). *Figurative Language*. New York: Cambridge University Press.

Darnovsky, M. (2013). A slippery slope to human germline modification. *Nature, 499,* 127.

Davis, K. C., Patel, D., Shafer, P., Duke, J., Glover-Kudon, R., Ridgeway, W., et al. (2018). Association between media doses of the *Tips From Former Smokers* campaign and cessation behaviors and intentions to quit among cigarette smokers, 2012–2015. *Health Education & Behavior, 45*(1), 52–60.

Dobson, S. J. A., & Jayaprakasan, K. M. (2018). Aetiology of recurrent miscarriage and the role of adjuvant treatment in its management: A retrospective cohort review. *Journal of Obstetrics and Gynaecology, 38*(7), 967–974.

Drope, J., Liber, A. C., Cahn, Z., Stoklosa, M., Kennedy, R., Douglas, C. E., et al. (2018). Who's still smoking? Disparities in adult cigarette smoking prevalence in the United States. *CA: A Cancer Journal for Clinicians, 68*(2), 106–115.

EBioMedicine. (2015). Banning psychoactive substances: A slippery slope. *EBioMedicine, 2,* 613–614.

Eiser, R. J., Stafford, T., Henneberry, J., & Catney, P. (2009). "Trust me, I'm a scientist (not a developer)": Perceived expertise and motives as predictors of trust in assessment of risk from contaminated land. *Risk Analysis, 29*(2), 288–297.

Feig, D. S. (2012). Avoiding the slippery slope: Preventing the development of diabetes in women with a history of gestational diabetes. *Diabetes/Metabolism Research and Reviews, 28,* 317–320.

Fernández, M. E., Diamond, P. M., Rakowski, W., Gonzales, A., Tortolero-Luna, G., Williams, J., et al. (2009). Development and validation of a cervical cancer screening self-efficacy scale for low-income Mexican American women. *Cancer Epidemiology, Biomarkers & Prevention, 18*(3), 866–875.
Finucane, T. E. (2012). Post hoc ergo propter hoc: Complications and death after gastrostomy placement. *Journal of the American Medical Directors Association, 13*(3), 197–198.
Fiske, S. T., & Dupree, C. (2014). Gaining trust as well as respect in communicating to motivated audiences about science topics. *Proceedings of the National Academy of Sciences of the United States of America, 111*(suppl. 4), 13593–13597.
Flammer, A. (2001). Self-efficacy. In N. J. Smelser & P. B. Baltes (Eds.), *International encyclopedia of the social & behavioral sciences* (pp. 13812–13815). Amsterdam and New York: Elsevier.
Fowler, F. J., Jr., Levin, C. A., & Sepucha, K. R. (2011). Informing and involving patients to improve the quality of medical decisions. *Health Affairs, 30*(4), 699–706.
Freed, G. L., Clark, S. J., Butchart, A. T., Singer, D. C., & Davis, M. M. (2011). Sources and perceived credibility of vaccine-safety information for parents. *Pediatrics, 127*(Suppl. 1), S107–S112.
Freedland, K. E., & Carney, R. M. (2009). Depression and medical illness. In I. H. Gotlib & C. L. Hammen (Eds.), *Handbook of depression* (2nd ed., pp. 113–141). New York and London: Guilford.
Gigerenzer, G., & Goldstein, D. G. (1996). Reasoning the fast and frugal way: Models of bounded rationality. *Psychological Review, 103*(4), 650–669.
Godlee, F., Smith, J., & Marcovitch, H. (2011). Wakefield's article linking MMR vaccine and autism was fraudulent. *BMJ, 342*, c7452.
Goswami, U., & Brown, A. L. (1990). Melting chocolate and melting snowmen: Analogical reasoning and causal relations. *Cognition, 35*(1), 69–95.
Graber, M. L., Franklin, N., & Gordon, R. (2005). Diagnostic error in internal medicine. *Archives of Internal Medicine, 165*(13), 1493–1499.
Green, A. E., Kenworthy, L., Gallagher, N. M., Antezana, L., Mosner, M. G., Krieg, S., et al. (2017). Social analogical reasoning in school-aged children with autism spectrum disorder and typically developing peers. *Autism, 21*(4), 403–411.
Green, A. E., Kenworthy, L., Mosner, M. G., Gallagher, N. M., Fearon, E. W., Balhana, C. D., et al. (2014). Abstract analogical reasoning in high-functioning children with autism spectrum disorders. *Autism Research, 7*(6), 677–686.
Grouse, L. (2016). Post hoc ergo propter hoc. *Journal of Thoracic Disease, 8*(7), E511–E512.
Guarini, M., Butchart, A., Smith, P. S., & Moldovan, A. (2009). Resources for research on analogy: A multi-disciplinary guide. *Informal Logic, 29*(2), 84–197.
Guignard, R., Gallopel-Morvan, K., Mons, U., Hummel, K., & Nguyen-Thanh, V. (2018). Impact of a negative emotional antitobacco mass media campaign on French smokers: A longitudinal study. *Tobacco Control, 27*(6), 670–676.
Gunning, J. (2008). The broadening impact of preimplantation genetic diagnosis: A slide down the slippery slope or meeting market demand. *Human Reproduction & Genetic Ethics, 14*(1), 29–37.
Hamblin, C. L. (1970). *Fallacies*. London: Methuen.
Handley, M. A., Nelson, K., Sanford, E., Clarity, C., Emmons-Bell, S., Gorukanti, A., et al. (2017). Examining lead exposures in California through state-issued health alerts for food contamination and an exposure-based candy testing program. *Environmental Health Perspectives, 125*(10), 104503.
Haroutounian, S., Ratz, Y., Ginosar, Y., Furmanov, K., Saifi, F., Meidan, R., et al. (2016). The effect of medicinal cannabis on pain and quality-of-life outcomes in chronic pain: A prospective open-label study. *Clinical Journal of Pain, 32*(12), 1036–1043.
Howard-Snyder, F., Howard-Snyder, D., & Wasserman, R. (2009). *The power of logic* (4th ed.). New York: McGraw Hill.
Huang, Y. M., Shiyanbola, O. O., & Smith, P. D. (2018). Association of health literacy and medication self-efficacy with medication adherence and diabetes control. *Patient Preference and Adherence, 12*, 793–802.
Hughes, H. K., Rose, D., & Ashwood, P. (2018). The gut microbiota and dysbiosis in autism spectrum disorders. *Current Neurology and Neuroscience Reports, 18*(11), 81.
Hurley, P. J. (2015). *A concise introduction to logic* (12th ed.). Stamford, CT: Cengage Learning.

Inungu, J., Mumford, V., Younis, M., & Langford, S. (2009). HIV knowledge, attitudes and practices among college students in the United States. *Journal of Health and Human Services Administration, 32*(3), 259–277.

Jalloh, M. F., Sengeh, P., Monasch, R., Jalloh, M. B., DeLuca, N., Dyson, M., et al. (2017). National survey of Ebola-related knowledge, attitudes and practices before the outbreak peak in Sierra Leone: August 2014. *BMJ Global Health, 2,* e000285. ► https://doi.org/10.1136/bmjgh-2017-000285.

Johnson, R. H. (2011). Informal logic and deductivism. *Studies in Logic, 4*(1), 17–37.

Kahane, H. (1971). *Logic and contemporary rhetoric: The use of reason in everyday life*. Belmont, CA: Wadsworth Publishing Company.

Kelley, D. (2014). *The art of reasoning: An introduction to logic and critical thinking* (4th ed.). New York: W. W. Norton.

Keogh, B. (2012). *Poly Implant Prothèse (PIP) breast implants: Final report of the expert group*. London: Department of Health.

Krawczyk, D. C., Kandalaft, M. R., Didehbani, N., Allen, T. T., McClelland, M. M., Tamminga, C. A., et al. (2014). An investigation of reasoning by analogy in schizophrenia and autism spectrum disorders. *Frontiers in Human Neuroscience, 8,* 517.

Krzemien, M., Jemel, B., & Maillart, C. (2017). Analogical reasoning in children with specific language impairment: Evidence from a scene analogy task. *Clinical Linguistics & Phonetics, 31*(7–9), 573–588.

LeBlanc, J. (1998). *Thinking clearly: A guide to critical reasoning*. New York: W. W. Norton.

Lee, A. S.-Y., & Gibbon, F. E. (2015). Non-speech oral motor treatment for children with developmental speech sound disorders. *Cochrane Database of Systematic Reviews*, Issue 3, Art. No.: CD009383.

Lee, M. J. (2018). College students' responses to emotional anti-alcohol abuse media messages: Should we scare or amuse them? *Health Promotion Practice, 19*(3), 465–474.

Lerner, B. H., & Caplan, A. L. (2015). Euthanasia in Belgium and the Netherlands: On a slippery slope? *JAMA Internal Medicine, 175*(10), 1640–1641.

Llewelyn, M. J., Fitzpatrick, J. M., Darwin, E., Tonkin-Crine, S., Gorton, C., Paul, J., et al. (2017). The antibiotic course has had its day. *BMJ, 358,* j3418.

Locke, J. (1959). *An essay concerning human understanding* (A. C. Fraser, Ed.). New York: Dover.

Loucks, E. B., Buka, S. L., Rogers, M. L., Liu, T., Kawachi, I., Kubzansky, L. D., et al. (2012). Education and coronary heart disease risk associations may be affected by early life common prior causes: A propensity matching analysis. *Annals of Epidemiology, 22*(4), 221–232.

McCartney, M. (2016). Media's misrepresentation of science. *British Medical Journal, 352,* i355.

McKinstry, B. (1992). Paternalism and the doctor-patient relationship in general practice. *The British Journal of General Practice, 42*(361), 340–342.

McNabola, A., & Gill, L. W. (2009). The control of environmental tobacco smoke: A policy review. *International Journal of Environmental Research and Public Health, 6*(2), 741–758.

Melvin, C. L., Jefferson, M. S., Rice, L. J., Cartmell, K. B., & Halbert, C. H. (2016). Predictors of participation in mammography screening among non-Hispanic Black, non-Hispanic White, and Hispanic women. *Frontiers in Public Health, 4,* 188.

Mill, J. S. (1882). *A system of logic ratiocinative and inductive, being a connected view of the principles of evidence, and the methods of scientific investigation*. New York: Harper & Brothers.

Munson, R., & Black, A. (2017). *The elements of reasoning* (7th ed.). Boston, MA: Cengage Learning.

Murray-Johnson, L., Witte, K., Liu, W.-Y., Hubbell, A. P., Sampson, J., & Morrison, K. (2001). Addressing cultural orientations in fear appeals: Promoting AIDS-protective behaviors among Mexican immigrant and African American adolescents and American and Taiwanese college students. *Journal of Health Communication, 6*(4), 335–358.

Nakayachi, K., & Cvetkovich, G. (2010). Public trust in government concerning tobacco control in Japan. *Risk Analysis, 30*(1), 143–152.

Oakley, J., & Cocking, D. (2005). Consequentialism, complacency, and slippery slope arguments. *Theoretical Medicine and Bioethics, 26*(3), 227–239.

Orbell, S., Szczepura, A., Weller, D., Gumber, A., & Hagger, M. S. (2017). South Asian ethnicity, socioeconomic status, and psychological mediators of faecal occult blood colorectal screening participation: A prospective test of a process model. *Health Psychology, 36*(12), 1161–1172.

Ozonoff, S., Heung, K., Byrd, R., Hansen, R., & Hertz-Picciotto, I. (2008). The onset of autism: Patterns of symptom emergence in the first years of life. *Autism Research, 1*(6), 320–328.

Pechmann, C., & Reibling, E. T. (2000). Anti-smoking advertising campaigns targeting youth: Case studies from USA and Canada. *Tobacco Control, 9*(Suppl. II), ii18–ii31.

Pennington, L., Parker, N. K., Kelly, H., & Miller, N. (2016). Speech therapy for children with dysarthria acquired before three years of age. *Cochrane Database of Systematic Reviews*, Issue 7, Art. No.: CD006937.

Pinto, R. C. (1995). Post hoc ergo propter hoc. In H. V. Hansen & R. C. Pinto (Eds.), *Fallacies: Classical and contemporary readings* (pp. 302–314). University Park: The Pennsylvania State University Press.

Rescher, N. (1980). *Scepticism: A critical reappraisal.* Oxford: Basil Blackwell.

Rhodes, F., & Wolitski, R. J. (1990). Perceived effectiveness of fear appeals in AIDS education: Relationship to ethnicity, gender, age, and group membership. *AIDS Education and Prevention, 2*(1), 1–11.

Richland, L. E., & Burchinal, M. R. (2013). Early executive function predicts reasoning development. *Psychological Science, 24*(1), 87–92.

Robinson, R. (1971). Arguing from ignorance. *The Philosophical Quarterly, 21*(83), 97–108.

Roeselers, G., Bouwman, J., & Levin, E. (2016). The human gut microbiome, diet, and health: "*Post hoc non ergo propter hoc*". *Trends in Food Science & Technology, 57,* 302–305.

Roskos-Ewoldsen, D. R., Yu, J. H., & Rhodes, N. (2004). Fear appeal messages affect accessibility of attitudes toward the threat and adaptive behaviors. *Communication Monographs, 71*(1), 49–69.

Rowe, T. (2015). The stress of pregnancy. *Journal of Obstetrics and Gynaecology Canada, 37*(5), 393–394.

Ruiter, R. A. C., Kessels, L. T. E., Peters, G.-J. Y., & Kok, G. (2014). Sixty years of fear appeal research: Current state of the evidence. *International Journal of Psychology, 49*(2), 63–70.

Saposnik, G., Redelmeier, D., Ruff, C. C., & Tobler, P. N. (2016). Cognitive biases associated with medical decisions: A systematic review. *BMC Medical Informatics and Decision Making, 16,* 138. ▶ https://doi.org/10.1186/s12911-016-0377-1.

Shi, J. J., & Smith, S. W. (2016). The effects of fear appeal message repetition on perceived threat, perceived efficacy, and behavioral intention in the extended parallel process model. *Health Communication, 31*(3), 275–286.

Sidgwick, A. (1883). *Fallacies: A view of logic from the practical side.* London: Kegan Paul, Trench.

Simms, N. K., Frausel, R. R., & Richard, L. E. (2018). Working memory predicts children's analogical reasoning. *Journal of Experimental Child Psychology, 166,* 160–177.

Simpson, J., & Done, D. J. (2004). Analogical reasoning in schizophrenic delusions. *European Psychiatry, 19*(6), 344–348.

Spielthenner, G. (2010). A logical analysis of slippery slope arguments. *Health Care Analysis, 18*(2), 148–163.

Steen, G., & Gibbs, R. (2004). Questions about metaphor in literature. *European Journal of English Studies, 8*(3), 337–354.

Tan, E., Wu, X., Nishida, T., Huang, D., Chen, Z., & Yi, L. (2018). Analogical reasoning in children with autism spectrum disorder: Evidence from an eye-tracking approach. *Frontiers in Psychology, 9,* 847.

Taylor, C. M., Emmett, P. M., Emond, A. M., & Golding, J. (2018). A review of guidance on fish consumption in pregnancy: Is it fit for purpose? *Public Health Nutrition, 21*(11), 2149–2159.

Todd, P. M., & Gigerenzer, G. (2000). Simple heuristics that make us smart. *Behavioral and Brain Sciences, 23*(5), 727–741.

Toulmin, S., Rieke, R., & Janik, A. (1984). *An introduction to reasoning.* New York: Macmillan.

Trowbridge, R. L. (2008). Twelve tips for teaching avoidance of diagnostic errors. *Medical Teacher, 30,* 496–500.

Tsoumanis, A., Hens, N., & Kenyon, C. R. (2018). Is screening for chlamydia and gonorrhoea in men who have sex with men associated with reduction of the prevalence of these infections? A systematic review of observational studies. *Sexually Transmitted Diseases, 45*(9), 615–622.

Tversky, A., & Kahneman, D. (1974). Judgement under uncertainty: Heuristics and biases. *Science, 185*(4157), 1124–1131.

Tversky, A., & Kahneman, D. (2004). Belief in the law of small numbers. In E. Shafir (Ed.), *Preference, belief and similarity: Selected writings by Amos Tversky* (pp. 193–202). Cambridge: MIT Press.

Ursell, L. K., Metcalf, J. L., Parfrey, L. W., & Knight, R. (2012). Defining the human microbiome. *Nutrition Reviews, 70*(Suppl. 1), S38–S44.

Vogel, A. P., Keage, M. J., Johansson, K, & Schalling, E. (2015). Treatment for dysphagia (swallowing difficulties) in hereditary ataxia. *Cochrane Database of Systematic* Reviews, Issue 11, Art. No.: CD010169.

Wada, K., & Smith, D. R. (2015). Mistrust surrounding vaccination recommendations by the Japanese government: Results from a national survey of working-age individuals. *BMC Public Health, 15,* 426.

Wakefield, A. J., Murch, S. H., Anthony, A., Linnell, J., Casson, D. M., Malik, M., et al. (1998). Ileal-lymphoid-nodular hyperplasia, non-specific colitis, and pervasive developmental disorder in children. *The Lancet, 351*(9103), 637–641.

Walton, D. N. (1985a). Are circular arguments necessarily vicious? *American Philosophical Quarterly, 22*(4), 263–274.

Walton, D. N. (1985b). *Arguer's Position.* Westport, CT: Greenwood Press.

Walton, D. N. (1987). The ad hominem argument as an informal fallacy. *Argumentation, 1*(3), 317–331.

Walton, D. N. (1991). *Begging the question: Circular reasoning as a tactic of argumentation*. New York: Greenwood Press.

Walton, D. N. (1992). *Plausible argument in everyday conversation*. Albany: SUNY Press.

Walton, D. N. (1996). *Argumentation schemes for presumptive reasoning*. Mahwah, NJ: Erlbaum.

Walton, D. N. (1997). *Appeal to expert opinion: Arguments from authority*. University Park: The Pennsylvania State University Press.

Walton, D. N. (2000). *Scare tactics: Arguments that appeal to fear and threats*. Dordrecht: Kluwer Academic.

Walton, D. N. (2008). *Informal logic: A pragmatic approach* (2nd ed.). New York: Cambridge University Press.

Walton, D. N. (2010). Why fallacies appear to be better arguments than they are. *Informal Logic, 30*(2), 159–184.

Walton, D. N. (2017). The slippery slope argument in the ethical debate on genetic engineering of humans. *Science and Engineering Ethics, 23*(6), 1507–1528.

Watson, J. C., & Arp, R. (2015). *Critical thinking: An introduction to reasoning well*. London and New York: Bloomsbury Academic.

Watts, I. (1807). *Logic: Or the right use of reason, in the inquiry after truth*. Edinburgh: Abernethy and Walker.

Weingart, S. N., Wilson, R. M., Gibberd, R. W., & Harrison, B. (2000). Epidemiology of medical error. *Western Journal of Medicine, 172*(6), 390–393.

Weinstein, N. D. (1980). Unrealistic optimism about future life events. *Journal of Personality and Social Psychology, 39*(5), 806–820.

Weinstein, N. D. (1984). Why it won't happen to me: Perceptions of risk factors and susceptibility. *Health Psychology, 3*(5), 431–457.

Whately, R. (1855). *Elements of logic*. Boston and Cambridge: James Munroe.

Witte, K., & Allen, M. (2000). A meta-analysis of fear appeals: Implications for effective public health campaigns. *Health Education & Behavior, 27*(5), 591–615.

Witte, K., Meyer, G., & Martell, D. (2001). *Effective health risk messages: A step-by-step guide*. Thousand Oaks, London, and New Delhi: Sage.

Woods, J. (1995). Appeal to force. In H. V. Hansen & R. C. Pinto (Eds.), *Fallacies: Classical and contemporary readings* (pp. 240–250). University Park: The Pennsylvania State University Press.

Woods, J. (2004). *The death of argument: Fallacies in agent-based reasoning*. Dordrecht: Kluwer Academic.

Woods, J. (2007). Lightening up on the ad hominem. *Informal Logic, 27*(1), 109–134.

Woods, J. (2008). Begging the question is not a fallacy. In C. Dégremont, L. Keiff, & H. Rükert (Eds.), *Dialogues, logics and other strange things: Essays in honour of Shahid Rahman* (pp. 523–544). London: College Publications.

Xi, B., Veeranki, S. P., Zhao, M., Ma, C., Yan, Y., & Mi, J. (2017). Relationship of alcohol consumption to all-cause, cardiovascular, and cancer-related mortality in U.S. adults. *Journal of the American College of Cardiology, 70*(8), 913–922.

Zhang, W., Zhang, X., Tian, Y., Zhu, Y., Tong, Y., Li, Y., et al. (2018). Risk assessment of total mercury and methylmercury in aquatic products from offshore farms in China. *Journal of Hazardous Materials, 354,* 198–205.

Index

A

B

C

D

E

F

G

H

I

J

L

M

CPSIA information can be obtained
at www.ICGtesting.com
Printed in the USA
LVHW082038040320
648985LV00001B/3

9 783030 285128